CLINICAL HANDBOOK FOR MEDICAL-SURGICAL NURSING

Critical Thinking in Patient Care

FIFTH EDITION

Priscilla LeMone, RN, DSN, FAAN
Associate Professor Emeritus
Sinclair School of Nursing
University of Missouri–Columbia
Columbia, MO

Karen Burke, RN, MS
Education Consultant
Oregon State Board of Nursing
Portland, Oregon

Jane Bostick, RN, PhD
Sinclair School of Nursing
University of Missouri–Columbia
Columbia, MO

Pearson

Boston Columbus Indianapolis New York San Francisco Upper Saddle River
Amsterdam Cape Town Dubai London Madrid Milan Munich Paris Montreal Toronto
Delhi Mexico City Sao Paulo Sydney Hong Kong Seoul Singapore Taipei Tokyo

Library of Congress Cataloging-in-Publication Data
LeMone, Priscilla, author.
  Clinical handbook for medical-surgical nursing : critical thinking in patient care / Priscilla
LeMone, RN, DSN, FAAN, Associate Professor Emeritus, Sinclair School of Nursing,
University of Missouri-Columbia, Columbia, MO, Karen Burke, RN, MS, Education
Consultant, Oregon State Board of Nursing, Portland, Oregon, Jane Bostick, RN, PhD, Sinclair
School of Nursing, University of Missouri-Columbia, Columbia, MO. -- Fifth edition.
    p. ; cm.
  Includes index.
  ISBN-13: 978-0-13-512515-1 (pbk.)
  ISBN-10: 0-13-512515-4
  1. Nursing--Handbooks, manuals, etc. 2. Surgical nursing--Handbooks, manuals, etc. I.
Burke, Karen M., author. II. Bostick, Jane E., author. III. LeMone, Priscilla. Medical-surgical
nursing. c2011. supplement (work) IV. Title.
  [DNLM: 1. Nursing Process--Handbooks. 2. Nursing Care--Handbooks. 3. Patient Care
Planning--Handbooks. 4. Perioperative Nursing--Handbooks. WY 49]
  RT51.G38 2012
  617'.0231--dc22

                                                                          2010047728

Notice: Care has been taken to confirm the accuracy of information presented in this book.
The authors, editors, and the publisher, however, cannot accept any responsibility for errors
or omissions or for consequences from application of the information in this book and make
no warranty, express or implied, with respect to its contents. The authors and publisher
have exerted every effort to ensure that drug selections and dosages set forth in this text
are in accord with current recommendations and practice at time of publication. However,
in view of ongoing research, changes in government regulations, and the constant flow of
information relating to drug therapy and drug reactions, the reader is urged to check the
package inserts of all drugs for any change in indications of dosage and for added warnings
and precautions. This is particularly important when the recommended agent is a new and/
or infrequently employed drug.

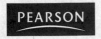

www.pearsonhighered.com

10 9 8 7 6 5 4 3 2 1
ISBN 10: 0-13-512515-4
ISBN 13: 978-0-13-512515-1

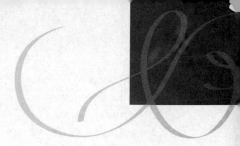

CONTENTS

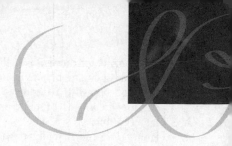

PREFACE

The *Clinical Handbook for Medical-Surgical Nursing: Critical Thinking in Patient Care* is a handy, pocket-sized reference for the care of patients with health problems often encountered in clinical situations. While primarily developed as a supplement to the fifth edition of *Medical-Surgical Nursing: Critical Thinking in Patient Care*, to which it is cross-referenced by chapter, the *Clinical Handbook* may also be used as a stand-alone reference text. It provides nursing students essential information in an easy-to-follow format, allowing them to respond quickly when a patient's condition changes or when they are assigned to a new patient.

ORGANIZATION

The *Clinical Handbook* covers the most common health problems nursing students are likely to encounter in medical-surgical nursing. The conditions appear in alphabetical order for quick retrieval of the most vital information.

KEY FEATURES

The *Clinical Handbook* presents varying amounts of information about each condition according to its prevalence and/or seriousness.

- **Overview** includes the definition of the condition, its classification within other categories, incidence, and basic pathophysiologic mechanisms.
- **Causes** list actual causes, when known, or provides a risk-factor assessment when appropriate.
- **Manifestations** appear in order of those most characteristic of the condition to those less frequently encountered.
- **Diagnostic Tests** include the most frequently used laboratory tests, diagnostic imaging tests, and/or other testing methods, as well as the significance of abnormal results.

- **Collaborative Management** lists the medications and treatments most commonly associated with each condition.
- **Selected Nursing Diagnoses with Interventions** list the nursing diagnoses of high priority, with related nursing interventions.
- **Home Care and Teaching** provides teaching topics and referral sources, as appropriate, for patients who are being discharged from a healthcare facility or who provide self-care at home.
- Cross-references guide students to more detailed information available in *Medical-Surgical Nursing: Critical Thinking in Patient Care*.

Every effort has been made to ensure that the *Clinical Handbook* is as accurate, current, and practical as possible so that nursing students can find ready answers to clinical problems.

ACKNOWLEDGMENTS

Our thanks to the editorial staff at Pearson Education for their guidance in the revision of the fifth edition of the *Clinical Handbook for Medical-Surgical Nursing: Critical Thinking in Patient Care*. We are grateful to the students who use the book to provide safe and knowledgeable patient care and to the faculty who have found it to be a useful teaching–learning tool in the clinical setting.

Priscilla LeMone, RN, DSN, FAAN
Associate Professor Emeritus
Sinclair School of Nursing
University of Missouri—Columbia
Columbia, MO

Karen M. Burke, RN, MS
Clatsop Community College
Astoria, OR

Jane Bostick, RN, PhD
Sinclair School of Nursing
University of Missouri–Columbia
Columbia, MO

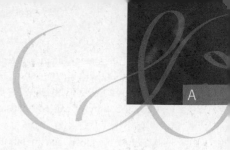

ACID–BASE DISORDERS

Overview

- A stable balance of acids and bases in the body is necessary for normal cellular metabolic function.

- The balance of acids and bases is maintained by buffers; the respiratory system, which eliminates or retains carbon dioxide (CO_2); and the kidneys, which eliminate or retain both hydrogen ions and bicarbonate (HCO_3).

- Buffers, which have a limited capacity to maintain acid–base balance, combine with hydrogen ions or release hydrogen ions to maintain pH within the normal range. The HCO_3–carbonic acid system is the major buffering system in the body. The normal ratio of HCO_3 (the primary base in the body) to carbonic acid (a major acid) is 20:1.

- Acid–base balance is evaluated using an arterial blood sample and arterial blood gas (ABG) analysis.

- Hydrogen ion concentration is measured by the pH. Body fluids are normally slightly alkaline with a pH of 7.35 to 7.45. A lower pH reflects a higher concentration of hydrogen ions and acidosis; a higher pH indicates a lower hydrogen ion concentration and alkalosis.

- The balance between acids and bases is evaluated using ABG values for dissolved CO_2, an acid-forming gas (a volatile acid), and the concentration of HCO_3, a base.

- Altered respiratory function affects ventilation and gas exchange, altering CO_2 elimination and acid–base balance. It can lead to either respiratory acidosis or respiratory alkalosis.

- Only the kidneys can compensate for respiratory disturbances of pH.

- Metabolic acidosis and metabolic alkalosis result from conditions that alter either the production or elimination of nonvolatile acids in the body.

- Both the respiratory and renal systems, if functioning optimally, can compensate for metabolic disturbances of pH.

- Acid–base status is monitored by serial ABGs and capnography, or measurements of exhaled CO_2. ABGs can identify an acid–base imbalance, the type of imbalance, and the presence of compensation. Capnography primarily is used to evaluate respiratory imbalances.

- The components of ABGs used to assess acid–base status are pH, dissolved CO_2 ($PaCO_2$), serum bicarbonate (HCO_3), and base excess (BE).

Causes

Acute Respiratory Acidosis

- Hypoventilation: muscle damage/paralysis, asphyxia, foreign body aspiration, chest wall/central nervous system trauma, opiate overdose, inadequate mechanical ventilation

- Impaired gas exchange: acute respiratory failure, acute respiratory distress syndrome, pulmonary edema, pneumonia, acute asthma

Chronic Respiratory Acidosis

- Hypoventilation: multiple sclerosis and other neuromuscular diseases, stroke (CVA)

- Impaired gas exchange: Chronic obstructive pulmonary disease (COPD), emphysema, chronic bronchitis, bronchiectasis, cystic fibrosis

Respiratory Alkalosis

- Hyperventilation: anxiety, fever, gram-negative sepsis, early salicylate intoxication, excessive mechanical ventilation

Metabolic Acidosis

- Acid gain: lactic acidosis (shock, cardiac arrest), ketoacidosis (diabetes, starvation), renal failure
- Base loss: diarrhea, intestinal suction, or abdominal fistulas

Metabolic Alkalosis

- Acid loss: vomiting, gastric lavage/nasogastric suction, administration of diuretics (loop or thiazides), and corticosteroids
- Base gain: excessive HCO_3 ingestion/infusion, milk-alkali syndrome

Manifestations

Acute Respiratory Acidosis

- Cardiac: tachycardia, ventricular fibrillation, cardiac arrest
- Skin/mucous membranes: warm, flushed skin
- Neurologic: blurred vision, altered mental status, decreasing level of consciousness (LOC)
- General: headache, irritability

Chronic Respiratory Acidosis

- Neurologic: impaired memory, personality changes
- General: weakness, dull headache, sleep disturbances with daytime sleepiness

Respiratory Alkalosis

- Cardiac: palpitations, dysrhythmias
- Respiratory: dyspnea, chest tightness
- Skeletal/muscular: tremors, tetany, positive Chvostek's and Trousseau's signs
- Neurologic: paresthesias (around mouth, hands, and feet); seizures, loss of consciousness
- General: anxiety, panic, dizziness, lightheadedness, tinnitus

Metabolic Acidosis

- Cardiac: dysrhythmias, bradycardia, cardiac arrest
- Respiratory: hyperventilation (Kussmaul's respirations), dyspnea
- GI: anorexia, nausea, vomiting, abdominal pain

- Skin/mucous membranes: warm, flushed skin
- Neurologic: decreasing LOC, stupor, and coma

- General: weakness, fatigue, general malaise, headache

Metabolic Alkalosis

- Cardiac: dysrhythmias, hypotension
- Respiratory: decreased respiratory rate and depth
- Neurologic: confusion, decreasing LOC, seizures
- Skeletal/muscular: hyperreflexia, twitching, tetany, Trousseau's sign

Diagnostic Tests

- Normal ABG values and changes in acid–base disorders are outlined in Tables 1 and 2, page 565.
- Exhaled CO_2 increases in hypermetabolic states and hypoventilation, and decreases when lung perfusion is impaired.

Interdisciplinary Care

For all types of acid–base disorders, treat the primary underlying cause.

Respiratory Acidosis

- Improve alveolar ventilation and use pulmonary hygiene (percussion and drainage) and adequate hydration to remove respiratory secretions; mechanical ventilation is used when necessary.
- Administer oxygen cautiously to patients with chronic respiratory conditions (COPD, emphysema, bronchitis) to avoid carbon dioxide narcosis.
- Naloxone is used to treat respiratory depression related to opiate overdose.

Respiratory Alkalosis

- A rebreather mask or breathing into a paper bag is used to increase $PaCO_2$; administer oxygen.
- Use sedation as necessary to slow the respiratory rate.

- Adjust ventilator settings to reduce the respiratory rate and tidal volume as indicated.

Metabolic Acidosis

- Intravenous (IV) or oral sodium HCO_3 or another alkalinizing solution such as lactate may be administered. IV fluids and insulin are given to treat diabetic ketoacidosis; alcoholic ketosis is treated with saline solutions and glucose.
- K^+ supplementation may be necessary to prevent hypokalemia with correction of acidosis.

Metabolic Alkalosis

- Fluids to restore normal fluid volume; sodium chloride and potassium chloride solutions to restore fluid and electrolyte balance and promote HCO_3 excretion.

Selected Nursing Diagnoses with Interventions

Decreased Cardiac Output

- Monitor vital signs, LOC, peripheral pulses, capillary refill, and electrocardiogram pattern.
- Report abnormal laboratory values (ABGs, serum electrolytes, blood urea nitrogen, and creatinine) to the physician.

Ineffective Breathing Pattern

- Provide reassurance. Instruct to maintain eye contact and breathe with you to slow respiratory rate.
- Help to breathe into a paper bag or rebreather mask.
- Adjust settings on mechanical ventilator as ordered.

Impaired Gas Exchange

- Frequently assess respiratory rate, depth, effort, oxygen saturation, and breath sounds.
- Place in semi-Fowler's, Fowler's, or high Fowler's position as tolerated.
- Administer oxygen as necessary to maintain oxygen saturation; closely monitor respiratory status.

Deficient Fluid Volume

- Monitor intake, output, daily weight, skin turgor, and mucous membranes.
- Administer oral or IV fluids as ordered.

Risk for Injury

- Monitor mental status and muscle strength. Report decreasing LOC or behavior changes such as restlessness, confusion, or agitation.
- Institute safety measures (maintain low bed position, remove clutter in room).
- Reorient to time, place, and circumstances as needed.

Community-Based Care

- Discuss underlying disorder (e.g., COPD, diabetes) and measures to prevent recurrence (e.g., control of diabetes mellitus, effect of antacids containing sodium HCO_3, treatment of diarrhea, avoiding respiratory infections).
- Maintain contact with primary care provider for conditions commonly associated with acid–base imbalances such as diabetes and COPD.
- Refer for diabetic education or home respiratory care services as appropriate.

For more information about acid–base disorders, see Chapter 10 in *Medical-Surgical Nursing,* Fifth Edition, by LeMone, Burke, and Bauldoff.

ACUTE CORONARY SYNDROME

Overview

- Acute coronary syndrome (ACS) is unstable cardiac ischemia. It includes unstable angina and acute myocardial ischemia.
- In ACS, coronary blood flow is acutely reduced, but not fully occluded, resulting in myocardial cell injury. With prompt restoration of blood flow, muscle tissue recovers.

- ACS is usually precipitated by rupture or erosion of atherosclerotic plaque with formation of a blood clot that does not fully occlude the vessel.
- Blood flow distal to the clot is severely impaired, leading to tissue ischemia. Injured myocardial cells contract less effectively, and cardiac output may fall. Lactic acid released from ischemic cells stimulates pain receptors, causing chest pain.
- An estimated 1.4 million Americans are admitted to the hospital annually with ACS. ACS is the most commonly identified cause of sudden cardiac death.

Causes
- Coronary heart disease, atherosclerosis

Manifestations
- Chest pain, usually substernal or epigastric, often radiating to the neck, left shoulder, and/or left arm
- Pain may occur at rest and typically lasts longer than 10 to 20 minutes; may be unrelieved by nitroglycerin
- Dyspnea, diaphoresis, pallor, and cool skin; nausea, lightheadedness
- Tachycardia and hypotension

Diagnostic Tests
- The electrocardiogram (ECG) may show T-wave inversion and elevation of the ST segment.
- Cardiac muscle troponins, cT_nT and cT_nI, may be elevated or within normal limits.
- Creatine kinase and creatine kinase-MB levels may be within normal limits or demonstrate transient elevation, returning to normal within 12 to 24 hours.

Interdisciplinary Care
- Nitrates and beta blockers are used to restore blood flow and reduce the cardiac workload. If chest pain is unrelieved by oral or buccal nitroglycerine, an intravenous infusion is started.

- Fibrinolytic drugs may be given to restore blood flow to ischemic cardiac muscle and can prevent permanent damage.

- Aspirin, other antiplatelet drugs, and heparin are given to inhibit blood clotting and reduce the risk of thrombus formation.

- Percutaneous coronary revascularization (PCR) or coronary artery bypass grafting may be used to restore coronary blood flow.

Selected Nursing Diagnoses with Interventions

Ineffective Tissue Perfusion: Cardiac

- Keep prescribed nitroglycerin tablets or spray at the bedside.

- Administer oxygen per nasal cannula at 4 to 6 L/min as ordered.

- Monitor for and treat or report chest pain as indicated.

- Assess knowledge and understanding of planned therapy. Clarify and reinforce knowledge, including expected sensations during planned procedures.

- Monitor vital signs and cardiac rhythm continuously during fibrinolytic drug infusion and following PCR. Treat dysrhythmias as ordered. Obtain a 12-lead ECG if signs of ischemia develop (ST elevation or depression, inverted T waves), and notify physician.

- Maintain intravenous nitroglycerin infusion. Administer anticoagulant and antiplatelet medications, nitrates, and calcium channel blockers as ordered.

- Following PCR, maintain bed rest with the head of the bed at 30 degrees or less. Prevent flexion of the leg on the affected side. Following sheath removal, follow protocol for pressure dressing or device or sandbag placement.

- Monitor distal pulses, color, movement, sensation, and temperature of the affected leg and insertion site every 15 minutes for the first hour, every 30 minutes for the next hour, every hour for the next 8 hours, and then every 4 hours.

- Monitor intake and output, serum electrolytes, blood urea nitrogen, creatinine, complete blood count, partial thromboplastin time, and cardiac enzymes. Report abnormal results to the physician.

- Monitor for bradycardia, lightheadedness, hypotension, diaphoresis, and loss of consciousness during sheath removal. Keep atropine at bedside during sheath removal.

Ineffective Protection

- Inquire about a history of intracranial hemorrhage, upper gastrointestinal bleeding, peptic ulcer disease, or known bleeding tendency.

- Observe for and report increased bruising, petechiae, purpura, apparent or occult bleeding (e.g., melena, hematemesis).

- For parenteral antiplatelet drugs, monitor complete blood count, clotting studies, vital signs, and ECG during therapy.

- Closely observe for and immediately report anaphylaxis or bleeding uncontrolled by pressure. Keep resuscitation equipment readily available.

- Maintain bed rest during infusion of antiplatelet or fibrinolytic drugs.

Community-Based Care

- Instruct to avoid nonsteroidal anti-inflammatory drugs or other over-the-counter drugs that may contain aspirin or a nonsteroidal anti-inflammatory drug if aspirin or another antiplatelet drug is prescribed.

- Report unusual bruising or excessive bleeding.

- Inform all care providers (including dental professionals) of use of these drugs.

- Provide written instructions for resumption of activities and follow-up care.

- Refer to cardiac rehabilitation program for risk factor and lifestyle management as indicated.

For more information about acute coronary syndrome, see Chapter 30 in *Medical-Surgical Nursing,* Fifth Edition, by LeMone, Burke, and Bauldoff.

ACUTE RESPIRATORY DISTRESS SYNDROME

Overview

- Acute respiratory distress syndrome (ARDS) is a severe form of respiratory failure characterized by noncardiac pulmonary edema and progressive refractory hypoxemia.

- The underlying pathophysiology of ARDS is acute lung injury due to a systemic inflammatory response to acute injury. Inflammatory responses and biochemical mediators damage the alveolar-capillary membrane, often within 24 hours of the initial insult.

- Damaged membranes allow plasma and blood cells into the interstitial space and alveoli. Surfactant is inactivated and surfactant-producing cells are damaged, leading to alveolar collapse, decreased lung compliance, increased work of breathing, and impaired gas exchange.

- With progression, hyaline membranes and fibrotic changes in lung tissue further impair gas exchange. Hypoxemia becomes *refractory* or resistant to improvement with supplemental oxygen. Carbon dioxide exchange is impaired, and respiratory acidosis develops.

- Significant tissue hypoxia leads to metabolic acidosis as well. Sepsis and multiple organ system dysfunction are the leading causes of death in ARDS. If the process is halted before this occurs, the long-term prognosis for recovery is good.

Causes

- Shock, gram-negative sepsis
- Aspiration, near-drowning
- Inhalation of smoke or toxic gases
- Pneumonia: viral, bacterial, fungal, *Pneumocystis carinii*
- Trauma: burns, head injury, lung contusion
- Disseminated intravascular coagulation; fat, air, or amniotic fluid emboli
- Multiple transfusions, cardiopulmonary bypass
- Drug overdose: heroin, methadone, aspirin
- Systemic disorders: pancreatitis, uremia

Manifestations

- Early: dyspnea, tachypnea, and anxiety
- Progressive respiratory distress: increasing tachypnea, intercostal retractions, use of accessory muscles of respiration
- Cyanosis

- Breath sounds initially clear; crackles (rales) and rhonchi develop later
- Mental status changes: agitation, confusion, and lethargy

Diagnostic Tests

- Arterial blood gases (ABGs): initial hypoxemia with PO_2 of less than 60 mmHg, and respiratory alkalosis due to tachypnea; mixed respiratory and metabolic acidosis later.
- Chest x-ray: diffuse infiltrates progressing to a "white out" pattern.
- Pulmonary function testing: decreased lung compliance with reduced vital capacity, minute volume, and functional vital capacity.
- Normal pulmonary artery pressures help distinguish ARDS from cardiogenic pulmonary edema.

Interdisciplinary Management

- Inhaled nitric oxide is used to reduce intrapulmonary shunting and improve oxygenation by dilating blood vessels in better-ventilated areas of the lungs.
- Surfactant therapy to reduce surface tension within the alveoli, decrease the work of breathing, improve lung compliance and gas exchange, and prevent atelectasis.
- Nonsteroidal anti-inflammatory drugs and corticosteroids may be prescribed.
- Endotracheal intubation and mechanical ventilation, often using positive airway pressure or support, to maintain adequate tissue oxygenation.
- Prone positioning with mechanical ventilation to prevent atelectasis in dependent lung tissue and improve oxygenation.
- Careful fluid replacement; enteral or parenteral feeding to maintain nutritional status and prevent tissue catabolism.
- Low-molecular weight heparin may be given to prevent thrombophlebitis or disseminated intravascular coagulation.

Selected Nursing Diagnoses with Interventions

Impaired Spontaneous Ventilation

- Assess and document respiratory rate, vital signs, and oxygen saturation hourly or more frequently as needed.

- Promptly report signs of respiratory distress (tachypnea, tachycardia, nasal flaring, use of accessory muscles, intercostal retractions, cyanosis, increasing restlessness, anxiety, or decreased level of consciousness), worsening ABGs, and oxygen saturation levels.
- Administer oxygen as ordered, monitoring response.
- Place in Fowler's or high Fowler's position.
- Minimize activities and energy expenditures by assisting with activities of daily living, spacing procedures and activities, and allowing uninterrupted rest periods.
- Avoid sedatives and respiratory depressant drugs unless mechanically ventilated.
- Prepare for endotracheal intubation and mechanical ventilation.
- Explain intubation and mechanical ventilation to the patient and family; provide reassurance that this is a temporary measure to reduce the work of breathing and allow rest. Explain that talking is not possible while the endotracheal tube is in place, and establish a means of communication.

Decreased Cardiac Output

- Frequently assess and record vital signs and level of consciousness after initiation of mechanical ventilation or addition of positive end expiratory pressure.
- Measure urine output hourly; weigh daily.
- Monitor pulmonary artery pressures, central venous pressure, and cardiac output every 1 to 4 hours.
- Assess heart and lung sounds every 2 to 4 hours or as indicated.
- Keep skin clean and dry; frequently reposition and provide skin care. Protect bony prominences and pressure points.
- Maintain intravenous fluids as prescribed.

Dysfunctional Ventilatory Weaning Response

- Assess vital signs every 15 to 60 minutes following changes in ventilator settings and during T-piece trials.
- Monitor ABGs, $ETCO_2$, and oxygen saturation following changes in ventilator settings.
- Fully explain all weaning procedures, including expected changes in breathing. Provide psychologic support.

- Start weaning processes in the morning, when well rested. Weaning may be discontinued overnight to allow adequate rest.
- Avoid giving drugs that may depress respirations during weaning.
- Provide pulmonary hygiene with percussion, vibration, and postural drainage as indicated.

Community-Based Care
- Provide factual information about ARDS and its cause.
- Maximal respiratory function following ARDS is usually achieved within 6 months; respiratory function may remain significantly impaired. This may necessitate changes in occupation, lifestyle, and family roles.
- Avoiding smoking and exposure to secondhand smoke and environmental pollutants is vital to prevent further lung damage.
- Obtain immunization for pneumococcal pneumonia and annual influenza immunizations to prevent further episodes of serious respiratory disease.
- Provide referrals to home health and respiratory care services as indicated, as well as for occupational therapy and counseling as needed.

For more information about acute respiratory distress syndrome, see Chapter 37 of *Medical-Surgical Nursing*, Fifth Edition, by LeMone, Burke, and Bauldoff.

ADRENOCORTICAL INSUFFICIENCY (ADDISON'S DISEASE)

Overview
- Adrenal cortical insufficiency results in inadequate levels of glucocorticoids, mineralocorticoids, and androgens.
- Adrenal insufficiency is divided into two categories:
  - *Primary:* due to adrenal gland destruction and a lack of adrenal hormones. Addison's disease, failure of adrenal cortex function, is the most common form leading to deficits of glucocorticoids, mineralocorticoids, and androgens, and elevated adrenocorticotropic hormone (ACTH) levels.

- *Secondary:* due to hypopituitarism, surgical removal of the pituitary, or rapid withdrawal of therapeutically administered glucocorticoids.
- Addisonian crisis is a serious, life-threatening response to acute adrenal insufficiency. Primary problems are severe hypotension, circulatory collapse, shock, and coma.

Causes

Primary Insufficiency

- Addison's disease (autoimmune)
- Bilateral adrenalectomy
- Infections (tuberculosis, septicemia), neoplasms, trauma, or hemorrhage of the adrenal glands

Secondary Insufficiency

- Hypopituitarism (decreased ACTH)
- Surgical removal of ectopic ACTH-secreting tumors (e.g., oat cell carcinoma of the lungs)
- Abrupt withdrawal of long-standing corticosteroid drug therapy

Manifestations

- Weakness, fatigue, fever
- Anorexia, nausea, vomiting, weight loss
- Myalgias, arthralgias
- Anxiety and irritability, emotional changes
- Hyperpigmentation (bronzed color) of skin (especially areas such as knuckles, elbows, and palmar creases) and mucous membranes
- Hypoglycemia
- Hypotension, orthostatic hypotension
- Scant axillary and pubic hair in women

Diagnostic Tests

- Plasma cortisol and aldosterone levels are decreased in primary or secondary forms.

- Serum ACTH level: increased in primary; decreased in secondary.
- A 24-hour urine evaluates for decreased cortisol excretion.
- ACTH stimulation testing shows decreased cortisol secretion in primary disease.
- Serum electrolytes: decreased sodium, increased potassium, and possibly increased calcium.
- Fasting blood glucose or fasting blood sugar may be low.

Interdisciplinary Management

- The primary treatment of Addison's disease is oral replacement of corticosteroids and mineralocorticoids, accompanied by increased dietary sodium.

Selected Nursing Diagnoses with Interventions

Deficient Fluid Volume

- Monitor intake and output and assess for signs of dehydration (tenting of skin; dry mucous membranes; dark, scant urine).
- Monitor cardiovascular status: Take and record vital signs including orthostatic BPs, assess character of pulses, and monitor sodium and potassium levels.
- Weigh daily at the same time and in the same clothing.
- Encourage an oral fluid intake of 3000 mL per day and to increase salt intake.
- Teach to sit and stand slowly and provide assistance as necessary to avoid orthostatic hypotension.

Risk for Ineffective Therapeutic Regimen Management

- Encourage the patient to verbalize concerns.
- Teach the patient and significant others the effects of the illness and how to provide care. Family stability, an awareness of the serious nature of the disease, and the effectiveness of treatment all promote compliance.

Community-Based Care

- Teach how to self-administer steroids.

- Emphasize the importance of wearing a MedicAlert bracelet or medal and carrying at all times an emergency kit for administering parenteral cortisone.
- Teach to exercise regularly and to maintain a generous fluid intake and a diet high in sodium and low in potassium.
- Discuss the effect of emotional or physical stressors on physical health and medication management.
- Emphasize the importance of continuing health care; refer to community health services and support groups for information and follow-up health care as appropriate.

For more information on adrenocortical insufficiency (Addison's disease), see Chapter 19 in *Medical-Surgical Nursing,* Fifth Edition, by LeMone, Burke, and Bauldoff.

ALZHEIMER'S DISEASE

Overview

- Alzheimer's disease (AD) is a chronic, progressive, degenerative disorder of the cerebral cortex that results in severe cognitive dysfunction.
- It accounts for about 50% to 70% of all cases of dementia, affecting approximately 4.5 million people.
- Familial AD follows an inheritance pattern; sporadic AD has no obvious inheritance pattern.
- Early onset AD affects people aged 30 to 60, is relatively rare, and often progresses more rapidly than late-onset AD, which affects people aged 65 and older.
- AD is characterized by the changes in neuronal proteins (tau), the presence of neurofibrillary tangles and amyloid plaques, and loss of neurons. Neuron loss produces deficits in neurotransmitters, including acetylcholine, norepinephrine, serotonin, somatostatin, and dopamine. The overall effect is impaired transmission of nerve impulses.
- Blood flow to affected areas of the brain is impaired, leading to atrophy of the brain (especially frontal, parietal, and medial temporal regions) with enlargement of the ventricles.

- Areas involved in short-term memory and cognition (the hippocampus and related structures) are affected first. With progression, loss of neurons in the cerebral cortex affects language skills and judgment. Frontal lobe involvement leads to emotional lability, agitation, and wandering. As all affected areas of the brain atrophy, the person becomes helpless and unresponsive.

- The onset is insidious; disease progresses relentlessly to total disability.

- Death usually occurs within 4 to 6 years of diagnosis, due to secondary complications such as aspiration pneumonia, malnutrition, trauma, or infection.

Causes

The exact cause is unknown but the following factors have been suggested.

- Genetics: gene defects on chromosomes 14, 19, or 21, leading to clumping and precipitation of insoluble amyloid as plaques; mitochondrial defects that alter cell metabolism and protein processing

- Biochemistry: lack of an enzyme (choline acetyltransferase) necessary for forming acetylcholine, a neurotransmitter; alterations in apolipoprotein E or protein kinase C

- Environmental: viral infection or exposure to an unknown toxin

- Immunologic: autoimmune response

Manifestations

Stage 1: No cognitive impairment

Stage 2: Very mild decline (may last 2 to 4 years)

- Forgetfulness

- Memory loss (especially for recent events)

- Difficulty learning new information; decreased ability to concentrate

- Lack of spontaneity, social withdrawal, loss of sense of humor

Stage 3: Mild cognitive decline (may last several years)

- Mental/behavioral changes including apathy, anxiety, depression, irritability, suspiciousness
- Progressive forgetfulness and memory loss
- Language disturbances: poor word choices, circumlocution, echolalia

Stage 4: Moderate cognitive decline

- Decreased capacity to perform complex tasks (buying groceries, paying bills)
- Reduced memory for personal history
- Subdued and withdrawn

Stage 5: Moderately severe cognitive decline

- Requires some assistance with activities of daily living, can usually eat and use the toilet
- Knows his or her name and the name of family members
- Inability to recall current address or telephone number
- Confusion about place, date, day, week, or season

Stage 6: Severe cognitive decline

- May forget names but can recognize familiar faces
- Progressive mental/behavioral deterioration: delusions, hallucinations, wandering (especially in late afternoon or early evening, labeled *sundowning*)
- Motor manifestations: apraxia, myoclonus, Parkinsonism
- Progressive self-care deficit
- Needs help with details of toileting; increasingly incontinent of feces and urine
- Apathy

Stage 7: Very severe cognitive decline (final stage)

- Total care needed for eating and toileting
- Inability to respond to environment, speak, or control movements
- Inability to recognize family, friends, or even self

Diagnostic Tests

- Mental status examination shows deficits in short-term memory, judgment, and cognition.
- Computed tomography scan and magnetic resonance imaging (MRI) show cortical atrophy and ventricular enlargement.
- Positron emission tomography shows reduced metabolic activity level of cerebral cortex; may be used to establish early diagnosis.

Interdisciplinary Management

- Tacrine (Cognex), donepezil (Aricept), and galantamine (Reminyl) are used to treat mild to moderate AD.
- Rivastigmine (Exelon) improves activities of daily living, decreases agitation and delusions, and improves cognitive function.
- Memantine (Namenda) improves cognitive function in moderate-to-severe AD.
- Antidepressant medications and low-dose psychotropic drugs may be used to manage behavior problems.

Selected Nursing Diagnoses with Interventions

Chronic Confusion

- Label rooms, drawers, and other items as appropriate.
- Keep environmental stimuli to a minimum. Decrease noise levels and speak in a calm, low voice. Take an unhurried approach.
- Limit questions to those that require a simple yes or no response.
- Orient to the environment, person, and time as able.
- Provide continuity in nursing staff.
- Repeat explanations simply and as needed to decrease anxiety.

Anxiety

- Assess for early behaviors of fatigue and agitation.
- Keep daily routine as consistent as possible.
- Schedule rest periods or quiet times throughout the day.

Hopelessness

- Assess the patient's and significant others' responses to the diagnosis and understanding of AD. Encourage expression of feelings.

- Provide realistic information about the disorder at the patient's level of understanding. The patient and family may need to have separate sessions.
- Avoid criticizing or judging expressed feelings.
- Support positive family bonds and enhance communication among family members.
- Promote positive regard.
- Encourage the patient to make as many decisions as possible.
- Encourage the patient and significant others to seek spiritual guidance or other strategies that previously inspired hope.

Caregiver Role Strain

- Teach the caregivers self-care techniques, such as taking rest periods and avoiding fatigue.
- Have the caregivers list and partake regularly in activities they enjoy, such as walking.
- Refer the caregivers to local AD support groups and to the national association. Suggest books on the topic.
- Refer the caregivers to Meals on Wheels, home health services, and other community services.

Community-Based Care

- Explain the disorder and its usual progression to the patient and caregivers.
- Review medication regimen and provide written instructions.
- Address safety considerations as well as the ability of caregivers to meet the patient's needs, such as maintaining hygiene and other activities of daily living.
- Suggest memory cues such as labeling drawers and rooms, and keeping the furniture and other items in each room in a consistent place.
- Suggest obtaining a MedicAlert bracelet or medal in case the patient wanders and is unable to provide verbal identification.
- Refer to community services, including long-term care facilities.
- A home safety inspection may be appropriate.

For more information on Alzheimer's disease, see Chapter 44 in *Medical-Surgical Nursing,* Fifth Edition, by LeMone, Burke, and Bauldoff.

For more information on Alzheimer's disease, see Chapter 44 in *Medical-Surgical Nursing,* Fifth Edition, by LeMone, Burke, and Bauldoff.

AMYOTROPHIC LATERAL SCLEROSIS (ALS, LOU GEHRIG'S DISEASE)

Overview

- Amyotrophic lateral sclerosis (ALS) is a chronic, progressive, disabling motor neuron disease leading to muscle atrophy and weakness.
- ALS is diagnosed in 1 to 2 people per 100,000 each year.
- Onset is middle to late adult age; incidence is two times higher in men than in women. ALS results from degeneration and demyelination of upper motor neurons (motor cortex and corticospinal tracts), motor nuclei of the brain, and lower motor neurons (anterior horn cells of spinal cord and cranial nerves), causing muscle atrophy with progressive weakness and paresis.
- Sensory, cognitive, and sphincter function remain intact throughout the disease.
- Death usually results within 2 to 5 years after onset, usually from respiratory failure.

Causes

- Approximately 5% to 10% of patients inherit ALS as an autosomal-dominant trait; the majority of cases occur randomly.
- In most instances, the cause of ALS is unknown; damage from free radicals, higher than normal glutamate levels, and autoimmune responses are being studied. Viral, environmental, and other factors are also being researched. Risk factors may include age, diet, and military service.

Manifestations

- Muscle weakness/fatigue; usually begins in distal, upper extremities
- Muscle fasciculations/spasticity, progressing to atrophy and flaccid paralysis

- Hyperreflexia
- Dysphagia, dysarthria (slurred speech), drooling
- Dyspnea, ineffective cough, shallow respirations

Diagnostic Tests

- No specific diagnostic tests are available.
- Electromyogram shows abnormal electrical activity of involved skeletal muscles.
- Nerve conduction studies are usually normal.
- Cerebrospinal fluid analysis shows increased protein content in some patients.
- Muscle biopsy shows atrophy of myofibrils; rules out primary muscle disease.

Interdisciplinary Management

- Medical care for patients with ALS is mainly supportive. Riluzole, a drug that inhibits glutamate release, may slow the progression of ALS. As the disease progresses, nutritional and ventilatory support may be primary considerations.

Selected Nursing Diagnoses with Interventions

Risk for Disuse Syndrome

- Assess current condition for baseline parameters, particularly skin over bony prominences, lung sounds, and vital signs.
- Lubricate and inspect skin. Obtain an alternating-pressure mattress.
- Institute active range-of-motion exercises as the patient is able. Perform passive range-of-motion exercises every 2 hours when the patient is turned.
- Maintain positive nitrogen balance and hydration status: monitor albumin levels, hemoglobin and hematocrit levels, and urine specific gravity.
- Monitor patient for manifestations of infection. Specifically, assess urine for color, odor, and consistency, especially if a urinary catheter is present.

Ineffective Breathing Pattern

- Monitor breathing pattern, air movement, and oxygen saturation.
- Turn at least every 2 hours.
- Elevate the head of the bed at least 30 degrees, suction as indicated, and provide oxygen.
- Assess temperature and lung sounds routinely. Obtain sputum culture as indicated.

Community-Based Care

- Initial teaching centers on explaining the disease process, expected course, and prognosis.
- As the disease progresses, teach caregivers how to suction the patient and perform the Heimlich maneuver to treat aspiration.
- Teach bowel care, considerations related to a urinary catheter, and prevention and manifestations of infection, emphasizing the need to promptly notify the healthcare provider if these occur.
- Refer to a social worker to determine home care needs and financial assistance as indicated.
- Refer to a mental health counselor to assist with coping as appropriate. An ALS support group may also be helpful.

For more information on amyotrophic lateral sclerosis, see Chapter 44 in *Medical-Surgical Nursing,* Fifth Edition, by LeMone, Burke, and Bauldoff.

ANAPHYLAXIS

Overview

- Anaphylaxis is an acute, life-threatening, systemic hypersensitivity reaction.
- It is mediated by IgE antibody on sensitized mast cells produced during previous exposure to the antigen.
- During the acute reaction, antigen and IgE binding release histamine and leukotrienes into the general circulation.
- Bronchospasm, massive vasodilation, and increased capillary permeability and leakage occur within seconds or minutes of exposure to the offending antigen.

- Anaphylaxis may progress rapidly to vascular collapse, shock, and possibly death.

Causes

- Usually associated with ingestion, infusion, and/or inhalation of significant amounts of antigen, the most common of which are as follows:
  - Antibiotics (especially penicillin)
  - Sulfonamides
  - Local anesthetics
  - Salicylates
  - Iodine drugs used in diagnostic tests
  - Hormones/enzymes
  - Vaccines/serums, immunoglobulin therapy
  - Foods, including seafood, eggs, berries, nuts, legumes (including peanuts), foods containing sulfites
  - Latex
  - Insect venom, including bees, hornets, wasps, yellow jackets, fire ants, spiders
  - Snake venom

Manifestations

- Onset occurs usually within minutes of exposure to the offending antigen; may persist for 24 hours.

General Manifestations

- Anxiety, sense of impending doom
- Weakness
- Urticaria
- Cutaneous wheals: well circumscribed, erythematous
- Angioedema
- Sweating

Cardiovascular Manifestations

- Hypotension

- Shock
- Cardiac dysrhythmia
- Possible cardiac arrest

Respiratory Manifestations
- Urticaria
- Nasal congestion, watery rhinorrhea
- Hoarseness, stridor
- Wheezing, "tight chest"
- Dyspnea, shortness of breath
- Respiratory failure

Gastrointestinal Manifestations
- Nausea
- Severe gastrointestinal cramps
- Diarrhea

Neurologic Manifestations
- Dizziness
- Drowsiness
- Headache
- Seizures

Diagnostic Tests
- Allergic skin testing may indicate antigenic substance; may also precipitate an acute anaphylactic response.
- Arterial blood gases are obtained during acute phase to assess respiratory impairment; the pH, PaO_2, and total oxygen saturation decrease, and the $PaCO_2$ increases in respiratory failure.
- Serum electrolytes: with progressive shock, glucose and sodium levels decrease and potassium levels increase.
- Differential white blood cell count: eosinophils are increased.

Interdisciplinary Management
- Intravenous (IV) fluid resuscitation with isotonic solution

- Oxygen therapy, usually by mask or nasal cannula
- Medications, including epinephrine to increase tissue perfusion and oxygenation, diphenhydramine to treat angioedema and urticaria, aminophylline drip for bronchospasm, and/or steroids for long-term care
- Possible emergency intubation or tracheostomy

Selected Nursing Diagnoses with Interventions

Ineffective Airway Clearance

- Ask all patients about allergies prior to administering any medications, using latex gloves, or hanging an IV.
- Assess for manifestations of anaphylaxis, including itching, edema, wheezing, dyspnea, cyanosis, anxiety, flushing, diaphoresis, hypotension, and bronchospasm.
- Assess airway. Prepare for possible emergency tracheostomy.
- Suction as needed.
- Administer oxygen as ordered.
- Administer epinephrine per orders: (1:1000) 0.3 to 0.5 mg/kg IM, SL, or inhaled, or (1:10,000) 0.5 mg in 10 mL IV slowly over 5 to 10 minutes.
- Administer diphenhydramine, 50 to 100 mg IM, per orders.
- Administer other medications such as an aminophylline drip or corticosteroids per physician prescription.
- Clearly mark all records with known allergies.

Decreased Cardiac Output

- Administer isotonic IV fluids to maintain cardiac output.
- Decrease further absorption of antigen as appropriate by placing tourniquet between injection/sting site and heart, if possible. Apply ice pack to injection/sting site. If antigen was ingested, administer gastric lavage.

Community-Based Care

- Instruct how to avoid the antigen/causative agent.
- Explain where to obtain and keep an anaphylaxis kit (EpiPen), and how to use it for emergencies.

- Provide information on obtaining and wearing a MedicAlert bracelet to inform potential caregivers and others of the known antigen.

- Stress the importance of having family members trained in cardiopulmonary resuscitation.

For more information on anaphylaxis, see Chapters 11 and 13 in *Medical-Surgical Nursing,* Fifth Edition, by LeMone, Burke, and Bauldoff.

ANEMIA

Blood loss (acute, chronic)

Nutritional (iron deficiency, vitamin B_{12} deficiency, folate deficiency)

Hemolytic (sickle cell, Thalassemia, acquired)

Bone marrow suppression (aplastic)

Overview

- Anemia is an abnormally low circulating red blood cell (RBCs) count, hemoglobin (Hgb) concentration, or both.

- Anemia reduces the oxygen-carrying capacity of the blood, leading to tissue hypoxia.

Causes

- Anemia is categorized by cause: blood loss, nutritional, hemolytic, and bone marrow suppression.

  1. Blood loss anemias result from acute or chronic bleeding. Acute blood loss reduces the number of circulating RBCs, the Hgb, and the hematocrit (Hct). Chronic blood loss depletes iron stores as RBC production increases to maintain the supply.

  2. Nutritional anemias result from nutrient deficits that affect RBC formation or Hgb synthesis. Common nutritional anemias include iron, vitamin B_{12}, and folic acid deficiency anemias. Vitamin B_{12} deficiency usually results from impaired gastrointestinal absorption of the nutrient due to lack of intrinsic factor (pernicious anemia).

  3. Hemolytic anemias result from premature destruction (lysis) of RBCs. Hemolysis may be caused by genetic disorders such as sickle cell anemia, thalassemia, and glucose-6-phosphate

dehydrogenase anemia, or by acquired conditions such as mechanical trauma to RBCs, autoimmune disorders, infections, immune responses, and drugs, toxins, or venoms.

4. Bone marrow suppression (aplastic anemia) affects production of RBCs, white blood cells, and platelets as normal bone marrow is replaced by fat.

Manifestations

- May be asymptomatic.
- Severity of manifestations depends on rate at which anemia develops and the extent of RBC reduction.
- General manifestations include the following:
  - Pallor of skin, mucous membranes, conjunctiva, and nail beds
  - Tachycardia, tachypnea
  - Fatigue, dyspnea on exertion, night cramps
  - Bone pain
  - Headache, dizziness, dim vision
- Acute blood loss also can produce signs of shock due to reduced volume.
- Table 3 (pages 566–567) summarizes the manifestations of specific types of anemia.

Diagnostic Tests

- Complete blood count is done to determine blood cell counts, Hgb, Hct, RBC indices, and RBC morphology (shape and size).
  1. The RBC count is reduced in some anemias.
  2. Total Hgb measures the weight (g) of Hgb in a volume (dL) of blood; it is low in anemia.
  3. The Hct, the percentage of total blood volume that is RBCs, is reduced in anemia.
- RBC indices include the following:
  1. Mean corpuscular volume, the average size of RBCs.
  2. Mean corpuscular Hgb, the weight of Hgb in the average RBC.
  3. Mean corpuscular Hgb concentration, average Hgb concentration in RBCs.

- Iron levels and total iron-binding capacity help identify iron-deficiency anemia, characterized by low serum iron concentration and increased total iron-binding capacity.

- Serum ferritin is an iron-storage protein that mobilizes stored iron when metabolic needs are higher than dietary intake.

- Hgb electrophoresis is used to evaluate hemolytic and genetic anemias.

- The Schilling test measures vitamin B_{12} absorption to identify pernicious anemia.

- Bone marrow aspiration may be used to diagnose aplastic anemia.

Interdisciplinary Management

- Iron replacement therapy (oral or parenteral) is used to treat iron-deficiency anemia.

- Parenteral vitamin B_{12} is given to treat vitamin B_{12} deficiency anemia.

- Folic acid is ordered for women of childbearing age, pregnant women, and patients with folic acid deficiency or sickle cell anemia.

- Hydroxyurea (Hydrea, Droxia), a drug that promotes fetal Hgb production, may be ordered for sickle cell disease as increased levels of fetal Hgb interfere with the sickling process and reduce the incidence of crises.

- Immunosuppressive therapy may be used to treat aplastic anemia.

- Dietary modifications are recommended for nutritional deficiency anemias.

- Blood transfusions may be indicated for anemia due to major blood loss and severe anemia regardless of cause.

Selected Nursing Diagnoses with Interventions

Activity Intolerance

- Help identify ways to conserve energy when performing necessary or desired activities.

- Help the patient and family establish priorities for tasks and activities.

- Assist in developing a schedule of alternating activity and rest periods throughout the day.

- Encourage 8 to 10 hours of sleep at night.
- Monitor vital signs before and after activity. Discontinue activity if chest pain, breathlessness, vertigo, palpitations, persistent tachycardia, bradycardia, tachypnea, dyspnea, or decreased systolic blood pressure develop.
- Instruct the patient not to smoke.

Impaired Oral Mucous Membrane

- Monitor condition of lips and tongue daily.
- Provide frequent oral hygiene and mouthwash of saline, saltwater, or half-strength peroxide and water to rinse the mouth every 2 to 4 hours.
- Apply a petroleum-based lubricating jelly or ointment to the lips after oral care.
- Encourage soft, cool, bland foods, and four to six small meals daily with high protein and vitamin content.

Risk for Decreased Cardiac Output

- Monitor vital signs, breath sounds, and apical pulse.
- Assess for pallor, cyanosis, and dependent edema.
- Report signs of decreased cardiac output to the physician.

Community-Based Care

- Explain nutritional strategies to address deficiencies.
- Describe prescribed medications, vitamins, or mineral supplements; their appropriate use; intended effect; possible adverse effects; and interactions with food or other medications.
- Relate energy conservation strategies.
- Explain other recommended treatment measures and follow-up.
- If the anemia is genetically transmitted, such as sickle cell anemia, explain its inheritance patterns, symptoms of crisis, and manifestations to report to the physician. Provide referrals for counseling to facilitate decisions about pregnancy as indicated.
- Refer for nutritional assistance and teaching, home health care, or assistance with self-care and home maintenance activities as indicated.

For more information about anemia, see Chapter 33 in *Medical-Surgical Nursing,* Fifth Edition, by LeMone, Burke, and Bauldoff.

Aneurysm

Overview

- An aneurysm is an abnormal dilation of a blood vessel usually affecting high-pressure vessels such as the aorta and large peripheral arteries.

- True aneurysms affect all three layers of the vessel wall. Most are *fusiform* (spindle shaped, tapered at both ends) and *circumferential* (involving entire vessel diameter).

- False aneurysms (traumatic aneurysms) are caused by a traumatic break in the vessel wall. They may be *saccular* (shaped like small out-pouchings on the vessel wall).

- *Dissecting* aneurysms develop when a break or tear in the tunica intima and media allows blood to dissect the layers of the vessel wall.

- Thoracic aortic aneurysms may affect either the ascending or descending aorta (more common).

- Abdominal aortic aneurysms usually develop below the renal arteries where the aorta branches to form the iliac arteries.

- Popliteal and femoral aneurysms are often bilateral.

- Dissection can occur anywhere along the aorta: Type A (proximal) dissection affects the ascending aorta; type B (distal) dissection is limited to the descending aorta.

- Thoracic dissection progresses proximally and distally, and may affect aortic valve function, occlude the branches of the aorta, or extend into the renal, iliac, or femoral arteries.

Causes

- Commonly caused by arteriosclerosis or atherosclerosis.

- Hypertension is a major contributing factor.

- Advanced age and smoking may contribute.

- Trauma, infection, inflammatory, and genetic disorders also may cause aneurysms.

Manifestations

- Frequently asymptomatic.
- Manifestations vary by the location, size, and rate of aneurysm growth.

   a. Thoracic: substernal, neck, or back pain; dyspnea, stridor, cough, dysphagia, hoarseness, edema of the face and neck, and distended neck veins; angina; confusion, dizziness

   b. Abdominal: pulsating mass in the mid and upper abdomen, bruit over the mass; mild to severe midabdominal or lower back pain; manifestations of peripheral arterial occlusion by emboli

   c. Aneurysm rupture: hemorrhage, hypovolemic shock, death

   d. Popliteal and femoral aneurysms: intermittent claudication (cramping or pain in the leg muscles brought on by exercise and relieved by rest), rest pain, numbness of lower extremities; palpable pulsating mass behind the knee or in the femoral area

   e. Aortic dissection: sudden, excruciating pain over the area of dissection; syncope, dyspnea, weakness; initial increase in blood pressure followed by rapid drop; absent peripheral pulses

Diagnostic Tests

- Chest x-ray, abdominal ultrasonography, transesophageal echocardiography, contrast-enhanced computed tomography, and magnetic resonance imaging are used to detect and evaluate an aneurysm, depending on the suspected location.
- Angiography uses contrast solution injected into the involved vessel to visualize the precise size and location of the aneurysm.

Interdisciplinary Management

- Treatment depends on the size and location of the aneurysm. Hemodynamic pressures and urine are monitored to assess organ perfusion.
- Drugs used in treating aneurysms may include long-term beta blockers and other antihypertensive drugs to control heart rate and blood pressure. Sodium nitroprusside is infused to reduce systolic pressure.

- Anticoagulant therapy (heparin, oral anticoagulants, or aspirin) may be used to reduce the risk of clot formation.

- Surgical treatment may include excision of the aneurysm with synthetic graft insertion; the aneurysm walls may be left intact and used to cover the graft.

- An endovascular stent (a metal sheath covered with polyester fabric) graft may be inserted percutaneously under fluoroscopy for patients who have a high surgical risk.

Selected Nursing Diagnoses with Interventions

Risk for Ineffective Tissue Perfusion

- Immediately report manifestations of impending rupture, expansion, or dissection: increased pain, discrepancy between upper and lower extremity blood pressures and peripheral pulses, increased mass size, change in level of consciousness or motor or sensory function.

- Implement interventions to reduce the risk of rupture: maintain bed rest with legs flat and a calm environment, prevent straining during defecation, instruct to avoid holding the breath while moving.

- Report manifestations of arterial thrombosis or embolism: absent peripheral pulses; a pale or cyanotic, cool extremity; severe, diffuse abdominal pain with guarding; or increased groin, lumbar, or lower extremity pain.

- Continuously monitor cardiac rhythm. Report complaints of chest pain or changes in electrocardiogram tracing. Administer oxygen as indicated.

- Immediately report changes in mental status or symptoms of peripheral neurologic impairment (weakness, paresthesias, paralysis).

- Continuously monitor arterial pressure and hemodynamic parameters as indicated.

- Monitor urine output hourly. Report output less than 30 mL/hr.

Anxiety

- Explain all procedures and treatments, using simple and understandable terms.

- Respond to all questions honestly, using a calm, empathetic, but matter-of-fact manner.

- Provide care in a calm, efficient manner.
- Spend as much time as possible with the patient. Allow supportive family members to remain with the patient when possible.

Community-Based Care

Depending on the treatment plan, teaching topics include the following:

- Hypertension control, including lifestyle and prescribed drugs
- The benefits of smoking cessation
- Manifestations of increasing aneurysm size or complications to report to the physician
- Wound care and preventing infection; manifestations of wound complications to report
- Prescribed anticoagulation, expected and unintended effects
- Measures to prevent constipation and straining at stool (e.g., increasing fluid and fiber intake)
- The importance of avoiding prolonged sitting, lifting heavy objects, engaging in strenuous exercise, and having sexual intercourse until approved by physician
- Referrals to home health agency or a community health service as necessary

For more information on aneurysms, see Chapter 32 of *Medical-Surgical Nursing,* Fifth Edition, by LeMone, Burke, and Bauldoff.

ANGINA PECTORIS

Overview

- Angina pectoris (angina) is chest pain resulting from reduced coronary blood flow and a temporary imbalance between myocardial blood supply and demand.
- The imbalanced supply and demand causes temporary and reversible myocardial ischemia. Ischemia may be caused by partial obstruction or spasm of a coronary artery or a thrombus.
- Coronary artery obstruction leads to cellular hypoxia of the myocardium supplied by that vessel. As a result, cells switch to anaerobic metabolism, which increases lactic acid

production and affects cell membrane permeability, releasing substances such as histamine, kinins, and enzymes that stimulate terminal nerve fibers and send pain impulses to the central nervous system.

- Pain radiates to the upper body because the heart and upper body share the same dermatome.
- Return of adequate circulation provides oxygen and nutrients to the cells and clears waste products, relieving pain.
- There are three primary types of angina:
  1. Stable angina: predictable, occurring with a predictable amount of activity or stress, and relieved by rest and nitrates; associated with physical exertion, exposure to cold, or stress
  2. Prinzmetal's (variant) angina: atypical angina that occurs unpredictably (unrelated to activity), and, often at night; caused by coronary artery spasm
  3. Silent myocardial ischemia (asymptomatic ischemia) may occur with activity or mental stress

Causes

- Coronary heart disease, atherosclerosis, or vessel constriction
- Hypermetabolic conditions (e.g., exercise, cocaine use, hyperthyroidism, and emotional stress)
- Anemia, heart failure, or pulmonary diseases

Manifestations

- Chest pain: precipitated by activity, strong emotion, or stress; a tight, squeezing, heavy pressure, or constricting sensation; substernal, may radiate to jaw, neck, or arm
- Typically lasts less than 15 minutes; relieved by rest
- Dyspnea, pallor, tachycardia, anxiety, and fear

Diagnostic Tests

- Electrocardiogram may be normal or show nonspecific changes in the ST segment and T wave. During periods of ischemia, the ST segment is depressed or downsloping, and the T wave may flatten or invert.

- Stress electrocardiography (exercise stress tests) monitors for electrocardiogram changes during progressive exercise.

- Radionuclide testing uses an intravenous radioisotope (e.g., thallium-201) to evaluate myocardial perfusion and left ventricular function. May be combined with pharmacologic stress testing.
- Multiple gated acquisition scanning uses technetium 99m to assess for injury and residual cardiac function.
- Echocardiography uses ultrasound to evaluate cardiac structure and function. Transesophageal echocardiography can also identify abnormal blood flow patterns, using a probe on the tip of an endoscope inserted into the esophagus.
- Coronary angiography allows visualization of the coronary arteries and any abnormalities by injecting radiographic dye into each coronary opening. Most lesions causing symptoms involve more than 70% narrowing.

Interdisciplinary Management

- Coronary heart disease risk factor management.
- Medications include the following:
  1. Nitrates to treat acute attacks (e.g., sublingual nitroglycerin or buccal spray) and prevent angina (e.g., oral or topical nitroglycerin)
  2. Beta blockers to prevent anginal attacks
  3. Calcium channel blockers for long-term prophylaxis of angina
  4. Platelet inhibitors to reduce the risk of myocardial infarction
- Nonsurgical procedures restore blood flow and oxygen to ischemic tissue, such as transluminal coronary angioplasty, laser angioplasty, coronary atherectomy, and intracoronary stents.
- Surgical procedures (coronary artery bypass grafting, minimally invasive coronary artery surgery) are used to bypass coronary artery obstruction; or transmyocardial laser revascularization provides collateral blood flow to ischemic muscle.

Selected Nursing Diagnoses with Interventions

Ineffective Tissue Perfusion: Cardiac

- Keep prescribed nitroglycerin tablets available for patient to use at onset of pain.

- Start oxygen at 4 to 6 L/min per nasal cannula or as prescribed.
- Space activities to allow rest between them.
- Encourage to implement and maintain a supervised progressive 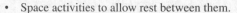 exercise program.
- Refer to a smoking cessation program as indicated.

Risk for Ineffective Therapeutic Regimen Management

- Assess knowledge and understanding of angina.
- Teach about angina and atherosclerosis as needed, building on current knowledge base.
- Stress importance of taking chest pains seriously while maintaining a positive attitude.
- Refer to a cardiac rehabilitation program.

Community-Based Care

- Explain prescribed medications, their purpose, appropriate use, anticipated and potential adverse effects; include importance of not discontinuing medications abruptly.
- Nitroglycerine use for acute angina: Always carry several tablets (not the entire supply); use prophylactically before activities that often cause chest pain; take tablet at first indication of pain rather than waiting to see if the pain develops; seek immediate medical assistance if three nitroglycerin tablets over 15 to 20 minutes do not relieve the pain.
- If cardiac surgery has been performed, include the following:
  1. Respiratory care, activity, and pain management
  2. Cardiac rehabilitation activities
  3. Manifestations and management of potential complications
- Discuss CHD and the relationship between pain and reduced blood flow to the heart muscle.
- Instruct to call 911 or go to the emergency department immediately for unrelieved chest pain.
- Nitroglycerine should be stored in a cool, dry, dark place; no more than a 6-month supply should be kept on hand.
- Refer to a cardiac rehabilitation program as appropriate.

For more information about angina pectoris, see Chapter 30 of *Medical-Surgical Nursing,* Fifth Edition, by LeMone, Burke, and Bauldoff.

ANTHRAX

Overview

- Anthrax is caused by an aerobic, gram-positive, spore-forming bacillus, the *Bacillus anthracis.*

- Anthrax is an infectious disease that may affect the skin, respiratory tract, gastrointestinal tract, or oropharynx.

- Aerosolized anthrax, resulting in inhalation anthrax, is considered a bioterrorism threat.

- Centers for Disease Control and Prevention guidelines for inhalation anthrax treatment protocols are followed for treatment of all types of anthrax.

- When antimicrobial therapy is prescribed to prevent inhalation anthrax, it must be taken for 60 days. Antimicrobial prophylaxis is indicated for the following:

  - Persons exposed to airspace with known contamination of aerosolized *B. anthracis.*

  - Persons exposed to an air space known to be the source of an inhalation anthrax case.

  - Persons along the transit path of an envelope or other vehicle containing *B. anthracis* that may have been aerosolized.

  - Unvaccinated laboratory workers exposed to confirmed *B. anthracis* cultures.

Cutaneous Anthrax

- Transmission is by direct skin contact with spores (as in soil) or by contact with infected animals or animal products (usually related to occupational exposure).

- The incubation period ranges from an immediate response to up to 1 day.

- Manifestations: localized itching followed first by a papular lesion that becomes vesicular and within 7 to 10 days a black eschar.

- Treatment:
  - Culture before beginning antimicrobial therapy.
  - Do not use extended-spectrum cephalosporins or trimethoprim/sulfamethoxazole, as anthrax may be resistant to these drugs.
  - Use standard precautions and avoid direct contact with wound or wound drainage.

Inhalation Anthrax

- Incubation period is usually less than 1 week but may be prolonged for as long as 2 months.

- Manifestations:
  - Initially: low-grade fever, nonproductive cough, malaise, fatigue, muscle aches, profound sweating, chest discomfort. Chest x-ray shows mediastinal widening and (often) pleural effusion.
  - Subsequent phase (1 to 5 days after manifestations begin): abrupt onset of high fever, severe respiratory distress with dyspnea and cyanosis, shock. Death may occur within 24 to 36 hours.

- Treatment:
  - Culture specimens appropriate to system affected, including blood, pleural fluid, cerebral spinal fluid before beginning antimicrobial therapy.
  - Initiate antimicrobial therapy immediately upon suspicion of anthrax. Do not use anthrax-resistant medications (see Cutaneous Anthrax).
  - Provide supportive care.
  - Follow standard contact precautions.

- Report suspected or confirmed anthrax cases immediately to your local or state department of health.

For more information about anthrax, see Chapters 7 and 36 in *Medical-Surgical Nursing,* Fifth Edition, by LeMone, Burke, and Bauldoff.

Appendicitis

Overview

- Appendicitis is inflammation of the vermiform appendix, a common cause of acute abdominal pain, and the most common reason for emergency abdominal surgery in the United States.

- The appendix is a blind, tubelike pouch attached to the cecum just below the ileocecal valve. Its function is not well understood; it regularly fills and empties with digested food.

- Obstruction of the proximal lumen of the appendix causes it to become distended with fluid secreted by its mucosa, increasing pressure within the appendix. This impairs its blood supply and causes inflammation, edema, ulceration, and infection. The appendix may rupture, resulting in bacterial peritonitis.

- In simple appendicitis, the appendix is inflamed but intact. Areas of tissue necrosis and microscopic perforations are present in gangrenous appendicitis. A perforated appendix shows evidence of gross perforation and contamination of the peritoneal cavity.

Causes

- Obstruction of the appendix by a fecalith, or hard mass of feces, is the usual cause; a calculus or stone, foreign body, inflammation, tumor, parasites (e.g., pinworms), or lymphoid tissue edema also may obstruct the appendix.

Manifestations

- Initial continuous mild generalized or upper abdominal pain; increasing pain intensity and localization to right lower quadrant of abdomen

- Pain that is aggravated by moving, walking, or coughing

- Localized and rebound tenderness at McBurney's point

- Low-grade temperature, anorexia, nausea, and vomiting

Diagnostic Tests

- White blood cell count shows elevated total white cell count (10,000 to 20,000/mm³), and increased immature white blood cells.
- Abdominal ultrasound is used to diagnose acute appendicitis, reducing the incidence of exploratory surgery.
- Pelvic examination is usually done on female patients of child-bearing age to rule out a gynecologic disorder or pelvic inflammatory disease.

Interdisciplinary Management

- Rapid diagnosis and treatment are important; diagnostic testing and preoperative treatment are limited.
- Oral food and fluids are withheld until a diagnosis is made.
- Appendectomy, surgical removal of the appendix, is the treatment of choice for acute appendicitis. Appendectomy may be performed using a laparoscopic approach or laparotomy (open approach).

Selected Nursing Diagnoses with Interventions

Risk for Infection

- Frequently assess abdominal status. Increasing generalized pain, a rigid, board-like abdomen, and abdominal distention may indicate developing peritonitis.
- Monitor vital signs, including temperature.
- Maintain intravenous infusion until oral intake is adequate.
- Assess wound, abdominal girth, and postoperative pain.

Acute Pain

- Assess character, location, severity, and duration of pain. Report unexpected changes in the nature of pain. Sudden relief of preoperative pain may signal rupture of the distended and edematous appendix.
- Administer analgesics as ordered.
- Assess effectiveness of medication following administration. Report unrelieved pain.

Community-Based Care

With uncomplicated appendectomy, the patient often is discharged either the day of surgery or the following day. Postoperative teaching includes the following:

- Wound or incision care, including hand hygiene
- Instructions to report fever, increased abdominal pain, swelling, redness, drainage, bleeding, or warmth of the operative site to the physician
- Activity limitations (e.g., lifting, driving), if any
- Returning to work

For more information about appendicitis, see Chapter 24 of *Medical-Surgical Nursing,* Fifth Edition, by LeMone, Burke, and Bauldoff.

ASTHMA

Overview

- Asthma, classified as a reactive airway disorder, is a chronic inflammatory disorder of the airways characterized by recurrent episodes of wheezing, breathlessness, chest tightness, and coughing.
- An acute inflammatory response triggered by factors such as allergens, respiratory tract infection, and exercise affects hyperreactive airways predisposed to bronchospasm.
- Sensitized mast cells in the bronchial mucosa release inflammatory mediators that stimulate parasympathetic receptors and bronchial smooth muscle to produce bronchoconstriction. They also increase capillary permeability, leading to mucosal edema, and stimulate mucus production.
- The attack is prolonged by activation of inflammatory cells such as basophils and eosinophils, which damage airway epithelium, produce mucosal edema, impair mucociliary clearance, and produce or prolong bronchoconstriction.
- Bronchoconstriction, edema and inflammation, and mucus secretion narrow the airway. Airway resistance increases, limiting airflow and increasing the work of breathing.

- Distal to the spastic airways, trapped air mixes with inspired air in the alveoli, reducing its oxygen tension and gas exchange across the alveolar-capillary membrane. Blood flow to distended alveoli is reduced. Resulting hypoxemia and increased lung volume due to trapping stimulate the respiratory rate, leading to tachypnea and respiratory alkalosis.
- Widespread airflow obstruction usually reverses spontaneously or with treatment.
- Status asthmaticus is severe, prolonged asthma that does not respond to routine treatment.

Causes
- Cause is unknown. Risk factors include allergies, genetic predisposition, air pollution, occupational exposure to industrial compounds, respiratory viruses; contributory factors include exercise and emotional stress.

Manifestations
- Abrupt or insidious onset of chest tightness, dyspnea, wheezing, and cough
- Tachycardia, tachypnea, prolonged expiration
- Diffuse wheezing and distant breath sounds
- Use of accessory muscles of respiration, intercostal retractions
- Fatigue, anxiety, apprehension
- Inaudible breath sounds with reduced wheezing and an ineffective cough may herald the onset of respiratory failure

Diagnostic Tests
- Pulmonary function tests are used to evaluate the degree of airway obstruction and its reversibility. The forced expiratory volume and peak expiratory flow rate (PEFR) evaluate the severity of an asthma attack and the effectiveness of treatment.
- Challenge or bronchial provocation testing uses an inhaled substance with pulmonary function tests to confirm the diagnosis of asthma by detecting airway hyperresponsiveness.

- Arterial blood gases are drawn during an acute attack to evaluate oxygenation, carbon dioxide elimination, and acid–base status. Common initial findings are hypoxemia with a low PO_2 and mild respiratory alkalosis due to tachypnea. Severe airflow obstruction causes significant hypoxemia and respiratory acidosis (pH less than 7.35 and PCO_2 greater than 42 mmHg), indicative of respiratory failure.
- Skin testing may be done to identify specific allergens if an allergic trigger is suspected.

Interdisciplinary Management

- Day-to-day asthma management focuses on controlling symptoms and preventing acute attacks.
  a. PEFR is used to evaluate bronchial hyperresponsiveness. Green (80% to 100% of personal best) indicates asthma that is under control; yellow (50% to 80%) indicates need for further medication or treatment; and red (50% or less) signals immediate need for a bronchodilator and possible medical treatment.
  b. Preventive measures include avoiding allergens and environmental triggers.
- Drugs for long-term asthma control include anti-inflammatory agents, long-acting bronchodilators, and leukotriene modifiers.
- Quick-relief medications, which provide prompt relief of bronchoconstriction and airflow obstruction, include short-acting adrenergic stimulants (rapid-acting bronchodilators), anticholinergic drugs, and methylxanthines.
- Inhalation of nebulized or aerosolized medication is the preferred route for administering most asthma medications.

Selected Nursing Diagnoses with Interventions

Ineffective Airway Clearance

- Assess respiratory status at least every 1 to 2 hours, including rate and depth, chest movement or excursion, breath sounds, PEFR, and cough effort and sputum.
- Monitor skin color, temperature, and level of consciousness.

- Report abnormal values and changes in arterial blood gases results and pulse oximetry readings.
- Place in Fowler's, high Fowler's, or orthopneic position to facilitate breathing and lung expansion.
- Administer oxygen and nebulizer treatments as ordered.
- Increase fluid intake.

Ineffective Breathing Pattern

- Assist with activities of daily living as needed.
- Provide rest periods between scheduled activities and treatments.
- Teach and assist to use techniques such as pursed-lip or abdominal breathing to control breathing pattern.

Anxiety

- Provide physical and emotional support. Remain with the patient during episodes of severe anxiety; schedule time every 1 to 2 hours to be with the patient who is mildly or moderately anxious. Answer call lights promptly.
- Listen actively to concerns; do not deny or negate the fear of dying or of being unable to breathe.
- Provide clear, concise directions and explanations about procedures.
- Include the patient in care planning and decisions as appropriate, without making excessive demands.
- Allow supportive family members to remain present.

Ineffective Therapeutic Regimen Management

- Assess level of understanding about asthma and the prescribed treatment regimen. Provide additional information and teaching as indicated.
- Assist to identify factors that contributed to the acute episode, as well as problems or difficulties integrating the treatment regimen into the patient's lifestyle.
- Refer to counseling, support groups, or self-help organizations.

Community-Based Care

- Suggest lifestyle changes to avoid specific triggers for asthma attacks (e.g., warming up before exercising, reducing the risk for respiratory infections, and using techniques to manage physical and psychologic stress).

A
- Use PEFR meter to monitor airway status; show how to manage the disease based on results.

- Explain prescribed medications, including the desired effect of each, potential adverse effects and their management, interactions with other drugs, and measures to avoid developing tolerance.

For more information about asthma, see Chapter 37 in *Medical-Surgical Nursing,* Fifth Edition, by LeMone, Burke, and Bauldoff.

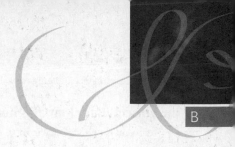

Bell's Palsy

Overview

- Bell's palsy, also known as facial paralysis, is characterized by unilateral weakness of the face.
- Bell's palsy produces acute unilateral flaccid paralysis of the muscles of facial expression.
- The disorder usually resolves spontaneously in a few weeks or months.
- It is seen at all ages, but is most common in people aged 20 to 60 years.

Causes

- This classic disorder is believed to be caused by the herpes simplex virus type 1 and herpes zoster virus.

Manifestations

- Onset is rapid, with initial numbness or stiffness of the affected side of the face.
- Aching pain, behind the ear or in the jaw, may precede facial weakness.
- Unilateral manifestations are as follows:
  - Drooping of affected side of the face
  - Inability to wrinkle the forehead, close eye, purse lips, puff out cheek
  - Drooping of mouth, with drooling
  - Loss or distortion of taste sensation
  - Excessive tearing

Diagnostic Test

- Magnetic resonance imaging may show swelling of the facial nerve.

B Interdisciplinary Management

- Treatment is unnecessary in most cases; 75% recover completely without treatment.
- A combination of antiviral therapy (e.g., acyclovir) and a corticosteroid drug may limit facial nerve damage.
- Eye protection is helpful, with lubricating drops and/or ointment and an eye patch, if closure is not possible.

Selected Nursing Diagnoses with Interventions

Risk for Imbalanced Nutrition: Less than Body Requirements

- Recommend soft diet and six small meals a day.
- Instruct patient to chew slowly on the unaffected side and avoid hot foods.
- Consume frequent, small, soft meals. Inspect and clean the mouth carefully after eating.

Risk for Injury

- Assess the degree of involvement and the resulting deficits.
- Nursing interventions are aimed primarily at teaching the patient and family about the disease and how to prevent injury and maintain nutrition.

Community-Based Care

- Inability to close the eyelid increases the risk of corneal dryness and abrasion. Use artificial tears four times a day and wear an eye patch at night and sunglasses or goggles when outdoors or when exposed to dust or sprays.
- Apply moist heat to the affected side of the face for comfort. Gently massage the affected side of the face and manually close the eyelid several times a day to maintain muscle tone. As function returns, wrinkle the forehead, open and close the eyes, and whistle several times daily.

- Seek medical follow-up care if the condition does not resolve spontaneously within a few months.

For more information on Bell's palsy, see Chapter 44 in *Medical-Surgical Nursing,* Fifth Edition, by LeMone, Burke, and Bauldoff.

BENIGN PROSTATIC HYPERPLASIA

Overview

- Benign prostatic hyperplasia (BPH) is an enlargement of the prostate gland.
- Manifestations of BPH typically develop after age 55. The risk of developing BPH is highest and symptoms develop earlier in African American men; native Japanese men have the lowest risk.
- The prostate enlarges through formation and growth of nodules (hyperplasia) and enlargement of glandular cells (hypertrophy).
- Manifestations of urinary obstruction generally are the earliest symptoms of BPH as the enlarging gland gradually obstructs the urethra.
- Obstruction and urinary retention increase the risk for urinary tract infection.

Causes

- Possible increased sensitivity to dihydrotestosterone, an androgen formed in the prostate from testosterone; altered testosterone-estrogen balance
- Risk factors: age, family history, race, and a diet high in meat and fats

Manifestations

- Urinary hesitancy (difficulty starting urine stream), frequency, nocturia
- Incomplete bladder emptying, dribbling after voiding
- Urinary retention, manifestations of urinary tract infection
- Urinary incontinence

- Enlarged prostate gland on rectal examination
- Complete obstruction: anuria, bladder pain, renal insufficiency

Diagnostic Tests

- Prostate-specific antigen is measured to help differentiate BPH from prostate cancer.
- Digital rectal examination reveals an enlarged prostate with a firm, rubbery surface.
- Uroflowmetry is useful to determine the peak urinary flow rate; a flow rate of less than 10 mL/second is indicative of obstruction.
- Ultrasonography may be used to estimate the size of the gland and assess postvoid urinary retention.

Interdisciplinary Management

- Mild prostate enlargement is treated with finasteride (Proscar) or dutasteride (Avodart), antiandrogen agents that reduce the size of the enlarged prostate.
- Alpha-adrenergic antagonists such as terazosin (Hytrin), doxazosin (Cardura), tamsulosin (Flomax), and alfuzosin (Uroxatral) block excessive smooth muscle contraction, relieving obstruction and increasing urine flow in BPH.
- These medications may be used in combination to relieve manifestations and prevent progression of BPH.
- Surgery for BPH includes transurethral incision of the prostate, transurethral resection of the prostate, and simple prostatectomy.
- Minimally invasive procedures such as balloon urethroplasty, laser or microwave hyperthermia, and intraurethral stents to maintain patency of the urethra can be done as outpatient procedures. These procedures preserve continence and potency.

Selected Nursing Diagnoses with Interventions

Deficient Knowledge

- Assess severity of symptoms.
- Teach methods to minimize symptoms and prevent infection.

- Advise to restrict alcohol intake, especially at night, to minimize problems with nocturia.

Risk for Imbalanced Fluid Volume (following Transurethral Resection of the Prostate)

- Assess for manifestations of fluid volume excess and dilutional hyponatremia.
- Monitor fluid balance. Weigh the patient daily at the same time each day.
- Restrict fluids and administer diuretics as prescribed.
- Administer replacement therapy as prescribed.

Community-Based Care

- Provide information about the disease process and treatment options.
- Maintain a fluid intake of 2 to 3 L per day of nonalcoholic beverages, unless contraindicated.
- Teach how to do Kegel exercises to reduce the risk for urinary incontinence.
- Provide detailed information about prescribed medications:
  - Antiandrogen agents may cause impotence, decreased libido, and decreased ejaculate volume; crushed tablets should not be handled by pregnant women, as the drug may be absorbed through the skin and be harmful to a male fetus.
  - Alpha-adrenergic antagonists may cause orthostatic hypotension; instruct to change positions slowly. Talk to a healthcare provider or pharmacist before taking over-the-counter medications for coughs, colds, or allergies.
- If blood is noticed in the urine, increasing fluid intake should clear the urine in one or two voidings. Notify the physician if blood in the urine continues, clots are noticed, or if the patient is unable to urinate.
- Avoid strenuous activity, sexual intercourse, heavy labor, and heavy lifting for 6 weeks postoperatively.
- If the patient is discharged with a catheter, provide catheter care instructions.

- Address concerns about sexuality following prostate surgery; refer to counseling or support services as indicated.

For more information on benign prostatic hyperplasia, see Chapter 48 in *Medical-Surgical Nursing,* Fifth Edition, by LeMone, Burke, and Bauldoff.

BLADDER CANCER

Overview

- Bladder cancer is a malignant tumor of the urinary bladder, the most common urinary system malignancy.
- Men are four times more likely to develop bladder cancer than women; it is the fourth most commonly occurring cancer and the eighth highest cause of cancer deaths in men.
- Most bladder tumors arise from transitional epithelium of the bladder mucosa.
- Most bladder tumors are superficial, noninvasive papillary lesions (*papillomas*) that bleed easily and frequently recur. Papillomas rarely become invasive, and the prognosis for recovery is good.
- Carcinoma *in situ*, which occurs less frequently, is a poorly differentiated flat tumor that invades directly and has a poorer prognosis.

Causes

The precise cause of bladder cancer is unknown; however, risk factors are as follows:

- Male gender, age > 60, residence in urban area
- Cigarette smoking
- Occupational exposure to dyes or solvents
- Chronic urinary tract infection or bladder calculi
- The parasite *Schistosoma haematobium,* endemic to Egypt and the Sudan

Manifestations

- Gross or microscopic hematuria

- Frequency, urgency, dysuria, nocturia
- Manifestations of obstruction, hydronephrosis, or renal failure

Diagnostic Tests

- Urinalysis to evaluate for hematuria
- Urine cytology to identify abnormal cells (tumor or pretumor cells)
- Ultrasound of the bladder to detect bladder tumors
- Intravenous pyelography to evaluate the structure and function of the kidneys, ureters, and bladder
- Cystoscopy and urethroscopy for direct visualization, assessment, and biopsy of lesions of the urethra, bladder, or ureters
- Computed tomography scan or magnetic resonance imaging to evaluate tumor invasion or metastasis

Interdisciplinary Management

- Surgery ranges from simple resection of noninvasive tumors to removal of the bladder and surrounding structures, including hysterectomy in women. A urinary diversion is created to provide for urine collection and drainage.
- Radiation may be used as adjunctive therapy to reduce tumor size prior to surgery, or for palliation in patients with inoperable tumors.
- Chemotherapy may be delivered by intravesicular (into the bladder) instillation or intravenous administration (less common). Agents such as Bacillus Calmette-Guérin (BCG Live, TheraCys) suspension, doxorubicin and mitomycin, cisplatin, methotrexate, and vinblastine may be used for intravesicular chemotherapy.

Selected Nursing Diagnoses with Interventions

Impaired Urinary Elimination

- Monitor amount, color, and clarity of urinary output from all catheters, stents, and tubes hourly for the first 24 hours postoperatively, then every 4 to 8 hours. Promptly report urine output of less than 30 mL per hour.
- Label all catheters, stents, and drainage containers. Maintain separate closed gravity drainage systems for each.

- Secure ureteral catheters and stents with tape to prevent kinking or occlusion. Maintain gravity flow by keeping drainage bag below the level of the kidneys.
- Encourage fluid intake of 3000 mL per day.
- Monitor urine output closely for first 24 hours after removal of stents or ureteral catheters.
- Encourage activity as tolerated.

Risk for Impaired Skin Integrity

- Assess peristomal skin for redness, excoriation, or signs of breakdown. Assess for urine leakage from catheters, stents, or drains. Apply protective skin barrier ointment or dressing as indicated.
- Change urine collection appliance as needed, removing any mucus from stoma.

Risk for Infection

- Use strict aseptic technique and appropriate procedure when irrigating catheters and stents and for dressing changes.
- Monitor for signs of infection.
- Teach the patient and his or her significant others manifestations of infection and self-care measures to prevent urinary tract infection.

Community-Based Care

- Explain urinary stoma and skin care, preventing urine reflux and infection, pouch emptying and change, and use of night drainage system.
- Maintain a fluid intake of at least 2 quarts per day.
- Explain manifestations of tumor recurrence.
- Return for diagnostic tests and follow-up physician visits as scheduled.
- Provide home health referral for continued teaching and assessment as indicated.
- Provide a list of local resources for required equipment or supplies.
- Provide information about national and local support groups, such as the United Ostomy Association and the American Cancer Society.

For more information on bladder cancer, see Chapter 27 in *Medical-Surgical Nursing,* Fifth Edition, by LeMone, Burke, and Bauldoff.

Bone Tumor, Primary

Overview

- Bone tumors are benign or malignant neoplasms arising from bone or bony structures.
- Malignant tumors most often affect the long bones (femur, tibia, humerus) and the knee.
- Bone tumors may arise from cartilage (chondrogenic), bone (osteogenic), collagen (collagenic), or bone marrow (myelogenic).
- Primary malignant tumors are rare, accounting for about 0.2% of all adult cancers and about 15% of pediatric cancers. Secondary bone tumors, arising from metastases of primary tumors of other tissue, are more common, most often associated with cancer of the prostate, breast, kidney, thyroid, and lung.
- Tumors arising in bone and cartilage are more common in males, whereas those arising in collagen and bone marrow are more common in females.
- Osteosarcoma is the most common malignant bone tumor; its incidence is highest in adolescents and in people aged 50 to 60.
- Malignant bone tumors often cause rapid bone destruction and metastasis (to lung or other bones).
- The course and prognosis depend on the specific type of tumor.

Causes

- Unknown; associated with rapid bone growth (adolescence) and Paget's disease

Manifestations

- Bone pain (most common): dull, more common at night
- Visible or palpable mass

- Pathologic fracture
- Impaired function, weakness, or limp
- Tenderness, redness, swelling over tumor site

B

Diagnostic Tests

- X-ray, computed tomography scan, or magnetic resonance imaging may show tumor location, size, and invasion of adjacent tissues.
- Biopsy (needle or percutaneous needle) determines the type of tumor present.
- Serum calcium and alkaline phosphatase (a bone enzyme) are usually elevated.

Interdisciplinary Management

- Chemotherapeutic agents or radiation therapy are administered to shrink the tumor before surgery, to control recurrence of tumor growth after surgery, or to treat metastasis of the tumor.
- Radiation therapy also may be used to control pain.
- The goal of surgery is to eliminate the bone tumor completely. Bone grafts often are used to replace missing bone, preserving the limb and preventing amputation.

Selected Nursing Diagnoses with Interventions

Risk for Injury

- Instruct patients in ways to avoid falls or injury to the tumor site.

Acute Pain, Chronic Pain

- Develop strategies for controlling both acute pain (from surgery, fracture, or inflammation) and chronic pain (from progression of the disease).
- Provide assistive devices (e.g., canes, walkers, crutches) when the patient ambulates.

Impaired Physical Mobility

- Begin muscle-strengthening and active and passive range-of-motion exercises immediately after surgery. A continuous passive motion (CPM) machine may be used after surgical procedures to either upper or lower extremities.

- For the patient who has had an amputation, encourage active range-of-motion exercises for all uninvolved joints.

- Encourage exercises that help strengthen the triceps muscles to assist in use of crutches or other devices.

- For the patient who has undergone amputation of a lower extremity, encourage quadriceps and gluteal setting exercises and leg raises.

Community-Based Care

- Provide pain management information, including dosage, desired and adverse effects, and timing to effectively manage pain.

- Teach activity and weight-bearing restrictions: how to use correctly assistive devices such as crutches, walkers, and a trapeze, and prescribed exercises for optimum range of mobility.

- Explain wound care, if appropriate. Provide a list of local resources for supplies.

- Refer to physical therapy for ambulation training and appropriate muscle group strengthening exercises.

- Refer the patient with an amputation to a prosthetic specialist.

- Instruct to notify the physician immediately if increased swelling, discoloration, or changes in sensation occur. Stress the importance of continuing monitoring and follow-up care with the oncologist.

- Discuss hospice services and support groups for patients with metastatic disease.

For more information on bone tumors, see Chapter 40 in *Medical-Surgical Nursing,* Fifth Edition, by LeMone, Burke, and Bauldoff.

BRAIN TUMOR (BENIGN AND MALIGNANT)

Overview

- Brain tumors are growths of abnormal cells in brain tissue, meninges, the pituitary gland, or blood vessels.

- Brain tumors may be benign or malignant, primary or metastatic, and intracerebral or extracerebral.

- Because brain tumors grow within the closed cranial vault, displacing or impinging on central nervous system structures, all can cause significant neurologic deficits and death.

- Brain tumors account for 2% of all cancer deaths.
- In adults, the highest incidence is between ages 50 to 70, and the most common tumor is glioblastoma multiforme, followed by meningioma and astrocytoma.
- Glioblastomas represent more than 50% of all primary intracranial lesions.

Causes

- The cause of brain tumors is unknown. Heredity is a possible factor.
- DNA mutations may affect oncogenes (speed up cell division) or tumor suppressor genes (slow cell division or cause cell death). Mutations may be genetic or may occur as cells continually divide, die, and are replaced.

Manifestations

- Onset is usually insidious.

General

- Headache, especially in morning
- Vomiting, with or without nausea
- Changes in cognition or consciousness, personality changes
- Seizures
- Manifestations of increased intracranial pressure

Focal

- Frontal lobe: impaired memory, cognition/judgment; personality/mood changes, apathy, lethargy, ataxia, apraxia, aphasia, incontinence
- Temporal lobes: abrupt changes in personality (affective/psychotic), mood, appetite, libido; hallucinations (auditory); partial-complex seizures; contralateral visual-field cuts; dilated pupils; contralateral hemiparesis
- Parietal lobes: receptive aphasia with contralateral hemianopia (left); spatial disorientation, constructional apraxia, and contralateral hemianopsia (right)
- Occipital lobe: seizures, visual agnosia, visual-field cuts

- Cerebellum: tremors, nystagmus, incoordination, ataxia, nuchal headache
- Cranial nerves: ptosis, diplopia, changes in sense of smell and ocular movement, ipsilateral drooping of face, loss of cough/swallow/gag reflex, tongue protrusion; unilateral hearing loss, tinnitus, ataxia (cranial nerve [CN] VIII); decreased facial sensation, facial weakness/paralysis (CN VII); schwannoma of CN VIII can compress CN VII and cause facial features

Diagnostic Tests

- Computed tomography scan or magnetic resonance imaging can show tumor location, size, shape, and the presence of cerebral edema or tissue shifts.
- Biopsy can distinguish between normal, benign, or malignant tissue.
- Brain scan may show increased radioisotope uptake, indicative of tumors; especially useful for meningiomas.
- Cerebral angiography may show effects of the tumor on cerebral perfusion patterns and tumor vascularity.
- Electroencephalogram may show localized abnormal brain wave function indicative of neoplastic growth.
- Positron emission tomography may show altered normal brain tissue metabolism versus abnormal brain neoplasm metabolism.
- X-ray of cranium may show tumor calcification or erosion of bony skull.

Interdisciplinary Management

- Various chemotherapeutic agents are used in the treatment of brain tumors. They may be administered intravenously, intra-arterially, intrathecally (into the spinal canal), intraventricularly, or implanted into the tumor during surgery. Convection-enhanced delivery (CED) is the continuous injection of chemotherapy (as a fluid) directly to the tumor site.
- Radiation therapy may be administered alone or as an adjunct to surgery.
- Neurosurgery is used to remove tumors, to reduce the size of a tumor, or for symptom relief.

Selected Nursing Diagnoses with Interventions

Anxiety

- Reinforce, clarify, and repeat information that has been provided.
- Encourage patient and significant others to verbalize feelings, questions, and fears; provide realistic information appropriate to their level of understanding.
- Arrange for a member of the clergy to visit if the patient so desires.
- Assess knowledge and response to hospitalization and impending surgery.
- Provide preoperative teaching. If possible, orient to the intensive care unit and introduce to personnel who provide postoperative care. Discuss the anticipated postoperative changes in appearance and behavior.
- Allow time for the patient and significant others to be together.

Risk for Infection

- Assess and report leakage of cerebrospinal fluid; prevent contamination of the area leaking cerebrospinal fluid.
- Use strict aseptic technique, keep the patient's hands away from dressings, and administer prescribed antibiotics.
- Assess and report manifestations of infection, including increased temperature, redness, swelling, drainage, pain, fever, chills, increasing headache, neck stiffness, photophobia, or positive Kernig's or Brudzinski sign.

Ineffective Protection

- Monitor for and promptly report manifestations of increased intracranial pressure, including restlessness, decreasing level of consciousness, headache, vomiting, seizures, decreasing sensory and motor function, changes in pupil size and reaction, changes in vital signs, and abnormal posturing.
- Implement interventions to decrease the risk of increased intracranial pressure:
  - Elevate the head of the bed 15 to 30 degrees unless contraindicated.
  - Avoid neck flexion or rotation.

- Do not take rectal temperatures.
- Avoid clustering activities that increase intracranial pressure, such as suctioning, turning, bathing.
- Administer prescribed antiemetics.
- Do not suction for more than 10 seconds at one time.
- Instruct to avoid—if possible—coughing, sneezing, and straining to have a bowel movement.
- Maintain prescribed fluid restrictions and administer prescribed diuretics.
- Maintain patency of drains or shunts.
- Implement interventions to prevent seizures or, if they occur, to prevent injury:
  - Pad side rails of bed.
  - Place bed in lowest position and keep side rails up.
  - Have oral airway and suction equipment immediately available.
  - Administer prescribed anticonvulsants.
  - If seizure occurs, maintain a patent airway, do not restrain patient, do not force anything into the patient's mouth, and provide physical and emotional support.

Community-Based Care

- Include caregivers as appropriate.
- Explain the disease process, treatment, and prognosis
- Teach safety measures for motor deficits, sensory deficits, lack of coordination, seizures, and cognitive deficits as appropriate.
- Provide medication information, including dosage and side effects.
- Explain nonpharmacologic comfort measures for nausea, vomiting, and pain.
- Teach alternative ways of communicating if aphasia is present, and compensatory measures if visual deficits are present.
- Stress the importance of reporting to the physician stiff neck, increasing headache, elevated temperature, new motor or sensory deficits, vision changes, or seizures.

- Provide information on how to purchase wigs and hairpieces if desired.

- Provide referrals to support groups and community resources such as the local chapter of the American Cancer Society.

- A referral to a rehabilitation service or home health nursing service may be appropriate.

For more information on brain tumors, see Chapter 42 in *Medical-Surgical Nursing,* Fifth Edition, by LeMone, Burke, and Bauldoff.

Breast Cancer

Overview

- Breast cancers are malignant neoplasms of breast tissues.

- They are the most common female cancer, and the second most common malignancy causing death in women.

- Malignancy in women less than 35 years of age is often familial and more serious.

- Incidence is lower in African American women than in European Americans; however, mortality rate is higher as it often is diagnosed at a later stage and survival rates are lower at all stages.

- Breast cancer is hormone dependent and does not develop in the absence of estrogen.

- It may remain noninvasive or invasive without metastasis for long periods of time.

- Breast cancer does occur in men, but is rare.

Causes

Genetics

- Family history of breast malignancy in first-degree family member (mother, sister, daughter, a male family member with breast cancer)

- Gene mutations: ATM (gene that repairs damaged DNA), p53 (tumor-suppressor gene), CHEK2 (greater risk if strong family history of breast cancer), PTEN (cell growth regulating gene)

- Mutation of BRCA1 gene on chromosome 17
- BRCA2, a gene on chromosome 13

Hormones

- Early menarche (< 11 years)/late menopause (> 55 years)
- Nulliparity or first child after age 30 years
- Estrogen replacement therapy or oral contraceptive use

Environment

- Radiation, especially if exposure occurs between 10 and 14 years of age
- High-fat diet; moderate to high alcohol intake

Other

- Age: rises continuously with age
- History of cancer in contralateral breast or endometrial/ovarian cancer
- Caucasian
- Middle/upper socioeconomic groups
- Obesity

Manifestations

- Breast lump is palpable if larger than 1 cm; lump characteristics include the following:
    - Hard or stony
    - Painless (most common)
    - Irregular in shape
    - "Fixed" or immovable
    - Often found in upper, outer quadrant
- Advanced disease may show the following:
    - Nipple retraction or discharge
    - Breast dimpling, contour changes, ulceration
    - Inflammation (redness, heat, edema)
    - Peau d'orange appearance
    - Palpable axillary lymph nodes

Diagnostic Tests

- Diagnostic mammography is used to help differentiate an identified lesion as benign or requiring further evaluation.

- Ultrasonography can differentiate cystic from solid lesions.

- Biopsy (fine needle, core needle, or surgical) is used to differentiate benign lesions from malignant ones.

- Scans of bone, brain, and liver can identify distant metastasis.

Interdisciplinary Management

- Surgical excisions range from removal of the lump itself, called a lumpectomy, to removal of the entire breast, the underlying chest muscles, and the lymph nodes under the arms, called a radical mastectomy.

- Radiation therapy is typically used following breast cancer surgery.

- Adjuvant chemotherapy has become the standard of care for the majority of breast cancer cases with axillary lymph node involvement. Hormonal therapy may be used to shrink the tumor or to delay postsurgical recurrence.

- Tamoxifen, a drug that interferes with estrogen activity, is used to prevent breast cancer in women at high risk and as adjunctive therapy for stage II, III, and IV breast cancer. Immunotherapy, using trastuzumab, is used to stop growth in tumors that express HER-2/neu receptor (an epidermal growth factor receptor-2 protein) on their cell surface.

Selected Nursing Diagnoses with Interventions

Anxiety

- Provide opportunities for the patient to express her thoughts and feelings, including immediate concerns about resuming home life and necessary changes.

- Assess knowledge of breast cancer; provide factual information about the disease and treatment options.

- Explain the surgical procedure, including what to expect in the preoperative and recovery periods.

- Explain that it is normal to have decreased sensation in the surgical area.

Decisional Conflict

- Provide an opportunity for questions, responding as simply and directly as possible. Make eye contact and pay attention to body language.

- Focus on immediate concerns and provide up-to-date written material for review.

- Listen in a nonjudgmental manner during the decision-making process.

- If the patient wishes, provide opportunities to meet other women who have had breast cancer surgery.

Anticipatory Grieving

- Listen attentively to expressions of grief and watch for nonverbal cues (failure to make eye contact, crying, silence).

- Explain that it is normal to have periods of depression, anger, and denial after breast surgery.

- If desired, involve the partner in helping the patient cope with grief. Remember that the partner may also be grieving.

Risk for Infection

- Assess the dressings for bleeding, drainage, color, and odor every 4 hours for 24 hours.

- Observe the incision and intravenous sites for pain, redness, swelling, and drainage. Assess drainage system for patency and adequate suction. Note color and amount of drainage.

- Use sterile technique to change dressings and intravenous tubing.

- Encourage a protein-rich diet. Refer for a dietary consultation as indicated.

- Teach wound and drainage system care.

- Instruct to promptly report manifestations of infection: fever, redness, or hardness at the surgical site, or purulent drainage.

- Advise that scaling, flaking, dryness, itching, rash, or dry desquamation of the involved skin may occur, particularly after radiation therapy.

- Instruct to avoid deodorants and talcum powder on the affected side until the incision is completely healed.

Risk for Disturbed Body Image

- Assess how the patient views her body.
- Explain that redness and swelling will fade with time.
- Include significant others if possible when discussing the plan of care and activities of daily living. Request consultation with a psychologist or other professional if the patient is interested.
- Offer referral to support groups with women experiencing similar problems.
- Encourage the patient to look at her incision when ready. Often the reality is not as frightening as imagined. Explain that fear of looking at it is normal.
- Inform that there is no rush in deciding about a prosthesis, reconstruction, or neither option.
- If interested, provide written material about breast reconstruction and encourage the patient to talk with a plastic surgeon and with women who have had reconstruction.

Community-Based Care

- Instruct to continue to perform breast self-examination (BSE).
- Develop a postoperative exercise program in consultation with the physician and physical therapist.
- Teach manifestations of metastasis to the lungs, liver, and bones and the importance of promptly reporting these signs to the physician.
- Review medications and the schedule of follow-up visits for care and treatment.
- Refer to breast cancer support groups for sharing thoughts, feelings, experiences, and information about treatments, side effects, insurance, and other practical aspects of living with breast cancer.
- Discuss options for reconstructive surgery or using a prosthesis. Provide information about these options, such as when reconstructive surgery can be considered and where to purchase a prosthesis.

For more information on breast cancer, see Chapters 48 and 49 in *Medical-Surgical Nursing,* Fifth Edition, by LeMone, Burke, and Bauldoff.

Bronchiectasis

Overview

- Bronchiectasis is characterized by permanent abnormal dilation of one or more large bronchi and destruction of bronchial walls.
- The destructive process is initiated by inflammation, usually due to recurrent airways infection.
- Bronchial walls are weakened and dilated due to inflammation and airway obstruction; pooling of secretions and further infection and inflammation result.
- Destruction may be focal, affecting a limited lung region, or diffuse and widespread.
- Bronchiectasis results in a chronic, obstructive pulmonary disease.

Causes

- Related to cystic fibrosis (50% of all cases)
- Infectious causes: severe pneumonia, tuberculosis, or fungal infections
- Lung abscess
- Exposure to toxic gases
- Abnormal lung or immunologic defenses
- Localized airway obstruction due to a foreign body or tumor

Manifestations

- Initially may be asymptomatic
- Chronic cough productive of large amounts of mucopurulent sputum
- Hemoptysis
- Recurrent pneumonia
- Wheezing and shortness of breath, rales and rhonchi on auscultation
- Malnutrition, right-sided heart failure, and cor pulmonale

Diagnostic Tests

- Chest x-ray may show characteristic changes associated with bronchiectasis.

- Computed tomography scans can provide a more precise view of airway destruction.
- Bronchoscopy identifies the source of secretions and/or bleeding.
- Pulmonary function tests reveal decreased vital capacity and expiratory flow.

Interdisciplinary Management

- Antibiotics are prescribed at the first indication of infection and may be used prophylactically.
- Inhaled bronchodilators may be ordered.
- Chest physiotherapy is a vital component of care to help mobilize secretions.
- Oxygen may be prescribed.
- Bronchoscopy may be used to clear retained secretions or obstruction.
- If lung destruction is localized and unresponsive to conservative management, surgical lung resection may be necessary.

Selected Nursing Diagnoses with Interventions

Ineffective Breathing Pattern

- Assess respiratory rate and pattern, arterial blood gases, and signs of hypoxia and hypercapnia.
- Maintain quiet, calm environment.

Ineffective Airway Clearance

- Maintain high Fowler's position.
- Administer medications as prescribed and monitor side effects.
- Provide adequate hydration, 2 to 3 L per day unless contraindicated.
- Perform chest physiotherapy, assessing breath sounds before and after treatment.

Impaired Gas Exchange

- Administer low-flow oxygen therapy.
- Assist with energy conservation; plan frequent rest periods.

Imbalanced Nutrition: Less than Body Requirements

- Provide frequent, small feedings
- Arrange dietary consultation to maintain nutritional intake.

Community-Based Care

- Teach how to use pursed-lip breathing, diaphragmatic breathing, and huff cough techniques.
- Explain appropriate use of all medications, including inhalers and nebulizers.
- Discuss stress management techniques such as relaxation and meditation.
- Advise to avoid respiratory irritants such as smoke, dust, and powders, and exposure to perceptibly ill people.
- Report manifestations of hypoxia and hypercapnia to physician.
- Provide referral to a smoking-cessation program as appropriate.
- Encourage to obtain pneumonia vaccine and annual influenza immunizations.
- Provide information about or referral to home care services (home maintenance, personal care, respiratory care) as appropriate.

For more information on bronchiectasis, see Chapter 37 in *Medical-Surgical Nursing,* Fifth Edition, by LeMone, Burke, and Bauldoff.

BRONCHITIS, ACUTE

Overview

- Acute bronchitis, inflammation of the bronchi, is relatively common in adults.
- Typically follows a viral upper respiratory infection.
- The inflammatory response causes vasodilation and edema of the mucosal lining of the bronchi, as well as exudate formation and increased mucus production. Ciliary function is impaired by damage to ciliated epithelium lining the respiratory tract.
- Mucosal irritation and increased mucous production initiates the cough reflex. Hyperirritability of the respiratory tract causes paroxysms of coughing and bronchospasm.

Causes

- Impaired immune defenses and cigarette smoking are risk factors for acute bronchitis.
- Infectious bronchitis can be caused by either viruses or bacteria that damage the respiratory mucosa.
- Inhalation of toxic gases or chemicals can lead to inflammatory bronchitis.

Manifestations

- Cough, initially nonproductive, later becoming productive; often in paroxysms
- Chest pain, substernal or chest wall pain
- Fever, general malaise
- Bronchovesicular breath sounds on auscultation

Diagnostic Test

- Chest x-ray can differentiate between bronchitis (no consolidation) and pneumonia (consolidation).

Interdisciplinary Management

- Pharmacologic agents include aspirin or acetaminophen to relieve fever and malaise. A broad-spectrum antibiotic may be prescribed, since bacterial infection is a common complication of acute viral bronchitis.
- An expectorant cough medication is recommended for use during the day and a cough suppressant is recommended at night to facilitate rest.

Selected Nursing Diagnoses with Interventions

Deficient Knowledge

- Explain use and effects of any prescribed medications; instruct to avoid alcohol and other central nervous system depressants if taking a narcotic cough suppressant.
- Teach the importance of smoking cessation, as appropriate.

Disturbed Sleep Pattern

- Use over-the-counter analgesics and cough preparations containing expectorants (during the day) and suppressants (during the night).

Community-Based Care

- Increase fluid intake to keep mucus thin and meet increased needs related to fever.
- Referral to a smoking cessation program may be appropriate.

For more information about acute bronchitis, see Chapter 36 in *Medical-Surgical Nursing,* Fifth Edition, by LeMone, Burke, and Bauldoff.

BRONCHITIS, CHRONIC

Overview

- Chronic bronchitis is a disorder of excessive bronchial mucous secretion characterized by a productive cough lasting 3 or more months in 2 consecutive years.
- It is a chronic inflammatory process causing vasodilation, congestion, and edema of the bronchial mucosa.
- Narrowed airways and excess secretions obstruct airflow—expiration in particular.
- Impaired ciliary function affects clearance of mucus and inhaled pathogens.
- Recurrent infection is common.
- An imbalance between ventilation and perfusion leads to hypoxemia, hypercapnia, and pulmonary hypertension, with possible right-sided heart failure.
- It is a component of chronic obstructive pulmonary disease and usually coexists with some degree of emphysema.

Causes

- Smoking, including passive smoke (the most common)
- Air pollution: incidence significantly higher in urban, industrial areas

- Occupational exposure to noxious dusts and gases
- Chronic airway infection
- Familial and genetic factors

B

Manifestations

- Chronic cough productive of copious amounts of thick, tenacious sputum; typically in the morning
- Dyspnea: first on exertion, later at rest
- Shortness of breath
- Respiratory rate normal to slightly increased
- Cyanosis
- Coarse rhonchi and wheezes on auscultation
- Possible manifestations of right-sided heart failure: distended neck veins, peripheral edema, liver engorgement, and enlarged heart

Diagnostic Tests

- Pulmonary function tests show increased residual volume; decreased vital capacity; decreased forced expiratory volume in one second.
- Arterial blood gases show severe hypoxemia and hypercapnia.
- Exhaled carbon dioxide (capnogram or $ETCO_2$) may be elevated, indicating impaired alveolar ventilation.
- Chest x-ray may show evidence of pulmonary infection.
- Complete blood count shows severe polycythemia (compensatory to low PaO_2).

Interdisciplinary Management

- Smoking cessation is vital.
- Drug treatment includes antibiotics, bronchodilators, and corticosteroids.
- Pulmonary hygiene measures include hydration, effective cough, percussion, and postural drainage.
- Acute exacerbation of the disease may necessitate oxygenation and positive pressure ventilation with a face mask or intubation and mechanical ventilation.

- Immunization with pneumococcal and influenza vaccines is recommended.

Selected Nursing Diagnoses with Interventions

Impaired Gas Exchange

- Assess respiratory rate and pattern, arterial blood gases, and signs of hypoxia and hypercapnia.
- Administer low-flow oxygen therapy (< 2 L/min) as prescribed.
- Maintain a quiet, calm environment; plan frequent rest periods; and assist with energy conservation.

Ineffective Airway Clearance

- Maintain high Fowler's position.
- Administer bronchodilators and corticosteroids as prescribed; monitor for side effects.
- Perform chest physiotherapy, assessing breath sounds before and after treatment.
- Encourage fluid intake of 2000 to 2500 mL per day unless contraindicated.

Compromised Family Coping

- Assess the effect of the illness on the family.
- Help the patient and family identify strengths for coping with the situation.
- Help family members recognize behaviors that may hinder effective treatment, such as continuing to smoke in the house.

Decisional Conflict: Smoking

- Assess knowledge and understanding of the choices involved and possible consequences of each.
- Acknowledge concerns, values, and beliefs; listen nonjudgmentally.
- Help plan a course of action for quitting smoking and adapt it as necessary.

Community-Based Care

- Use effective breathing, coughing, and relaxation techniques.

- Maintain adequate fluid intake, at least 2.0 to 2.5 quarts of fluid daily.

- Avoid respiratory irritants, including cigarette smoke (both primary and secondary), other smoke sources, dust, aerosol sprays, air pollution, and very cold, dry air.

- Prevent exposure to infection, especially upper respiratory infections.

- Use prescribed exercise program, maintaining activities of daily living and balancing rest and exercise.

- Identify early signs of an infection or exacerbation and the importance of seeking medical attention.

- Explain prescribed medications, their expected and unintended effects, and other prescribed therapies such as nebulizers and home oxygen.

- Refer to support groups, pulmonary rehabilitation programs, and smoking cessation programs as available.

- Refer to community agencies or services such as home health services, homemaker services, or Meals on Wheels as appropriate.

- Encourage pneumonia vaccine and annual immunization against influenza.

For more information on chronic bronchitis, see Chapter 37 of *Medical-Surgical Nursing,* Fifth Edition, by LeMone, Burke, and Bauldoff.

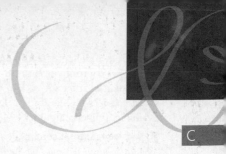

Calcium Imbalance

Hypercalcemia

Hypocalcemia

Overview

- Calcium is one of the most abundant ions in the body.
- Normal adult total serum calcium concentration is 8.5 to 10.0 mg/dL.
- About 99% of total body calcium is bound to phosphorus in bones and teeth.
- The remaining 1% is in extracellular fluid (ECF). About half of the extracellular calcium is ionized (free) and physiologically active. Ionized calcium is essential for the following:

  Stabilizing cell membranes

  Regulating muscle contraction and relaxation

  Maintaining cardiac function

  Blood clotting

- The interaction of parathyroid hormone (PTH), calcitonin, and calcitriol (a vitamin D metabolite) regulates serum calcium levels.

  1. Low serum calcium levels stimulate PTH secretion. PTH mobilizes skeletal calcium stores, increases calcium absorption in the intestines, and promotes calcium reabsorption by the kidneys.

  2. Calcitriol stimulates release of calcium from bone, intestinal calcium absorption, and renal calcium reabsorption.

  3. Calcitonin, secreted by the thyroid gland in response to high serum calcium levels, has the opposite effect of PTH. It inhibits calcium movement out of bone, reduces intestinal calcium absorption, and promotes renal calcium excretion.

- Acid–base balance affects serum calcium levels. Alkalosis (pH > 7.45) promotes protein binding of calcium, reducing the amount of ionized (active) calcium. Conversely, in acidosis (pH < 7.35), calcium is released from protein, increasing available ionized calcium.

- Hypocalcemia, total serum calcium level < 8.5 mg/dL (critical value < 6.0 mg/dL) may be due to decreased total body calcium stores or low levels of extracellular calcium with normal amounts of calcium stored in bone.

- Systemic effects of hypocalcemia are caused by decreased ECF levels of ionized calcium. Neuromuscular cell membranes are affected and the nervous system becomes more excitable. Paresthesias (altered sensation) and muscle spasms (tetany) develop. Cell membrane changes in the heart can lead to dysrhythmias; cardiac muscle fiber contractility decreases, leading to decreased cardiac output.

- Hypercalcemia, serum calcium > 10.0 mg/dL (critical value > 13.0 mg/dL), represents excess ionized calcium in ECF.

- Hypercalcemia decreases neuromuscular excitability, leading to muscle weakness, depressed deep tendon reflexes, and reduced gastrointestinal (GI) motility. Hypercalcemia affects the cardiac conduction system, leading to bradycardia and heart blocks. Renal urine concentration is impaired, leading to sodium and water loss and increased thirst.

- Increased cerebrospinal fluid calcium levels affect mental status and behavior.

Causes

Hypocalcemia

- Parathyroidectomy or neck surgery
- Acute pancreatitis
- Inadequate dietary intake
- Lack of sun exposure or weight-bearing exercise
- Massive transfusion of banked blood: citrate (an anticoagulant and preservative in stored blood) binds with calcium, temporarily reducing available ionized calcium

- Drugs: loop diuretics, calcitonin
- Hypomagnesemia, alcohol abuse

Hypercalcemia

- Hyperparathyroidism
- Some cancers (breast and lung, multiple myeloma)
- Prolonged immobilization
- Paget's disease
- Excess milk or antacid intake
- Renal failure

Manifestations

Hypocalcemia

- Neuromuscular:
  1. Tetany: paresthesias (numbness and tingling around mouth, distal extremities), muscle spasms, laryngospasm, and possible seizures
  2. Chvostek's sign: tapping over facial nerve just in front of ear to produce ipsilateral facial muscle contraction
  3. Trousseau's sign: blood pressure cuff on upper arm inflated to above systolic pressure for 3 minutes to produce carpal spasm (palmar flexion with finger spasms)
- Behavioral: anxiety, confusion, psychoses
- Cardiovascular: decreased cardiac output; hypotension; dysrhythmias
- GI: abdominal cramping, diarrhea

Hypercalcemia

- Neuromuscular: muscle weakness, fatigue; decreased deep tendon reflexes
- Behavioral: personality changes; altered mental status; decreasing level of consciousness
- GI: abdominal pain; constipation; anorexia, nausea, vomiting

- Cardiovascular: dysrhythmias; hypertension
- Renal: polyuria, thirst

Diagnostic Tests

Hypocalcemia

- Total serum calcium is < 8.5 mg/L. Ionized calcium levels may be estimated or measured using ion-selective electrodes. Direct measurement requires placing the blood specimen on ice and immediate analysis.
- Serum magnesium and phosphate levels affect calcium balance; hypomagnesemia (< 1.6 mg/dL) and hyperphosphatemia (> 4.5 mg/dL) may be present. There is an inverse relationship between phosphorus and calcium (as phosphate levels rise, calcium levels fall).
- PTH is measured to identify possible hyperparathyroidism.
- Electrocardiogram (ECG) may show effects of hypocalcemia, such as a prolonged ST segment and QT interval.

Hypercalcemia

- Serum electrolytes show total serum calcium > 10.0 mg/dL.
- Serum PTH levels are measured to identify hyperparathyroidism.
- ECG changes include a shortened QT interval, shortened and depressed ST segment, and widened T wave; bradycardia or heart block may be present.

Interdisciplinary Management

Hypocalcemia

- Oral or intravenous (IV) calcium; severe hypocalcemia is treated with IV calcium to prevent life-threatening problems such as airway obstruction. IV calcium solutions must be administered slowly and care taken to avoid extravasation, which can lead to tissue necrosis and sloughing.
- A diet high in calcium-rich foods for chronic hypocalcemia or low total body stores of calcium as indicated.

Hypercalcemia

- Acute hypercalcemia: intravenous fluids along with a loop diuretic to promote elimination of excess calcium; calcitonin to rapidly lower serum calcium levels; IV sodium phosphate or potassium phosphate to bind with ionized calcium

- Drugs to inhibit bone resorption, such as pamidronate (Aredia) and etidronate (Didronel); glucocorticoids to lower serum calcium levels by inhibiting intestinal calcium absorption and bone resorption

- Low-calcium diet

- Increased fluid intake to reduce risk of renal calculi

Selected Nursing Diagnoses with Interventions

Hypocalcemia
Risk for Injury

- Frequently monitor airway and respiratory status. Report stridor (high-pitched, harsh inspiratory sound) or increased respiratory rate or effort to the physician.

- Monitor heart rate and rhythm, blood pressure, and peripheral pulses.

- Continuously monitor ECG during IV calcium replacement.

- Provide a quiet environment. Institute seizure precautions such as raising the side rails and keeping an airway at the bedside.

Hypercalcemia
Risk for Injury

- Institute safety precautions for confusion or other mental status changes.

- Monitor cardiac rate and rhythm. Treat and/or report dysrhythmias as indicated. Prepare for possible cardiac arrest; keep emergency resuscitation equipment readily available.

- Observe for digitalis toxicity: vision changes, anorexia, altered heart rate and rhythm. Monitor serum digitalis levels.

- Promote fluid intake. Encourage fluids such as prune or cranberry juice to help maintain acid urine.

- Use caution when turning, positioning, transferring, or ambulating as indicated.

Risk for Excess Fluid Volume

- Closely monitor intake, output, and daily weight.
- Frequently assess vital signs, respiratory status, and heart sounds.
- Place in semi-Fowler's to Fowler's position.
- Administer diuretics as ordered, monitoring response.

Community-Based Care

Hypocalcemia

- Manage risk factors to prevent future episodes of hypocalcemia.
- Explain prescribed medications, including calcium supplements.
- Teach preventive measures such as increasing intake of foods high in calcium (dairy products, broccoli, collard greens, tofu), supplements (calcium carbonate), and vitamin D intake (sunlight, milk, liver, eggs).
- Teach signs and symptoms of decreased calcium: tetany and carpopedal spasm.
- Provide a list of foods high in calcium and sources of vitamin D if recommended.
- Maintain follow-up care as scheduled.

Hypercalcemia

- Avoid excess intake of calcium-rich foods and antacids; discontinue use of calcium and vitamin D supplements.
- Take prescribed drugs to prevent excess calcium resorption; teach their dose, use, and desired and possible adverse effects.
- Increase fluid intake to 3 to 4 quarts per day.
- Increase intake of foods that increase urine acidity (meats, fish, poultry, eggs, cranberries, plums, prunes).
- Increase dietary fiber to prevent constipation.
- Maintain weight-bearing physical activity to prevent hypercalcemia.
- Early manifestations of hypercalcemia should be reported to care provider.
- Recommended schedule for monitoring serum electrolyte levels.

For more information about calcium imbalance, see Chapter 10 in *Medical-Surgical Nursing,* Fifth Edition, by LeMone, Burke, and Bauldoff.

CANCER

Overview

- Cancer results when normal cells mutate into abnormal, deviant cells that then perpetuate within the body. Loss of cell differentiation (specialized structure and function) is a characteristic of cancer.
- Clones of abnormal cells form nests of malignant neoplasms (tumors).
- Malignant cells invade surrounding tissues, and may break away from the primary tumor to metastasize to distant sites in the body.
- Cancers tend to grow rapidly; crowd, invade, and destroy normal tissue; recur, if removed; and metastasize to distant tissues via the blood or lymph.
- Primary malignant neoplasms are those that grow in the tissue of origin.
- Secondary (metastatic) neoplasms grow in tissues distant from the tissue of origin.
- Types of cancer include the following:
  - **Carcinomas** (nonglandular epithelial tissue)
  - **Adenocarcinomas** (glandular epithelial tissue)
  - **Sarcomas** (connective tissue, muscle, bone)
  - **Leukemias** (blood cells, usually white blood cells [WBCs])
  - **Lymphomas/myelomas** (lymphatic cells, tissues, organs)
  - **Seminomas** (embryonic structures)
  - **Melanoma** (melanocytes)
  - **Meningioma** (meninges)
- Cancer (all types combined) is the second leading cause of death in the United States.
- Untreated cancer is usually fatal.

Causes

- Genetics: inherited oncogenes (cancer-promoting genes) or inherited lack of tumor-suppressor genes.

- Viruses: can carry mutations into cells and insert abnormal genes in the human genome; viruses known to have an associated cancer risk include several herpes type viruses, human cytomegalovirus, Epstein-Barr virus, hepatitis B virus, papillomavirus, and human T-lymphotropic viruses.

- Environment: many pollutants, chemicals, gases, toxins, and exposure to radiation are known to initiate or promote cell transformation.

- Lifestyle: stress, diet and obesity, occupation, socioeconomic status, sun exposure, and use of substances such as tobacco, alcohol, and recreational drugs contribute to the risk for cancer.

Manifestations

- Disease specific
- Generally asymptomatic in early stages
- Late manifestations: pain, anorexia, weakness, weight loss/cachexia, frequent infection

Diagnostic Tests

- Tumor markers are substances detectable in serum or body fluids that may indicate the presence or activity of malignant cells.

- X-ray imaging, computed tomography scans, magnetic resonance imaging, ultrasonography, radioisotope scans, angiography, tagged antibodies, and direct visualization (e.g., colonoscopy, endoscopy) may be used to detect tumors or tumor metastases.

- Laboratory tests may be used to screen for some malignancies, evaluate general health status, and identify effects of malignancy (e.g., neoplastic syndromes).

- Cytologic examination is carried out on specimens from biopsied tissues, tumors, body secretions, or body fluids.

Grading

- Measures the degree of cell disorganization (differentiation)

- Uses a scale (usually I to IV) with higher numbers indicating the least differentiation and thus most disorganized malignant cells

Staging

- Categorizes the extent of the disease
- The TNM system is an internationally recognized staging system. Each specific neoplastic disease will have different criteria regarding these categories:

  T—tumor size (primary site)

  N—node involvement (regional)

  M—metastasis, absence or presence (at distant site)

Interdisciplinary Management

- Chemotherapy: use of cytotoxic chemicals to decrease tumor size, to prevent or treat suspected metastases, and, in some cancers, to effect a cure. Chemotherapy disrupts the cell cycle in various phases by interrupting cell metabolism and replication. It also works by interfering with the ability of malignant cells to synthesize needed enzymes and chemicals. Phase-specific drugs work during specific phases of the cell cycle; non-phase-specific drugs work through the entire cell cycle.
- Surgery: used for diagnosis and staging of more than 90% of all cancers and for primary treatment of more than 60% of cases. Ideally, the entire tumor is removed, often along with adjacent tissues and regional lymph nodes.
- Radiation therapy: used to kill the tumor, to reduce its size, to decrease pain, or to relieve obstruction. Lethal injury to DNA is believed to be the primary mechanism by which radiation kills cells.
- Immunotherapy (or biotherapy): modifies biologic processes that support tumor growth, often by enhancing immune responses.
- Bone marrow transplantation: used to stimulate nonfunctioning marrow or replace diseased bone marrow. It is used to treat leukemias and other hematologic cancers.
- Pharmacologic management of pain includes opioid and nonopioid analgesics as well as adjuvant medications to enhance the effect of the analgesic.

Selected Nursing Diagnoses with Interventions

Anxiety

- Assess level of anxiety.
- Establish a therapeutic relationship.
- Encourage to acknowledge and express feelings.
- Review the coping strategies used in the past and build on past successful behaviors.
- Identify community resources for helping to manage anxiety-producing situations.
- Provide specific information about the disease, its treatment, and what may be expected.
- Provide a safe, calm, and quiet environment for the patient in panic. Administer antianxiety medications if prescribed.

Disturbed Body Image

- Assist the patient and significant others to cope with the loss or change in appearance by providing a supportive environment, encouraging expression of feelings, giving matter-of-fact responses to questions, identifying new coping strategies, and enlisting family and friends in reaffirming the patient's worth.
- Teach the patient and/or significant others to participate in the care of the affected body area.
- Teach specific strategies for minimizing physical changes, such as dressing to enhance appearance, using an ice cap or tight headband during chemotherapy treatments to decrease the amount of drug that reaches the hair follicles, and referring the patient to support programs.

Anticipatory Grieving

- Use therapeutic communication skills to provide an open environment for the patient and significant others to express their feelings and discuss their concerns.
- Answer questions about illness and prognosis honestly, while encouraging hope.
- Encourage continued work and participation in enjoyable activities for as long as possible.

- Encourage the dying patient to update his or her will, sign an advance directive and a durable power of attorney, and make funeral and burial plans to help maintain a sense of control.

Risk for Infection

- Monitor vital signs including temperature.
- Monitor WBC counts frequently, especially for the patient receiving chemotherapy that is known to cause bone marrow suppression.
- Teach the patient and significant others to avoid crowds, small children, and people with infections when the WBC count is low and to practice scrupulous personal hygiene.
- Teach to protect the skin and mucous membranes from injury.
- Encourage to consume a diet high in protein, minerals, and vitamins, especially vitamin C.

Imbalanced Nutrition: Less than Body Requirements

- Assess current eating patterns and identify factors that impair food intake.
- Evaluate the degree of malnutrition by monitoring total serum protein and albumin values.
- Calculate nitrogen balance and creatinine-height index. Calculate skeletal muscle mass and compare findings with normal ranges.
- Take anthropometric measurements and compare to standards.
- Teach principles of good nutrition; adapt diet to medical restrictions and current preferences.
- Encourage small, frequent meals. Cold and highly seasoned foods may appeal to patients with reduced sense of taste. Manage nausea and vomiting by administering antiemetic drugs and encouraging small, frequent, low-fat meals; avoiding liquids with meals; and sitting upright for an hour after meals.
- Advise use of nutritional supplements such as Ensure Plus or Isocal.
- Teach the patient and significant others to keep a food diary to document intake.
- Teach the patient and significant others to administer parenteral nutrition via a central line or other vascular access device. Teach safety measures and care of the vascular access device. Provide an emergency phone number for help.

Other nursing diagnoses may be appropriate. See listings for each specific type of cancer.

Community-Based Care

- Explain the specific type of cancer and the treatment options available.

- Teach relaxation techniques, stress management, and meditation.

- Provide information about prescribed medications and side effects.

- Show how to use any equipment placed in the home.

- Explain when to see the doctor for follow-up care.

- Assist in making arrangements for transportation for follow-up appointments for medical care, chemotherapy, and/or radiation.

- Encourage the patient to contact the American Cancer Society and other local cancer support groups.

- Make sure the patient has the equipment and supplies needed for home care, and provide information on where to obtain further supplies. For the patient needing complex care, a referral to a home health nurse is appropriate.

- Stress the importance of long-term medical follow-up care.

- Provide the patient and significant others with written information and a phone number to call for concerns and questions. Phone calls to the patient for several days after the patient arrives home are also appropriate.

- For the patient with terminal disease, hospice care may be appropriate and should be discussed with the patient and significant others.

For more information on cancer, see Chapter 14 in *Medical-Surgical Nursing,* Fifth Edition, by LeMone, Burke, and Bauldoff. In addition, specific cancers are discussed in various chapters in this textbook.

CANDIDIASIS (MONILIASIS, YEAST INFECTION, THRUSH)

Overview

- Candidiasis is an infection of the mucous membranes, nails, skin, or blood by fungi of the *Candida* genus.

- Mucous membranes of the vagina, oropharynx (thrush), esophagus, and gastrointestinal tract are most frequently infected.
- *Candida* organisms are part of the normal vaginal environment, causing problems only when they multiply rapidly in response to antibiotic therapy, increased estrogen levels, fecal contamination, or other factors.
- Occasionally, the organisms may infect the blood (candidemia) and various organ systems (brain, kidney, lung).
- Candidemia is most common in immunocompromised patients, such as those with human immunodeficiency virus/acquired immune deficiency syndrome, malignancy, diabetes, sepsis, trauma/burn injury, and history of IV drug use.
- The prognosis depends on the site and extent of infection as well as the state of the patient's resistance.

Causes

- Many *Candida* species are normal body flora that overgrow if the environment changes, as during antibiotic therapy and hyperglycemia, or during immunosuppression (*opportunistic* infection).
- *Candida albicans* is the most common species, but several others (glabrata, guilliermondii, krusei, parapsilosis, tropicalis) can cause deep infection and death in immunocompromised patients.

Manifestations

- Manifestations depend on the area of infection.
- Oral lesions appear as discrete or confluent patches in the mouth and throat and on the tongue.
- Vulvovaginal candidiasis causes intense pruritus—a creamy white, curdy discharge—and dysuria and dyspareunia.
- Skin infection appears as red, macerated areas and/or pustules, usually around nail beds (paronychia), glans penis (balanitis), or anus; drier areas may be red, papular, and scaly.
- Infected nails are red, swollen, or crumbling.
- Esophageal infection usually causes dysphagia.
- Systemic infection may produce general manifestations of fever, chills, rash, and prostration, or manifestations specific to the

infected organ system, such as meningitis, pneumonia, renal insufficiency, endocarditis, arthritis, osteomyelitis, myositis, or brain abscess.

Diagnostic Tests

- Wet smear (of mucous membrane, skin, nail scrapings) may show pseudophyphae; should be confirmed with culture (not diagnostic alone for superficial lesions).
- Biopsy is needed for deeper lesions.
- Culture of blood, cerebrospinal fluid, joint fluid may be done.

Interdisciplinary Management

- Over-the-counter antifungal creams and suppositories are available for vaginal yeast infections.
- Oral antifungal agents such as fluconazole, ketoconazole, clotrimazole troches, and nystatin troches are used to treat thrush.
- Deep or systemic *Candida* infections are treated with a systemic antifungal agent such as amphotericin B, flucytosine, or fluconazole (Diflucan) administered either orally or parenterally, depending on the drug and the infected system.

Selected Nursing Diagnoses with Interventions

Deficient Knowledge

- Explain the disease process and its transmission, prevention, and treatments.
- The patient with a vaginal yeast infection should be told about the importance of having her partner evaluated and treated for infection.

Impaired Skin Integrity

- Administer prescribed antifungal agents as appropriate to site. Cover antifungal products in moist areas with a moisture barrier cream.
- Monitor for signs of systemic infection.
- Suggest the use of cool compresses, vinegar douches, and sitz baths to alleviate the discomfort of vaginal yeast infections.

Imbalanced Nutrition: Less than Body Requirements

- Provide small, frequent feedings to the patient with thrush. Provide good oral hygiene and lidocaine-based mouthwash prior to eating.

Community-Based Care

- Instruct on the disease process, prevention, and treatment, including administration of antifungals and side effects.

- For the patient with a vaginal yeast infection, consume daily 8 oz. of yogurt containing live active cultures to help restore normal vaginal flora.

- Explain the importance of treating the patient's sexual partner as appropriate.

- Follow-up care is required for recurrence of symptoms.

For more information on candidiasis, see Chapters 12 and 50 in *Medical-Surgical Nursing,* Fifth Edition, by LeMone, Burke, and Bauldoff.

CARDIOMYOPATHY

Overview

- Cardiomyopathies are disorders of the heart muscle that affect both systolic and diastolic function.

- May be either primary or secondary; primary cardiomyopathies are idiopathic; secondary cardiomyopathies result from processes such as ischemia, infectious disease, toxins, connective tissue or metabolic disorders, or nutritional deficiencies.

- Categorized by pathophysiology and presentation as dilated, hypertrophic, and restrictive.

  1. Dilated cardiomyopathy is the most common type, usually affecting middle-aged males. Its incidence is higher in African Americans than in Whites. Heart chambers dilate, and ventricular contraction is impaired, decreasing cardiac output. Left ventricular dilation is prominent; right ventricle may be enlarged. Extensive interstitial fibrosis (scarring) and necrotic myocardial cells may be seen. Prognosis is poor.

2. Hypertrophic cardiomyopathy is characterized by decreased left ventricular compliance and myocardial muscle hypertrophy. Intraventricular septal hypertrophy impairs ventricular filling and outflow, decreasing cardiac output. May cause sudden cardiac death.

3. Restrictive cardiomyopathy is characterized by rigid ventricular walls that impair diastolic filling. Myocardial and endocardial fibrosis causes ventricular stiffness and rigidity, impairing filling, and decreasing cardiac output. Prognosis is poor.

Causes

- Dilated: toxins, metabolic conditions, infection; alcohol and cocaine abuse, chemotherapeutic drugs, pregnancy, systemic hypertension; genetically transmitted in an autosomal-dominant, autosomal-recessive, or X-linked pattern
- Hypertrophic: genetically transmitted in an autosomal-dominant pattern
- Restrictive: myocardial fibrosis and infiltrative processes, such as amyloidosis

Manifestations

Dilated Cardiomyopathy

- Manifestations of heart failure (biventricular), including dyspnea on exertion, orthopnea, paroxysmal nocturnal dyspnea, weakness, fatigue, peripheral edema, and ascites; S_3 and S_4 heart sounds, possible murmur; possible dysrhythmias; arterial emboli

Hypertrophic Cardiomyopathy

- Dyspnea, angina, and syncope; ventricular dysrhythmias, possible atrial fibrillation; fatigue, dizziness, and palpitations; harsh, crescendo-decrescendo systolic murmur, possible S_4; sudden cardiac death

Restrictive Cardiomyopathy

- Manifestations of heart failure and decreased tissue perfusion; dyspnea on exertion, exercise intolerance; elevated jugular venous pressure; S_3, S_4 common

Diagnostic Tests

- Echocardiography assesses chamber size and thickness, ventricular wall motion, valvular function, and systolic and diastolic function of the heart.

- ECG demonstrates cardiac enlargement and detects dysrhythmias.

- Chest x-ray shows cardiomegaly and possible pulmonary congestion.

- Hemodynamic studies assess cardiac output and pressures in the heart chambers and pulmonary vascular system.

- Radionuclear scans identify changes in ventricular volume and mass.

- Cardiac catheterization and coronary angiography evaluate coronary perfusion; the structure and function of cardiac chambers, valves, and great vessels; pressure relationships; and cardiac output.

- Myocardial biopsy examines myocardial cells for infiltration, fibrosis, or inflammation.

Interdisciplinary Management

- Strenuous physical exertion is restricted to prevent dysrhythmias or sudden cardiac death.

- Dietary and sodium restrictions may help diminish manifestations.

- Medications to treat heart failure, including ACE inhibitors, vasodilators, and digitalis; beta blockers may be used with caution. Anticoagulants to reduce the risk of thrombus formation and embolization.

- Cardiac transplant is the definitive treatment for dilated cardiomyopathy, but is not a viable option for restrictive cardiomyopathy, because the underlying process continues and eventually affects the transplanted organ.

- Surgical resection of excess intraventricular muscle may be done in obstructive hypertrophic cardiomyopathy.

- An implantable cardioverter-defibrillator may be inserted to treat potentially lethal dysrhythmias.

Selected Nursing Diagnoses with Interventions

Decreased Cardiac Output

- Assist to conserve energy while encouraging self-care.
- Support coping skills and adaptation to required lifestyle changes.

Ineffective Breathing Pattern

- Monitor vital signs, oxygen saturation, lung sounds, and manifestations of heart failure.
- Place in semi-Fowler's or Fowler's position.
- Administer oxygen as ordered.

Community-Based Care

- Teach about the disease process, expected outcomes, and treatment options such as an implantable cardioverter-defibrillator or cardiac transplant.
- Explain the prescribed drug regimen, its rationale, and intended and possible adverse effects.
- If appropriate, include the genetic transmission of hypertrophic cardiomyopathy, and screening of close relatives (parents and siblings).
- Provide information about cardiac transplantation if it is an option.
- Discuss the toxic and vasodilator effects of alcohol; encourage abstinence.
- Review activity restrictions and dietary changes to reduce manifestations and prevent complications.
- Lifetime immunosuppression following cardiac transplant is needed to prevent transplant rejection. Teach about the increased risk for infection associated with immunosuppression and measures to reduce this risk.
- Explain what symptoms to report to the physician or to seek immediate care for.
- Encourage family members to learn cardiopulmonary resuscitation procedures; provide a list of available training sites.
- Refer the patient and family for home and social services and counseling as indicated.

For more information about cardiomyopathy, see Chapter 31 of *Medical-Surgical Nursing,* Fifth Edition, by LeMone, Burke, and Bauldoff.

CARPAL TUNNEL SYNDROME

Overview

- Carpal tunnel syndrome is a disorder in which the medial nerve is compressed within the carpal tunnel of the wrist.

Causes

- Occupational risk factors: any job requiring repetitive hand movements (e.g., computer workers, assembly line workers, switchboard operators)
- Any condition that causes swelling or obstruction of the wrist (e.g., rheumatoid arthritis, tendinitis, pregnancy, renal failure, diabetes mellitus, hypothyroidism/myxedema, amyloidosis, or trauma)

Manifestations

- Pain in thumb, forefinger, middle finger, and half of fourth finger; more severe at night and in morning; possibly radiating to shoulder
- Paresthesia, numbness, tingling, burning
- Weakness, clumsiness, decreased ability to clench fist
- Positive compression test—application of inflated blood pressure cuff to elicit manifestations
- Positive Tinel's sign—a tingling sensation over the palm of the hand after lightly percussing over the medial nerve at the wrist
- Positive Phalen's test—flexion of both wrists to 90 degrees while pressing dorsal aspects of hands together to elicit pain or paresthesia

Diagnostic Test

- Electromyogram shows median nerve conduction velocity delayed > 5 milliseconds.

Interdisciplinary Management

- Medications usually include nonsteroidal anti-inflammatory drugs. The physician may opt to inject corticosteroids into the joint.
- Splint and avoid use of the affected extremity.
- Surgery entails resection of the carpal ligament to enlarge the tunnel.

Selected Nursing Diagnoses with Interventions

Acute Pain

- Ask the patient to rate the pain on a scale of 0 to 10 before and after interventions.
- Encourage the use of immobilizers.
- Apply ice and/or heat to promote comfort.
- Administer nonsteroidal anti-inflammatory drugs as ordered. Monitor for adverse effects such as gastric discomfort or evidence of gastrointestinal bleeding.

Impaired Physical Mobility

- Provide care to alleviate pain.
- Consult the physical therapist for exercises per physician's prescription.
- Suggest occupational rehabilitation to the patient and physician.

Community-Based Care

- Explain the condition, its causes, and treatment, including medication regimen.
- Suggest ways to avoid further injury.
- Instruct to avoid hot temperatures to the affected hand.
- Discuss measures to prevent carpal tunnel syndrome in people with high-risk occupations, including use of wrist supports with computer keyboard and mouse, and appropriate keyboard height.
- A hand and forearm splint may help relieve pain, particularly when worn at night.
- Tell the patient who has undergone surgery to avoid heavy lifting with the affected hand for at least 4 to 6 weeks.

For more information on carpal tunnel syndrome, see Chapter 39 in *Medical-Surgical Nursing,* Fifth Edition, by LeMone, Burke, and Bauldoff.

CATARACT

Overview

- A cataract is opacity of the lens of the eye.
- Cataracts are usually associated with aging (senile).
- As the lens ages, its fibers and proteins change and degenerate, losing clarity. The process usually begins at the periphery of the lens, gradually spreading to the central portion. Opacity reduces the amount of light reaching the retina and the clarity of transmitted images.
- It is the most common cause of age-related vision loss in the world.

Causes

- Senile: occurs due to age-related changes in water and protein content
- Genetic: primary or accompanying many other genetic disorders
- Congenital: most often secondary to intrauterine exposure to rubella, but also to herpes simplex virus, varicella zoster virus, cytomegalovirus, and syphilis
- Traumatic: may be unilateral; blunt, penetrating blows; burns
- Toxic: heavy smoking, chemicals (naphthalene), drugs (corticosteroids, ergot, phenothiazines)
- Radiation: long-term ultraviolet B exposure (sunlight), ionizing, infrared
- Accompanying other eye disorders: detached retina, glaucoma, retinitis, uveitis
- Secondary to metabolic disorders, such as diabetes mellitus

Manifestations

- Painless, gradual loss of visual acuity (clouding, blurring, distortion)

- Milky white lens
- Reports of headlight glare at night; better vision in dim light

Diagnostic Tests

- Indirect ophthalmoscopy shows a dark area in red reflex.
- Slit-lamp examination shows opacity.
- Visual acuity tests correlate amount of lens involved to function.

Interdisciplinary Management

- Surgical removal of the affected lens with implantation of an intra-ocular lens is the usual treatment for cataracts. Most cataracts are removed by laser outpatient surgery, using a local anesthetic. No medical therapies are available to prevent or treat them.

Selected Nursing Diagnoses with Interventions

Decisional Conflict: Cataract Removal

- Explain the slow progression of the condition, and help the patient determine the extent to which the cataract is affecting his or her daily life. Provide information and support to help the patient decide when to proceed with surgery.
- Provide preoperative teaching regarding the surgery and expected outcomes and limitations.

Readiness for Enhanced Self-Health Management

- Instruct to protect the operative eye following surgery: Use eye-glasses or sunglasses during the day and an eye shield at night to avoid inadvertent damage to eye sutures while sleeping.
- Discuss measures to avoid coughing, sneezing, heavy lifting, bending at waist, and sleeping on operative side for prescribed period.
- Teach to administer eye drops and ointments as ordered.
- Advise to avoid washing the hair until several days after the surgery and prevent getting water into the eyes during showering.

Community-Based Care

- Teach all patients to avoid tobacco use and to wear sunglasses, even on cloudy days, to reduce the risk of cataracts.

- A home safety assessment is appropriate for this patient to prevent accidents.

- Remind the patient of the importance of follow-up visits with the ophthalmologist.

- Instruct to abstain from driving, operating machinery, or participating in sports activities until allowed by the physician. Advise to use caution when ambulating until vision has stabilized.

For more information on cataracts, see Chapter 46 in *Medical-Surgical Nursing,* Fifth Edition, by LeMone, Burke, and Bauldoff.

CERVICAL CANCER

Overview

- Cervical cancer is readily diagnosed, and if treated early, has the greatest cure rate of all female reproductive cancers. Many women with cervical cancer survive for 5 years or more.

- Cervical cancer is classified as precancerous, preinvasive (cancer *in situ*), or invasive.

- Precancerous cervical changes usually spontaneously regress; a very small percent progress to invasive malignancy.

- Invasive carcinoma represents extension of the malignancy through the basement membrane, separating superficial cells from deeper tissues below; metastasis is via lymphatics.

- Most cervical cancers are squamous cell carcinoma.

- Distant metastasis is to liver, lungs, and bone.

- Death rates have dropped dramatically over the past 40 years owing to the widespread use of the Pap smear as a screening tool.

Causes

Human papillomavirus infection is the greatest risk factor for cervical cancer. Other risk factors include the following:

- First sexual intercourse before age 16

- Multiple sexual partners or male sexual partners who have multiple sexual partners

- History of sexually transmitted infections, especially human papillomavirus

- Smoking
- Poor nutritional status
- Family history of cervical cancer
- Exposure to diethylstilbestrol *in utero*

Manifestations

- Preinvasive and early invasive carcinomas are asymptomatic.
- Abnormal bleeding or spotting after intercourse is a common early sign (bloody or brown vaginal discharge); this may increase to intermenstrual or heavy menstrual bleeding.
- Referred lumbosacral back pain, and urinary symptoms also may develop.
- Manifestations of advanced carcinoma include bowel/bladder dysfunction or fistula formation; severe pelvic pain; bone pain; anorexia/weight loss/cachexia; fatigue.

Diagnostic Tests

- Pap smear, recommended yearly as the safest method of preventing invasive cervical cancer, shows abnormal desquamated cervical cells that can be categorized into classes (I to V) of increasing severity.
- Colposcopy magnifies cervix, and application of iodine dye (Schiller's test) isolates areas of abnormal-appearing tissue for biopsy.
- Biopsy determines degree of cellular neoplasia and depth of lesion.
- Loop electrosurgical excision procedure allows simultaneous diagnosis and treatment of dysplastic lesions found on colposcopy.
- Computed tomography and magnetic resonance imaging scans are used to locate distant metastasis.

Interdisciplinary Management

- Dysplastic lesions found on colposcopy can be removed in an outpatient procedure with a wire loop electrode. Other methods of biopsy and removal of lesions include electrocautery, cryosurgery, or carbon dioxide laser therapy.
- Surgical interventions include conization, vaginal hysterectomy, and radical hysterectomy. Pelvic exenteration, used for recurring

cancers, involves removal of some or all of the pelvic organs, and may require urinary diversion and colostomy.

- Radiation therapy is used alone or with surgery to treat the late stages of cervical cancer.

Selected Nursing Diagnoses with Interventions

Anxiety

- Assess level of anxiety, concerns about sexual functioning, and adjustment to altered body image.
- Assess level of pain and administer prescribed pain medications.
- Refer to a sex therapist to assist the patient in coping with the psychologic and physical changes associated with cervical cancer and its treatment.

Risk for Infection

- Provide pre- and postoperative care as appropriate for pelvic surgeries.
- After surgery, assess for potential complications such as wound infection, hemorrhage, pneumonia.
- Implement a sanitary pad count for vaginal procedures.
- Provide information about complications, including signs of infection that should be reported immediately to the physician.

Community-Based Care

- For all women, emphasize the importance of regular pelvic examinations and Pap smears.
- Discuss risk factors for cervical cancer and measures to reduce the risk.
- Encourage women to have their daughters vaccinated with Gardasil (or Cervarix as an alternative).
- Discuss the disease process, its causes, treatment, and prognosis, along with medications and their dosage and side effects.
- Teach self-care as appropriate. For instance, the patient with a total exenteration will require teaching for colostomy care and possible referral to an enterostomal specialist.

- Explain the importance of monitoring the amount, type, and duration of vaginal discharge.
- Explain the need for long-term follow-up care.

For more information on cervical cancer, see Chapter 49 in *Medical-Surgical Nursing,* Fifth Edition, by LeMone, Burke, and Bauldoff.

CHLAMYDIAL INFECTION

Overview

- Chlamydia is the most prevalent sexually transmitted infection (STI) in the United States.
- More common in women aged 15 to 25 years.
- The infections caused by Chlamydia include acute urethral syndrome, nongonococcal urethritis, mucopurulent cervicitis, and pelvic inflammatory disease (PID).
- Chlamydial infection during pregnancy may lead to premature delivery and/or postpartum endometritis.
- Newborns delivered vaginally to infected mothers may acquire chlamydial infection, including conjunctivitis and pneumonitis.
- Complications of chlamydia in women include PID, infertility, and ectopic pregnancy. In men, its complications include epididymitis, prostatitis, sterility, and Reiter's syndrome.
- In immunocompromised patients, chlamydia can cause pneumonia.

Causes

- Multiple strains of *Chlamydia trachomatis*
- Almost always transmitted sexually, orally, or congenitally from mother to newborn

Manifestations

- Frequently asymptomatic
- Cervicitis: yellow mucopurulent discharge, cervical edema, fragility, and eventually erosion

- PID: tenderness or pain of abdomen and pelvic region, fever, chills, bleeding/discharge, lymphadenopathy, signs and symptoms of urethritis, infertility
- Urethritis: erythema, dysuria, frequency, pruritus, purulent discharge
- Epididymitis: scrotal edema and pain
- Prostatitis: low back pain, painful ejaculation, signs and symptoms of urethritis
- Proctitis: rectal ulceration, rectal pain, mucous discharge, bleeding, tenesmus

Diagnostic Tests

- Routine screening for sexually active adolescents and young adults is recommended.
- Identification of polymorphonuclear leukocytes on Gram stain of urethral (males) or cervical discharge provides presumptive evidence of infection.
- Tests for antibodies to chlamydia, such as direct fluorescent antibody test and an enzyme-linked immunosorbent assay, are less specific than tissue cultures but more rapid and readily available.
- Polymerase chain reaction or ligase chain reaction tests are highly sensitive, specific tests that can be performed on urine and vaginal swab specimens.

Interdisciplinary Management

- The drugs of choice for chlamydia in men and nonpregnant women are oral azithromycin or doxycycline. For pregnant women, erythromycin is the alternative therapy. Both sexual partners should be treated at the same time.
- Sexual abstinence during treatment is advised to facilitate a cure.

Selected Nursing Diagnoses with Interventions

Acute Pain/Chronic Pain

- Assess level of pain. Teach use of medications and nonpharmacologic measures to reduce pain.

Anxiety

- Provide a supportive, nonjudgmental environment for the patient to discuss feelings and ask questions. Allow time and privacy to address concerns.
- Help the patient to focus on the present situation as a means of identifying coping mechanisms needed to reduce anxiety.

Sexual Dysfunction

- Encourage open communication between the patient and his or her sexual partner(s).
- Stress the need to comply with the treatment regimen, to refer partner(s) for examination and treatment, and to use condoms to avoid reinfection.

Community-Based Care

- Explain the complications of untreated chlamydial infection.
- Avoid sexual activity until the chlamydia has been eradicated.
- Provide a pamphlet or other literature on STIs, their prevention, and treatment.
- Discuss safer sex practices to reduce future risk of STIs.

For more information on chlamydial infection, see Chapter 50 in *Medical-Surgical Nursing,* Fifth Edition, by LeMone, Burke, and Bauldoff.

CHOLECYSTITIS

Cholelithiasis

Cholecystitis

Overview

- Cholelithiasis is the formation of gallstones (calculi).
- Cholecystitis is inflammation of the gallbladder, usually caused by obstruction of the cystic duct by a gallstone.
- Gallstones form when several factors interact: abnormal bile composition, biliary stasis, and inflammation of the gallbladder.

- Most gallstones consist primarily of cholesterol. They form in the gallbladder, and then may migrate into the ducts, causing cholangitis (duct inflammation) or cholecystitis.
- Cystic duct obstruction increases pressure within the gallbladder, leading to ischemia of the gallbladder wall and mucosa. Chemical and bacterial inflammation follow; necrosis and perforation are potential complications.

Causes

Although the cause of cholelithiasis and cholecystitis is unknown, the following risk factors are identified:

- Age, female gender
- Family history of gallstones
- Native American or Northern European heritage
- Obesity, hyperlipidemia
- Very-low-calorie diets
- Oral contraceptives; cholesterol-lowering drugs
- Biliary stasis: pregnancy, fasting, prolonged parenteral nutrition
- Cirrhosis; ileal disease or resection; sickle cell anemia; glucose intolerance

Manifestations

- Early: epigastric fullness or mild gastric distress after eating a large or fatty meal
- Cholecystitis: Abrupt onset of severe, steady epigastric or right upper quadrant pain which may radiate to the back, right scapula, or shoulder, often precipitated by eating
- Anorexia, nausea, and vomiting
- Fever, chills
- Right upper quadrant tenderness to palpation
- Possible jaundice; manifestations of pancreatitis

Diagnostic Tests

- Ultrasonography of the gallbladder identifies the presence of stones and assesses gallbladder emptying.

- Oral cholecystogram demonstrates the gallbladder's ability to concentrate and excrete bile.
- Gallbladder scans are used to diagnose cystic duct obstruction and cholecystitis.

Interdisciplinary Management

- Laparoscopic cholecystectomy (removal of the gallbladder) is treatment of choice for symptomatic cholelithiasis or cholecystitis. Risk of complications is low. Some patients require traditional cholecystectomy via laparotomy. Common bile duct exploration may accompany cholecystectomy.
- Shock wave lithotripsy may be used to dissolve large gallstones. High-risk patients may undergo percutaneous cholecystotomy, drainage of the gallbladder, to postpone or replace surgery.
- Medications include ursodiol (Actigall) or chenodiol (Chenix) to dissolve the gallstones. Drug therapy is expensive and is continued indefinitely to prevent recurrent stone formation.

Selected Nursing Diagnoses with Interventions

Pain

- Discuss the relationship between fat intake and the pain. Teach ways to reduce fat intake.
- Withhold oral food and fluids during episodes of acute pain. Insert nasogastric tube and connect to low suction if ordered.
- For severe pain, administer narcotic analgesia as ordered.
- Place in Fowler's position.

Imbalanced Nutrition: Less than Body Requirements

- Assess nutritional status, including diet history, height and weight, and skinfold measurements.
- Evaluate laboratory results, including serum bilirubin, albumin, glucose, and cholesterol levels. Report abnormal results.
- Refer to a dietitian or nutritionist for diet counseling to promote healthy weight loss and reduce pain episodes.

Risk for Infection

- Promptly report abrupt, transient pain relief as it may signal gall-bladder rupture.

- Monitor vital signs including temperature every 4 hours. Promptly report vital sign changes or temperature elevation.

- Assess abdomen every 4 hours and as indicated (e.g., when pain level changes abruptly).

- Assist to cough and use incentive spirometer every 1 to 2 hours while awake. Splint abdominal incision during coughing.

Community-Based Care

- Explain the role of bile and the function of the gallbladder.

- Provide appropriate preoperative teaching for the planned procedure, including the possibility of open cholecystectomy if a laparoscopic procedure is planned.

- Teach postoperative self-care to manage pain and prevent complications.

- If the patient will be discharged with a T-tube, provide instructions about T-tube care.

- Following cholecystectomy, a low-fat diet may be initially recommended. Refer the patient and food preparer to a dietitian to review low-fat foods.

- If surgery is not an option, teach about medications to dissolve stones, their use, and adverse effects (diarrhea is a common side effect).

- Discuss manifestations of complications to report to the physician.

For more information about cholecystitis and cholelithiasis, see Chapter 25 of *Medical-Surgical Nursing,* Fifth Edition, by LeMone, Burke, and Bauldoff.

CHRONIC OBSTRUCTIVE PULMONARY DISEASE

Overview

- Chronic obstructive pulmonary disease (COPD) is chronic airflow obstruction due to chronic bronchitis and/or emphysema.

- COPD affects an estimated 11.3 million Americans. It is more common in Whites than in African Americans, and in men than in women. It is the fourth leading cause of death in the United States.

- It is characterized by slowly progressive airways obstruction and periodic exacerbations, often related to respiratory infection. Airways and lung parenchyma show progressive destructive changes.

- COPD typically includes components of both chronic bronchitis and emphysema; chronic asthma is also often present. These processes cause airway narrowing, increased resistance to airflow, and slow, difficult expiration. Gas exchange is impaired by a mismatch between alveolar ventilation and blood flow or perfusion.

- See Asthma, Chronic Bronchitis, and Emphysema for more information.

Causes

- Cigarette smoking is the primary cause. Cigarette smoke impairs ciliary movement, inhibits alveolar macrophage function, causes hypertrophy of mucous secreting glands, produces airway destruction, and constricts smooth muscle, thus increasing airway resistance.

- Contributing factors include air pollution, occupational exposure to noxious dusts and gases, airway infection, and familial and genetic factors.

- Chronic lung diseases such as cystic fibrosis and occupational lung disease also may lead to COPD.

Manifestations

- Typically absent or minor early in the disease
- Productive cough, typically in the morning
- Dyspnea on exertion progressing to severe dyspnea even at rest
- Exercise intolerance

Diagnostic Tests

- Pulmonary function testing typically shows increased total lung capacity and residual volume, and decreased forced expiratory volume and forced vital capacity.

- Ventilation/perfusion scanning demonstrates the extent of ventilation/perfusion mismatch.

- Serum alpha$_1$-antitrypsin levels may be drawn to screen for deficiency, particularly with a positive family history, early onset, women, and nonsmokers.

- Arterial blood gases show mild to marked hypoxemia and possible hypercapnia with respiratory acidosis. Oxygen saturation levels are low.

- Exhaled carbon dioxide (capnogram or ETCO$_2$) is elevated when ventilation is inadequate, and decreased when pulmonary perfusion is impaired.

- Complete blood count often shows increased red blood cells and hematocrit (erythrocytosis); polycythemia, increased numbers of all blood cells, may be evident.

- Chest x-ray may show diaphragmatic flattening due to hyperinflation.

Interdisciplinary Management

- Smoking cessation is vital. Nicotine patches or gum and an antidepressant (e.g., bupropion [Wellbutrin, Zyban]) or varenicline (Chantix) improve the chances of success.

- Immunization against pneumococcal pneumonia and yearly influenza vaccine is important to reduce the risk of respiratory infections.

- A broad-spectrum antibiotic is prescribed if infection is suspected; prophylactic antibiotics may be prescribed for patients with more than four exacerbations per year.

- Bronchodilators improve airflow and reduce air trapping. Oral theophylline may be given to stimulate the respiratory drive, strengthen diaphragmatic contractions, and improve cardiac output.

- Corticosteroid therapy may improve symptoms and reduce the severity of exacerbations.

- Pulmonary hygiene (percussion and postural drainage) improves clearance of airway secretions.

- Regular aerobic exercise to gradually increase exercise tolerance is recommended. Breathing exercises slow the respiratory rate and relieve accessory muscle fatigue.

- Oxygen therapy improves exercise tolerance, mental functioning, and quality of life in advanced COPD. With acute exacerbation, intubation and mechanical ventilation may be necessary.
- Lung transplantation or lung reduction surgery may be used for advanced disease.

Selected Nursing Diagnoses with Interventions

Ineffective Airway Clearance

- Assess respiratory rate and pattern, cough and secretions (color, amount, consistency, and odor), and breath sounds every 1 to 2 hours as indicated.
- Promptly report changes in arterial blood gases, oxygen saturation, skin color, or mental status.
- Weigh daily, monitor fluid volume status.
- Encourage fluid intake of at least 2000 to 2500 mL per day unless contraindicated.
- Place in Fowler's, high Fowler's, or orthopneic position.
- Assist with coughing and deep breathing at least every 2 hours while awake.
- Refer to a respiratory therapist, and assist with or perform percussion and postural drainage as needed.
- Provide endotracheal, oral, or nasopharyngeal suctioning as necessary.
- Provide rest periods between treatments and procedures.
- Correlate timing of expectorant and bronchodilator medications with respiratory treatments.

Impaired Gas Exchange

- Provide supplemental oxygen as ordered.
- Prepare for intubation and mechanical ventilation if respiratory status deteriorates.

Imbalanced Nutrition: Less than Body Requirements

- Assess nutritional status, including diet history, weight for height, and skinfold measurements.
- Monitor laboratory values, including serum albumin and electrolyte levels.

- Consult with a dietitian to plan meals and nutritional supplements that meet caloric needs.
- Provide frequent, small feedings with between-meal supplements.
- Keep snacks at the bedside.

Compromised Family Coping

- Assess the effect of the illness on the family.
- Help family members recognize behaviors and attitudes that may hinder effective treatment, such as continuing to smoke in the house.
- If dysfunctional family relationships interfere with measures to enhance coping, advocate for the patient, reaffirming his or her right to make decisions.
- Arrange a social services consultation.

Decisional Conflict: Smoking

- Assess knowledge and understanding of the choices involved and possible consequences of each.
- Acknowledge concerns, values, and beliefs; listen nonjudgmentally.
- Help plan a course of action for quitting smoking and adapt it as necessary.
- Demonstrate respect for decisions and the right to choose.
- Refer to a counselor or other professional as needed.

Community-Based Care

- Teach pursed-lip breathing:
  1. Inhale through the nose with the mouth closed.
  2. Exhale slowly through pursed lips, as though whistling or blowing out a candle, making exhalation twice as long as inhalation.
- Teach diaphragmatic or abdominal breathing:
  1. Place one hand on the abdomen, the other on the chest.
  2. Inhale, concentrating on pushing the abdominal hand outward while the chest hand remains still.
  3. Exhale slowly, while the abdominal hand moves inward and the chest hand remains still.

- Teach controlled cough technique:
    1. Following prescribed bronchodilator treatment, inhale deeply and hold breath briefly.
    2. Cough twice, the first time to loosen mucus, the second to expel secretions.
    3. Inhale by sniffing to prevent mucus from moving back into deep airways.
    4. Rest. Avoid prolonged coughing to prevent fatigue and hypoxemia.
- Teach huff coughing:
    1. Inhale deeply while leaning forward.
    2. Exhale sharply with a "huff" sound to help keep airways open while mobilizing secretions.
- Instruct in ways to avoid respiratory irritants and prevent exposure to infection.
- Explain the importance of pneumococcal vaccine and annual influenza immunization.
- Discuss prescribed exercise, maintaining activities of daily living, and balancing rest and exercise.
- Advise to maintain fluid and nutrient intake (e.g., small, frequent meals and nutritional supplements).
- Identify early signs of infection or exacerbation; explain the importance of promptly seeking medical attention.
- Explain prescribed medications and therapies (e.g., oxygen, postural drainage), including purpose, proper use, and expected effects.
- Teach the importance of wearing a MedicAlert tag and carrying a list of medications at all times in case of an emergency.
- Provide referrals to services such as home health, activities of daily living and home maintenance assistance, respiratory therapy and home oxygen services, and agencies such as Meals on Wheels, senior services, as indicated.

For more information about chronic obstructive pulmonary disease, see Chapter 37 of *Medical-Surgical Nursing,* Fifth Edition, by LeMone, Burke, and Bauldoff.

Cirrhosis

Overview

- Cirrhosis is a progressive, irreversible disorder that eventually leads to liver failure.

- Types of cirrhosis:

  1. Alcoholic (Laënnec's) cirrhosis, the end result of alcoholic liver disease, is the most common type. Alcohol increases triglyceride and fatty acid synthesis and decreases the formation and release of lipoproteins in the liver, causing fatty infiltration of hepatocytes (fatty liver). Inflammatory cells infiltrate the liver, causing necrosis, fibrosis, and destruction of functional liver tissue.

  2. Biliary cirrhosis is caused by obstructed bile flow. Retained bile damages and destroys liver cells, leading to inflammation, fibrosis, and formation of regenerative nodules.

  3. Posthepatic cirrhosis is the end result of progressive liver damage due to chronic hepatitis B or C. The liver is shrunken and nodular, with extensive liver cell loss and fibrosis.

- Functional liver tissue is destroyed and replaced by fibrous scar tissue. Fibrous tissue forms constrictive bands that disrupt blood and bile flow within liver lobules. Blood no longer flows freely through the liver, causing increased pressure in the portal venous system (portal hypertension).

- Portal hypertension causes shunting of blood to adjoining lower pressure vessels. Veins in the esophagus, rectum, and abdomen become engorged and congested. Congestion of portal system vessels leads to the following:

  1. Splenomegaly, which increases the rate of blood cell destruction, leading to anemia, leukopenia, and thrombocytopenia.

  2. Ascites, the accumulation of plasma-rich fluid in the abdominal cavity. Hypoalbuminemia and increased aldosterone secretion contribute to ascites formation.

  3. Esophageal varices, enlarged, thin-walled veins that form in the submucosa of the esophagus. These thin-walled varices may rupture, causing massive hemorrhage. Thrombocytopenia, platelet deficiency, and impaired production of clotting factors by the liver contribute to the risk for hemorrhage.

- As hepatocytes and liver lobules are destroyed, liver functions are lost and liver failure develops.

- Hepatic encephalopathy results from accumulation of neurotoxins such as ammonia in the blood. Ammonia, a by-product of protein metabolism, normally is converted to urea by the liver. Liver failure impairs this conversion, and ammonia accumulates in the blood.

- Hepatorenal syndrome, renal failure associated with advanced cirrhosis, may develop, leading to azotemia, sodium and potassium retention, oliguria, and hypotension.

Causes

- Long-term alcohol abuse
- Chronic hepatitis B or C
- Prolonged obstruction of the biliary system
- Chronic severe right heart failure

Manifestations

Liver Failure

- Skin: dry, pigmented, itchy; spider angiomas; purpura/ecchymoses; possible jaundice
- Peripheral edema
- Hematologic: anemia, bleeding tendency
- Gastrointestinal: anorexia, nausea, vomiting; constipation or diarrhea; abdominal ache; hematemesis/ melena
- Respiratory: pleural effusion, dyspnea, hypoxemia
- Endocrine: testicular atrophy, gynecomastia, menstrual irregularities, reduced body hair
- Central nervous system: asterixis (hand-flapping tremor); personality changes; agitation, restlessness, impaired judgment, slurred speech; confusion, disorientation, incoherence; deep coma
- Hepatorenal syndrome: azotemia, oliguria, hyponatremia, and hypotension

Portal Hypertension

- Varices (esophageal, gastric, rectal); may hemorrhage

- Splenomegaly
- Ascites

Diagnostic Tests

- Liver function studies (ALT, AST, alkaline phosphatase, and GGT) may be elevated, but elevations may not indicate extent of liver damage. Bilirubin levels are usually elevated in severe cirrhosis.
- Complete blood count shows anemia, thrombocytopenia, and leukopenia.
- Coagulation studies show a prolonged prothrombin time.
- Serum albumin level is low; serum ammonia levels are elevated; glucose and cholesterol levels frequently are abnormal.
- Abdominal ultrasound evaluates liver size, detects ascites, and identifies liver nodules.
- Esophagoscopy may be done to detect esophageal varices.
- Liver biopsy may be done to distinguish cirrhosis.

Interdisciplinary Management

- Medications include diuretics and medications such as lactulose and neomycin to reduce the ammonia production. Vitamin supplements and antacids may also be indicated. Nadolol (Corgard) and isosorbide (ISMO, Imdur, Monoket) may be used to prevent rebleeding of esophageal varices. Ferrous sulfate and folic acid are given to treat anemia. Vitamin K may be used to reduce bleeding. Medications that are metabolized by the liver are avoided.

- Surgery may be indicated for biliary cirrhosis to restore duct patency and relieve obstruction. Sclerotherapy may be done to treat esophageal varices. Paracentesis to remove fluid from the abdominal cavity may be done for severe ascites. Transjugular intrahepatic portosystemic shunt is used to relieve portal hypertension and its complications. Liver transplantation provides the only chance for cure of cirrhosis.

- Dietary support is an essential part of care. Sodium intake is restricted to < 2 g/day, and fluids are restricted as necessary. If hepatic encephalopathy develops, protein is restricted to 60 g/day; otherwise, protein is allowed as tolerated. Parenteral nutrition is used as needed. Vitamin and mineral supplements are ordered based on laboratory values.

Selected Nursing Diagnoses with Interventions

Excess Fluid Volume

- Weigh daily. Assess for jugular vein distention, measure abdominal girth daily, and check for peripheral edema. Monitor intake and output.

- Monitor for signs of impaired renal function, such as oliguria, a fixed specific gravity, central edema (around the eyes and of the face), and increasing serum creatinine and blood urea nitrogen levels.

- Provide a low-sodium diet (500 to 2000 mg/day) and restrict fluids as ordered.

Risk for Acute Confusion

- Assess level of consciousness and mental status. Observe for signs of early encephalopathy: changes in handwriting, speech, and asterixis.

- Closely monitor patients who have had a gastrointestinal bleed for signs of hepatic encephalopathy.

- Avoid hepatotoxic medications and central nervous system depressant drugs.

- Provide low-protein diet as prescribed.

- Administer medications or enemas as ordered to reduce nitrogenous products.

- Orient to surroundings, person, and place; provide simple explanations and reassurance.

Risk for Bleeding

- Monitor vital signs; report tachycardia or hypotension.

- Institute bleeding precautions.

- Monitor coagulation studies and platelet count. Report abnormal results.

- Carefully monitor for rebleeding of esophageal varices.

- Carefully monitor respiratory status when a triple lumen nasogastric tube is in place. Keep the head of the bed elevated to 45 degrees.

Impaired Skin Integrity

- Use warm water rather than hot when bathing.

- Prevent dry skin: Apply an emollient or lubricant as needed, avoid soap or preparations with alcohol, and do not rub skin.

- If indicated, apply mittens to the hands to prevent scratching.

- Turn frequently, use an alternating-pressure mattress, and frequently assess skin condition.

Imbalanced Nutrition: Less than Body Requirements

- Weigh daily. Instruct to weigh at least weekly at home.

- Provide small meals with between-meal snacks.

- Unless protein is restricted, promote protein and nutrient intake with supplements such as Ensure or Instant Breakfast.

- Arrange for consultation with a dietitian for diet planning while hospitalized and at home.

Community-Based Care

- Teach the importance of maintaining nutrition and vitamin and mineral supplements.

- Reinforce with the patient and significant others the importance of avoiding alcohol ingestion.

- Discuss the medication regimen, effects, and side effects.

- Stress the importance of avoiding over-the-counter medications unless approved by the physician.

- Include significant others in care and teaching, especially when the etiologic agent is alcohol abuse. Provide referrals for home care, including follow-up visits to community health agencies and, if needed, Alcoholics Anonymous or similar rehabilitation and support groups.

- Stress the importance of continued care. Discuss signs and symptoms to report immediately to the physician, such as personality changes or blood in vomitus or stool.

- Refer to a nutritionist, social worker, and/or psychologist as indicated.

For more information on cirrhosis, see Chapter 25 in *Medical-Surgical Nursing,* Fifth Edition, by LeMone, Burke, and Bauldoff.

Colorectal Cancer

Overview

- Colorectal cancer, malignancy of the colon or rectum, is the third most common cancer and cause of cancer deaths in the United States.

- Most colorectal malignancies are adenocarcinomas that begin as adenomatous polyps.

- Most tumors occur in the rectum and sigmoid colon.

- Colorectal cancer grows slowly and spreads by direct extension to involve all bowel layers and neighboring structures.

- Metastasis to regional lymph nodes is the most common form of tumor spread. Cancerous cells may also spread via the lymphatic system or circulatory system to the liver, lungs, brain, bones, and kidneys.

Causes

The specific cause of colorectal cancer is unknown. Risk factors include the following:

- Age over 50
- Genetic factors: family history of the disease; familial adenomatous polyposis
- Inflammatory bowel disease (ulcerative colitis and Crohn's disease)
- Diet high in calories, meat proteins, and fats and low in fruits and vegetables, folic acid, and calcium
- Use of aspirin and other nonsteroidal anti-inflammatory drugs

Manifestations

- Occult or frank rectal bleeding
- Black, tarry stools
- Manifestations of anemia
- Weight loss
- Change in bowel habits: alternating diarrhea and constipation; narrow or ribbonlike stools

- Palpable abdominal mass
- Cramping or vague lower abdominal pain

Diagnostic Tests

- Complete blood count may show anemia from chronic blood loss and tumor growth.
- Fecal occult blood (by guaiac or hemoccult testing) detects blood in the feces.
- Carcinoembryonic antigen is a tumor marker used to estimate prognosis, monitor treatment, and detect cancer recurrence.
- Sigmoidoscopy or colonoscopy is used to detect and visualize tumors, as well as for tissue biopsy.
- Computed tomography scan, magnetic resonance imaging, or ultrasonic examination may be used to assess tumor depth and involvement of other organs.
- Tissue biopsy confirms cancerous tissue and evaluates cell differentiation.

Interdisciplinary Management

- Surgical resection of the tumor, adjacent colon, and regional lymph nodes is the standard treatment for colorectal cancer. Surgical resection of the bowel may be followed by a colostomy for diversion of fecal contents.
- Radiation therapy may be used in addition to surgery or to slow the progression of inoperable tumors.
- Chemotherapeutic agents such as oral levamisole and intravenous fluorouracil are used postoperatively as adjunctive therapy.

Selected Nursing Diagnoses with Interventions

Acute Pain

- Use a standard pain scale to document level of pain.
- Assess analgesic effectiveness 1/2 hour after administration. Monitor for pain relief and adverse effects.
- Assess the incision for inflammation or swelling; assess drainage catheters and tubes for patency.

- Assess abdomen for distention, tenderness, and bowel sounds.
- Assist with adjunctive relief measures.

Imbalanced Nutrition: Less than Body Requirements

- Assess nutritional status, using height and weight, skinfold measurements, body mass index calculation, and laboratory data including serum albumin.
- Assess readiness for oral intake after surgery or procedures using statements of hunger, presence of bowel sounds, passage of flatus, and minimal abdominal distention.
- Monitor and document food and fluid intake.
- Weigh daily.
- Maintain total parenteral nutrition and central intravenous lines as ordered.

Anticipatory Grieving

- Work to develop a trusting relationship with the patient and family.
- Listen actively, encouraging the patient and family to express their fears and concerns.
- Encourage discussion of the potential impact of loss on individual family members, family structure, and family function. Assist family members to share concerns with one another.
- Refer to cancer support groups, social services, or counseling as appropriate.

Risk for Sexual Dysfunction

- Provide opportunities for the patient and family to express feelings about the cancer diagnosis, ostomy, and effects of other treatments.
- Provide consistent colostomy care.
- Encourage expression of sexual concerns. Provide privacy and caregivers who have established trust with the patient and family and are comfortable in discussions about sexual concerns.
- Reassure the patient and significant other that the effect of physical illness and prescribed interventions on sexuality usually is temporary.
- Refer the patient and partner to social services or a family counselor for further interventions.

- Arrange for a visit from a member of the United Ostomy Association.

Community-Based Care

- Teach home management and care of the colostomy pouch and stoma. Provide suggestions for incorporating care into routine activities of daily living.

- Teach manifestations of postoperative complications, such as wound infection and intestinal obstruction.

- Provide referrals to an enterostomal therapy nurse, dietitian, home health nurse, and psychologist as appropriate.

- Refer to local chapters of the United Ostomy Association and the American Cancer Society.

- Provide locations of local suppliers of ostomy appliances.

- Provide information about hospice and home care as appropriate for advanced tumors.

For more information on colorectal cancer, see Chapter 24 in *Medical-Surgical Nursing,* Fifth Edition, by LeMone, Burke, and Bauldoff.

CONDYLOMA ACUMINATA (GENITAL WARTS)

Overview

- Condyloma acuminata are genital warts caused by one of more than 40 types of human papillomaviruses (HPVs).

- The incubation period ranges from 3 weeks to 18 months.

- HPV is a risk factor for cervical cancer, and is associated with cancer of the penis, anus, vagina, and vulva.

Causes

- Infection of skin and/or mucous membrane with various strains of HPV (6, 11, 30, 42–45, 51, 54)

- Transmitted by sexual contact; facilitated by trauma at inoculation site

- Increased susceptibility in immunocompromised patients

Manifestations

- Characteristic leafy-looking warts
- Warts located on external genitalia, perineum, anus, and/or vagina or cervix
- Itching, bleeding
- Secondary infection
- Possibly asymptomatic, and growths not noticed by the patient

Diagnostic Tests

- Visual inspection can identify most lesions.
- Pap smear may show atypical cells of the cervix.
- Colposcopy magnifies skin or mucous membranes for closer inspection.

Interdisciplinary Management

There is no treatment available to cure the disease; treatment is symptomatic.

- Gardasil is available to protect against the four types of HPV that cause most cervical cancers and genital warts. The Centers for Disease Control and Prevention currently recommends immunization of all previously unvaccinated women through age 26. Topical medications used to treat genital warts include podofilox and podophyllin.
- Warts may be removed by cryotherapy, electrocautery, or surgical excision. Carbon dioxide laser surgery is common for removal of extensive warts.

Selected Nursing Diagnoses with Interventions

Deficient Knowledge

- Discuss the need for prompt treatment and for sexual abstinence until lesions have healed.
- Discuss the need for examination and treatment of sexual partners.
- Stress to the female patient the increased risk of cervical cancer and the importance of an annual Pap smear.

Fear

- Allow expression of specific fears and feelings about wart treatment. Explain the planned procedure, approximate recovery time, and possible complications and ways to avoid them.

- Encourage verbalization of fears related to changes in and limitations of sexual activity.

Community-Based Care

- Provide information about the disease, prevention, treatment, and necessary follow-up care.

- Stress the importance of abstaining from sexual activity until all warts have been removed from the patient and the sexual partner.

- Schedule a follow-up visit with the physician 3 months after treatment.

- Encourage the female patient with cervical dysplasia related to HPV to obtain a Pap smear within 6 months following treatment.

- Discuss safer sex practices to reduce the risk of contracting sexually transmitted infections.

For more information on condyloma acuminata, see Chapter 50 in *Medical-Surgical Nursing,* Fifth Edition, by LeMone, Burke, and Bauldoff.

CORONARY HEART DISEASE

Overview

- Coronary heart disease (CHD) is heart disease caused by impaired blood flow to the myocardium.

- Accumulation of atherosclerotic plaque in the coronary arteries is the usual cause of CHD.

- Atherosclerosis is characterized by atheroma (plaque) formation in large and midsize arteries. The protruding lesion gradually impairs blood flow and vasodilation in response to increased oxygen demands.

- Myocardial cells become ischemic when the blood and oxygen supply is inadequate to meet metabolic demands. Cellular adenosine triphosphate stores are quickly depleted, affecting contractility. Lactic acid accumulates, and cells are damaged. Continued ischemia results in cell necrosis and death (infarction).

- CHD is divided into two categories:
    1. Chronic ischemic heart disease includes stable and vasospastic angina, and silent myocardial ischemia. See Angina Pectoris.
    2. Acute coronary syndromes include unstable angina and myocardial infarction (MI). See Acute Coronary Syndrome and Myocardial Infarction.

Causes

The causes of CHD and atherosclerosis are not known, but identified risk factors are as follows:

- Nonmodifiable: age, male gender, race, and genetic factors
- Modifiable diseases and conditions:
    - Hypertension, diabetes mellitus, hyperlipidemia
    - Elevated homocystine levels and the metabolic syndrome
    - In women, premature menopause, oral contraceptive use, and hormone replacement therapy
- Modifiable lifestyle factors:
    - Cigarette smoking
    - Obesity (body weight greater than 30% over ideal body weight), increased body mass index, and central fat distribution
    - Physical inactivity
    - Diet

Manifestations

- Often asymptomatic
- Angina: chest pain, dyspnea, anxiety
- MI: severe chest pain, dyspnea, nausea, diaphoresis, feeling of impending doom

Diagnostic Tests

- Total serum cholesterol and lipid profile are used to diagnose hyperlipidemia. Elevated lipid levels are associated with an increased risk of atherosclerosis.

- Exercise electrocardiogram testing is positive for CHD if myocardial ischemia is detected on the electrocardiogram, chest pain develops, or excess fatigue, dysrhythmias, or other symptoms necessitate stopping the test.

- Electron beam computed tomography can reveal coronary artery plaque and other abnormalities.

Interdisciplinary Management

- Care focuses on aggressive risk factor management to slow the atherosclerotic process and maintain myocardial perfusion, including smoking cessation, reducing dietary saturated fat and cholesterol, increasing fiber intake, weight loss, regular physical exercise, and hypertension and diabetes management.

- Drug therapy to lower total serum cholesterol and low-density lipoprotein levels and to raise high-density lipoprotein levels is an integral part of CHD management. The statins, lovastatin (Mevacor), pravastatin (Pravachol), simvastatin (Zocor), and others, are first-line drugs for treating hyperlipidemia.

- Patients at high risk for MI are often started on prophylactic low-dose aspirin therapy.

Selected Nursing Diagnoses with Interventions

Imbalanced Nutrition: More than Body Requirements

- Encourage assessment of food intake and eating patterns to help identify areas that can be improved.

- Discuss American Heart Association and therapeutic lifestyle change dietary recommendations, emphasizing the role of diet in heart disease. Provide guidance regarding specific food choices with healthy alternatives.

- Refer to clinical dietitian for diet planning and further teaching. Suggest cookbooks that offer low-fat recipes to encourage healthier eating, and provide American Heart Association and American Cancer Society recipe pamphlets and information on low-fat eating.

- Encourage gradual but progressive dietary changes.

- Encourage reasonable goals for weight loss. Provide information about weight loss programs and support groups such as Weight Watchers and Take Off Pounds Sensibly.

Ineffective Health Maintenance

- Discuss risk factors for CHD, stressing that changing or managing those factors that can be modified reduces the overall risk for the disease.

- Discuss the immediate benefits of smoking cessation. Provide resource materials from the American Heart Association, the American Lung Association, and the American Cancer Society. Refer to a structured smoking cessation program to increase the likelihood of success in quitting.

- Help identify specific sources of psychosocial and physical support for smoking cessation, dietary, and lifestyle changes.

- Discuss the benefits of regular exercise for cardiovascular health and weight loss. Help identify favorite forms of exercise or physical activity. Encourage planning for 30 minutes of continuous aerobic activity (i.e., walking, running, bicycling, swimming) four to five times a week. Encourage identification of an "exercise buddy" to help maintain motivation.

Community-Based Care

- Provide information and teaching about prescribed medications such as cholesterol-lowering drugs.

- Discuss the relationship between hypertension, diabetes, and CHD.

- Encourage participation in a cardiac rehabilitation program.

- Assist the patient to make healthy choices, and reinforce positive changes.

- Emphasize the importance of regular follow-up appointments to monitor progress.

For more information about coronary heart disease, see Chapter 30 in *Medical-Surgical Nursing,* Fifth Edition, by LeMone, Burke, and Bauldoff.

CROHN'S DISEASE

Overview

- Crohn's disease (regional enteritis) is a chronic, relapsing inflammatory disorder affecting the gastrointestinal tract.

- It usually affects the terminal ileum and ascending colon; any portion of the gastrointestinal (GI) tract can be affected. A patchy pattern of involvement with areas of inflammation and normal mucosa is characteristic.
- Crohn's disease involves all layers of the intestinal wall, causing a "cobblestone appearance" as fissures and ulcers surround islands of intact mucosa over edematous submucosa.
- Affected bowel walls become fibrotic, thickened, and inflexible; inflammation can lead to obstruction, abscesses, and fistulas between loops of bowel or bowel and other organs.
- Malabsorption and malnutrition may develop due to impaired nutrient absorption and chronic protein and blood loss.
- Peak incidence is between age 15 and 35, with a second peak between age 60 and 80.
- Long-standing Crohn's disease significantly increases the risk of intestinal cancer.

Causes

The etiology of Crohn's disease is unknown, but is thought to be autoimmune. Identified risk factors are as follows:
- Family history of the disease
- Jewish heritage
- Possibly infectious agents

Manifestations

- Continuous or episodic diarrhea with liquid or semiformed stools that typically do not contain blood
- Abdominal pain and tenderness, may be relieved by defecation
- Palpable right lower quadrant mass
- Systemic manifestations: fever, fatigue, malaise, weight loss, anemia
- Anorectal lesions
- Nausea, vomiting, and epigastric pain

Diagnostic Tests

- Colonoscopy provides visual evidence of Crohn's disease. Biopsy of bowel mucosa may differentiate the disease from cancer and other inflammatory bowel disorders.

- Upper GI series with small bowel follow-through and a barium enema can show changes such as ulcerations, strictures, or fistulas.
- Complete blood count shows anemia and leukocytosis; the sedimentation rate is elevated during periods of acute inflammation.
- Serum albumin, folic acid, and levels of most vitamins are decreased due to malabsorption, malnutrition, protein loss, and chronic inflammation.

Interdisciplinary Management

- Medications: anti-inflammatory drugs such as sulfasalazine and corticosteroids; immunosuppressive agents and immune modifiers. Metronidazole (Flagyl), an antibiotic with anti-inflammatory effects may help prevent remission. Antidiarrheal preparations may be used.
- All food is withheld during an acute exacerbation. Nutrition is maintained using enteral or total parenteral nutrition. An elemental diet such as Ensure, which provides all essential nutrients, may be prescribed. Lactose intolerance is common; milk and milk products may be eliminated.
- Surgical intervention is limited to patients with complications such as bowel obstruction.

Selected Nursing Diagnoses with Interventions

Imbalanced Nutrition: Less than Body Requirements

- Weigh daily and maintain accurate intake, output, and dietary records.
- Monitor the results of laboratory studies that indicate nutritional status.
- Provide the prescribed diet: high kilocalorie, high protein, low fat, with restricted dairy intake if lactose intolerance is suspected.
- Provide parenteral nutrition as necessary.
- Arrange for dietary consultation. Provide for food preferences as allowed.
- Administer prescribed nutritional supplements.
- Include significant others in teaching and dietary discussions.

Diarrhea

- Monitor and record the frequency and characteristics of bowel movements.
- Measure abdominal girth and auscultate bowel sounds every shift as indicated.
- Administer antidiarrheal medications as prescribed.
- Limit food intake if the diarrhea is acute, to allow the bowel to rest.

Community-Based Care

- Teach the patient and significant others about the disease, prescribed medications, and dietary management. Include manifestations of complications and their appropriate management.
- Present information on stress management and the importance of adequate rest.
- Instruct to avoid GI stimulants such as nicotine, caffeine, pepper, and alcohol.
- If the patient is to be discharged with a central catheter and home parenteral nutrition, provide written and verbal instructions on catheter care and troubleshooting as well as administration of total parenteral nutrition.
- Refer the patient with parenteral nutrition to home health and intravenous therapy services.
- Refer to the local chapter of the Crohn's and Colitis Foundation for support services.

For more information on Crohn's disease, see Chapter 24 of *Medical-Surgical Nursing,* Fifth Edition, by LeMone, Burke, and Bauldoff.

CUSHING'S SYNDROME

Overview

- Cushing's syndrome is a syndrome of excess glucocorticoid activity resulting in widespread metabolic, cardiovascular, neurologic, and immunologic changes.
- It can be primary or secondary, and is usually iatrogenic.
- Primary (adrenal form): results from excess steroid secretion from the adrenal gland itself; most common in women 20 to 40 years of age.

- Secondary (pituitary form): due to increased secretion of adrenocorticotropic hormone (ACTH) from the pituitary gland (Cushing's disease), or an ectopic focus.
- Iatrogenic (ectopic form): glucocorticoid therapy is commonly given for hypersensitivity reactions, autoimmune disease, or for severe inflammatory conditions; it produces exactly the same manifestations as disease forms.

Causes

- Primary: benign adrenal adenoma (85%); adrenal carcinoma
- Secondary: benign pituitary adenomas; hypothalamic-pituitary dysfunction; ectopic secretion of ACTH as in oat cell carcinoma, pancreatic carcinoma; carcinoid of thymus
- Iatrogenic: long-term glucocorticoid therapy (prednisone, prednisolone, Solu-Medrol)

Manifestations

- Protein catabolism: muscle atrophy/weakness, capillary fragility (ecchymosis), osteoporosis (decreased bone matrix), striae, poor wound healing
- Fat metabolism: central obesity, moon face, buffalo hump, rotund trunk, thin extremities
- Carbohydrate metabolism: glucose intolerance, secondary diabetes mellitus
- Fluid and electrolytes: sodium retention/potassium wasting, fluid retention, edema, weight gain
- Cardiovascular: hypertension, arteriosclerosis, decreased stress response
- Immunologic: reduced inflammatory/immunologic response, increased infection rate
- Neurologic: memory loss, poor concentration, mood swings, frank psychosis
- Reproductive: oligo/amenorrhea, virilism, hirsutism, and acne in women; impotence in men

Diagnostic Tests

- Plasma cortisol level is elevated in both primary and secondary types.

- A 24-hour urine test for cortisol is elevated in both primary and secondary types.
- Low-dose dexamethasone suppression test identifies Cushing's syndrome, but not type.
- High-dose dexamethasone suppression test is positive if pituitary-hypothalamic dysfunction is present; negative if disease is secondary to an ACTH-secreting adenoma.
- Plasma ACTH level is increased with ACTH-secreting neoplasms (pituitary or ectopic); reduced if primary.
- Visualization studies (ultrasound, angiography, computed tomography scan) may reveal adrenal, pituitary, or ectopic neoplasms.

Interdisciplinary Management

- Medications may be used as an adjunct to surgery or radiation or for patients with inoperable malignancies. Mitotane suppresses the activity of the adrenal cortex and decreases peripheral metabolism of corticosteroids. Metyrapone inhibits cortisol synthesis by the adrenal cortex. Other agents that block steroid synthesis include etomidate, ketoconazole, and aminoglutethimide. Somatostatin analog (Octreotide) suppresses ACTH secretion in some patients.
- Radiation therapy may be indicated to destroy the pituitary gland. Lifelong replacement of pituitary hormones is then necessary.
- Surgical removal of the pituitary gland is indicated when Cushing's syndrome is the result of a pituitary disorder. Lifelong replacement of pituitary hormones is then necessary. When Cushing's is caused by an adrenal cortex tumor, an adrenalectomy may be performed.

Selected Nursing Diagnoses with Interventions

Fluid Volume Excess

- Weigh daily at the same time and in the same clothes.
- Record intake and output each shift; monitor output compared to intake.
- Monitor blood pressure, pulse rate and rhythm, respiratory rate, and breath sounds.
- Assess for peripheral edema and jugular vein distention.
- Teach the patient and significant others the reasons for restricting fluids and the importance of limiting fluids if instructed.

Risk for Injury

- Maintain a safe environment (e.g., reduce clutter, maintain adequate lighting).
- Teach home safety measures.
- Monitor for signs of fatigue.
- Encourage the patient to use assistive devices for ambulation or to ask for help if needed. Nonskid slippers or shoes are also appropriate.

Risk for Infection

- Place in a private room and limit visitors.
- Monitor vital signs, including temperature, every 4 hours.
- Use principles of medical asepsis and sterile asepsis when providing care.
- If wounds are present, assess the color, odor, and consistency of wound drainage. Also assess for increased pain in and around the wound.
- Teach the patient to increase intake of protein and vitamins A and C.

Disturbed Body Image

- Encourage the patient to express feelings and to ask questions about the disorder and its treatment.
- Assist to identify strengths and previous coping strategies. Enlist the support of significant others in reaffirming the patient's worth.
- Discuss signs of progress in controlling symptoms (e.g., decreased facial edema).

Community-Based Care

- Teach the importance of home safety and tips for ensuring a safe home environment (e.g., nonskid rugs, shower rails).
- Teach the importance of maintaining the prescribed dietary supplements and fluid restrictions as instructed.
- Because patients often require medications for the rest of their lives, and dosage changes are likely, teach the importance of taking medications as indicated, and of having regular health assessments to maximize wellness.

- For patients with iatrogenic Cushing's, emphasize the importance of gradually discontinuing corticosteroid therapy (if possible) to avoid the risk of acute adrenal insufficiency with severe hypotension, circulatory collapse, shock, and coma.
- Provide information on obtaining a MedicAlert tag and stress the importance of wearing it.
- Refer to social services or a community health service as appropriate because of the complexity of the treatment and care required.

For more information on Cushing's syndrome, see Chapter 19 in *Medical-Surgical Nursing,* Fifth Edition, by LeMone, Burke, and Bauldoff.

Cystic Fibrosis

Overview

- Cystic fibrosis (CF) is an autosomal-recessive disorder that leads to abnormal exocrine gland secretions in the respiratory, gastrointestinal, and reproductive tracts.
- CF can lead to chronic obstructive pulmonary disease and death from respiratory complications in childhood and early adulthood, although improved disease management has prolonged the life span of people with CF.
- The hallmark pathophysiologic effects of CF include the following:
  1. Excess respiratory tract mucus production with impaired ciliary clearance
  2. Pancreatic enzyme deficiency and impaired digestion
  3. Abnormal elevation of sodium and chloride concentrations in sweat
- Respiratory effects lead to atelectasis, frequent infection, bronchiectasis, and dilation of distal airways.
- Severe airway obstruction and chronic hypoxemia lead to pulmonary hypertension, right heart failure, and cor pulmonale.

Cause

- CF is a genetic disorder transmitted in an autosomal-recessive pattern. About 5% of Caucasians in the United States carry the CF trait.

Manifestations

- Recurrent pneumonia, exercise intolerance
- Chronic cough
- Clubbing of digits
- Barrel chest
- Hyperresonant percussion tone; basilar crackles on auscultation
- Distended neck veins, ascites, and peripheral edema
- Abdominal pain and steatorrhea
- Small stature

Diagnostic Tests

- The pilocarpine iontophoresis sweat chloride test is used to establish the diagnosis; sodium and chloride levels in sweat are significantly elevated.
- Arterial blood gases and oxygen saturation levels show hypoxemia.
- Pulmonary function studies reveal reduced airflow, reduced forced vital capacity, and reduced total lung capacity.
- Ventilation-perfusion studies show reduced alveolar-capillary diffusion.

Interdisciplinary Management

- Immunization against respiratory infections is vital, including annual influenza vaccine and measles and pertussis boosters as needed.
- Drug therapy includes bronchodilator inhalers, antibiotic therapy for acute pulmonary infections, and dornase alfa, recombinant human DNAse, to break down excess DNA in the sputum, decreasing its viscosity.
- Chest physiotherapy with percussion and postural drainage promotes airway clearance, controlled huff cough, and autogenic drainage techniques.
- Liberal fluid intake and high-protein, high-fat, high-kilocalorie diet with vitamin and mineral supplements are prescribed, along with possible enteral or parenteral nutrition.
- Genetic screening of family members for the CF gene is encouraged.

- Lung transplantation currently offers the only definitive treatment for CF.

Selected Nursing Diagnoses with Interventions

Ineffective Airway Clearance

- Encourage fluid intake of 2.5 to 3 L per day unless contraindicated by heart failure.
- Place in Fowler's position.
- Encourage activity as tolerated.
- Assist with or provide percussion and postural drainage.

Imbalanced Nutrition: Less than Body Requirements

- Provide small meals with concentrated calories and between-meal snacks.
- Provide pancreatic enzyme supplements with meals as ordered.
- Space respiratory treatments between meals to promote appetite.

Community-Based Care

Education of the patient and family is vital to promote optimal health. Include the following topics when teaching for home care:

- Respiratory care techniques, including percussion, postural drainage, and controlled cough techniques
- Specific breathing and coughing exercises and procedures
- The importance of avoiding respiratory irritants, such as cigarette smoke, air pollution, and occupational dusts and gases
- Measures to prevent respiratory infection, such as maintaining immunizations and optimal general health, and avoiding exposure to large crowds and infected people
- Diet strategies to maintain nutrition and minimize gastrointestinal symptoms
- Community agencies and support groups
- Genetic transmission of CF; counseling, and possible genetic testing

For more information about cystic fibrosis, see Chapter 37 of *Medical-Surgical Nursing,* Fifth Edition, by LeMone, Burke, and Bauldoff.

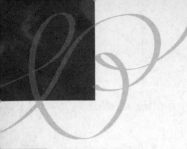

Decubitus Ulcers (Pressure Ulcers, Bedsores)

Overview

- Decubitus ulcers are defined as cellular necrosis of skin, subcutaneous, and/or deep tissues.
- They are usually localized over bony prominences.
- Pressure ulcers develop from external pressure that compresses blood vessels, and from friction and shearing forces that tear and injure vessels.
- The older adult is at increased risk for developing pressure ulcers because the dermis is thinner, with decreased vascularity, decreased sebaceous gland activity, and decreased strength and elasticity.

Causes

- Reduced mobility (common in bed- or wheelchair-bound patients)
- Altered level of consciousness, sensory perception
- Inadequate nutrition
- Susceptible skin/subcutaneous tissue due to edema, infection, fever, incontinence, cachexia, or obesity

Manifestations

- Stage I: skin redness (does not temporarily blanch when area is pressed by a finger)
- Stage II: cracked or peeling skin (partial-thickness loss)
- Stage III: broken skin with subcutaneous damage and exudate (full-thickness loss *without* bone tendon or muscle exposure)
- Stage IV: deep ulcer, through fascia to muscle, tendon, and bone; often includes undermining and tunneling (full-thickness loss *with* bone tendon, or muscle exposure)

Diagnostic Tests

- Culture and sensitivity will identify pathogens and the appropriate antibiotic.

Interdisciplinary Management

- Medications include antibiotics to eradicate any infection present and a variety of topical products to aid healing.

- Surgical debridement may be necessary if the ulcer is deep, if subcutaneous tissues are involved, or if an eschar (scab or dry crust) has formed over the ulcer. Large wounds may require skin grafting.

Selected Nursing Diagnoses with Interventions

Risk for Impaired Skin Integrity/Impaired Skin Integrity

The interventions listed are used to identify adults at risk and treat those with stage I ulcers.

- Assess patients who are bed- and chairbound, and those who are unable to reposition themselves.

- Assess patients on admission to acute care and rehabilitation hospitals, nursing homes, home care programs, and other healthcare facilities.

- Use a validated risk assessment tool.

- Conduct a systematic skin inspection at least once a day, paying particular attention to the bony prominences.

- Clean the skin at the time of soiling and at routine intervals, as frequently as the patient's needs dictate. Use lukewarm water, a mild cleansing agent, and gentle pressure.

- Minimize environmental factors leading to skin drying, such as low humidity and exposure to cold or dry heat. Treat dry skin with moisturizers.

- Do not massage over bony prominences.

- Minimize skin exposure to moisture due to incontinence, perspiration, or wound drainage.

- To minimize skin injury due to friction and shearing forces, use proper positioning, transferring, lifting, and turning techniques. Lubricants, protective films, protective dressings, and protective padding may also reduce friction injuries.

- Assess factors involved in inadequate dietary intake of protein or kilocalories. Offer nutritional supplements.

- Maintain the patient's current level of activity, mobility, and range of motion.

- For the patient who is on bed rest or is immobile, reposition every 2 hours; use positioning devices such as pillows or foam wedges to protect bony prominences; maintain the head of the bed at the lowest degree of elevation consistent with the patient's medical condition; and place any at-risk patient on a pressure-reducing device, such as a foam, static air, alternating air, gel, or water mattress.

- For patients who are chairbound, use pressure-reducing devices and reposition the patient every hour. Teach patients who can do so to shift their weight every 15 minutes.

Community-Based Care

- Teach the importance of position changes and range-of-motion exercises. Encourage the patient to participate in each as much as possible.

- Show the proper technique for prescribed dressing changes.

- Explain how to maintain a well-balanced diet.

- Teach signs of healing as well as signs of further skin breakdown.

- Referral to a home health agency can help the family through the lengthy healing process.

- Referral to a wound care center for treatment of nonhealing wounds may also be indicated.

For more information about decubitus ulcers, see Chapter 16 in *Medical-Surgical Nursing*, Fifth Edition, by LeMone, Burke, and Bauldoff.

DIABETES INSIPIDUS

Overview

- Diabetes insipidus (DI) is a deficiency of, or reduced sensitivity to, antidiuretic hormone (ADH).

- DI is characterized by excessive diuresis of very dilute urine (hypotonic polyuria).

- ADH is made in the hypothalamus and is stored and secreted from the posterior pituitary gland. ADH release is increased with stimulation of osmoreceptors (hyperosmolality), volume receptors (hypovolemia), and baroreceptors (decreased blood pressure). ADH normally promotes the reabsorption of pure water in distal renal tubules (distal convoluted and collecting tubules). When ADH is deficient, distal tubules are relatively impermeable to water, and urine volume increases.
- Untreated, DI can result in dehydration, hypovolemia, and possibly shock.

Causes

Central (Neurogenic) DI
- Deficiency of ADH secretion
- Genetic defect: autosomal-recessive Wolfram syndrome
- Neoplasms of hypothalamus or pituitary gland
- Hypothalamic or pituitary trauma secondary to head injury or surgery
- Hypoxia or ischemia (cardiopulmonary arrest, shock, hemorrhage)
- Pregnancy/postpartum Sheehan's syndrome

Nephrogenic DI
- Reduced response (sensitivity) to ADH at the renal tubules
- Genetic defect: X-linked recessive defect in ADH receptors in renal tubules
- Electrolyte disturbance
- Drugs: lithium, demeclocycline, methoxyflurane
- Medical conditions: amyloidosis, postrenal obstruction, sickle cell anemia

Manifestations
- Polyuria: 3 to 20 L/day; the greater the volume, the more dilute the urine
- Polydipsia/thirst: usually matches polyuria
- Almost colorless, clear, waterlike urine
- Dehydration, hypovolemia: if unable to meet fluid needs

Diagnostic Tests

- Plasma osmolality > 300 mOsm/L
- Urine osmolality < 50 to 200 mOsm/L
- Urine specific gravity < 1.005
- ADH challenge test: response to ADH (antidiuresis) negative if nephrogenic; positive if central

Interdisciplinary Management

- Primary treatment is correction of the underlying cause.
- Other interventions include administering intravenous hypotonic fluids, increasing oral fluids, and replacing ADH for neurogenic DI.

Selected Nursing Diagnoses with Interventions

Risk for Injury

- Institute safety precautions if the patient is dizzy and/or weak.
- Ensure access to bathroom, urinal, or bedpan.
- Provide meticulous skin and mouth care with alcohol-free emollient products after bath, and a soft toothbrush.
- Encourage verbalization of feelings and assist in development of coping strategies.

Deficient Fluid Volume

- Monitor fluid intake and output hourly, comparing amount of intake to amount of output.
- Monitor vital signs frequently.
- Weigh the patient daily, in the same clothes and at the same time each day.
- Monitor urine specific gravity.
- Monitor serum electrolytes and blood urea nitrogen.
- Monitor laboratory values for hypernatremia.

Community-Based Care

- Explain how to maintain adequate fluid intake to prevent dehydration.
- Explain the importance of reporting immediately to the physician signs of dehydration and hypovolemia.

- Show how to keep a record of daily weights, intake and output, and urine specific gravity; show how to use a hydrometer to measure urine specific gravity.

- Instruct about the need for long-term hormone therapy, the importance of taking medications as prescribed, and the importance of not stopping medications abruptly. Describe the effects and side effects of the medications.

- Teach the patient and significant others how to give subcutaneous and intramuscular injections of ADH and how to use nasal applicators.

- Stress the importance of long-term medical follow-up care.

- Explain to patients the importance of carrying medications with them at all times.

- Provide information on how to obtain a MedicAlert tag and stress the need to wear it at all times.

- Refer the patient to social services or a psychologist if appropriate.

For more information on diabetes insipidus, see Chapter 19 in *Medical-Surgical Nursing*, Fifth Edition, by LeMone, Burke, and Bauldoff.

DIABETES MELLITUS

Overview

- Diabetes mellitus (DM) is a group of chronic metabolic disorders characterized by inappropriate hyperglycemia.

- It results from a deficiency of, or resistance to, the hormone insulin.

- Insulin is normally secreted from the beta islet cells of the pancreas in response to increased blood glucose levels. Adequate insulin is necessary for glucose transport into insulin-dependent cells (muscle, adipose tissue); anabolic synthesis of glycogen (liver, muscle), cellular proteins (muscle), and triglycerides (adipose tissue); and maintenance of normal blood glucose concentration.

- Inadequate insulin effect leads to chronic hyperglycemia, with acute and chronic complications.

- Acute complications of type 1 DM include hypoglycemia (in people taking exogenous insulin) and diabetic ketoacidosis.
- An acute complication of type 2 DM is hyperosmolar hyperglycemic state (HHS).
- Chronic complications of DM include vasculopathy (nephropathy, retinopathy, peripheral) and neuropathy (sensory, motor, autonomic).
- DM is the sixth leading cause of death in the United States, primarily from the cardiovascular effects resulting in coronary artery disease and stroke.
- DM is the leading cause of renal failure, blindness, and nontraumatic amputations.

Causes

Type 1 Diabetes Mellitus

- Type 1 DM results from destruction of pancreatic islet beta cells, almost always from an autoimmune process.
- Precipitating factors include a genetic predisposition, an environmental trigger such as a viral infection (mumps, rubella, or coxsackievirus B4), or chemical toxin. An abnormal immune response that targets normal islet beta cells follows, destroying them.
- Produces an absolute insulin deficiency, necessitating exogenous insulin therapy.
- Affects approximately 5% to 10% of people with DM.

Type 2 Diabetes Mellitus

- Results from insufficient insulin to maintain normal blood glucose levels.
- Exact cause unknown; theories include limited beta cell response to hyperglycemia, peripheral insulin resistance, and abnormalities of insulin receptors.
- Type 2 is associated with obesity that decreases the number of available insulin receptor sites in skeletal muscle and adipose tissues.
- Unlike type 1 DM, there is sufficient insulin present to prevent fat breakdown.
- Incidence is higher among Hispanics, Native Americans, and African Americans.

Other Types
- Genetic beta cell defects
- Genetic insulin-action defects
- Exocrine pancreatic disorders
- Drug or chemical induced
- Infections
- Gestational DM

Manifestations

Short-Term Manifestations
- Hyperglycemia
- Polyuria
- Polydipsia
- Polyphagia (more common in type 1)
- Fatigue, weakness
- Weight loss (type 1)
- Blurred vision, frequent skin infections

Long-Term Manifestations
- Angiopathy of small vessels (microangiopathy) or large vessels (macroangiopathy)
- Microangiopathy:
  - Retinopathy, may progress to blindness
  - Nephropathy, may progress to renal failure
- Macroangiopathy:
  - Coronary heart disease (CHD), may result in acute coronary syndrome or myocardial infarction
  - Cerebral vascular disease, may result in stroke
  - Peripheral vascular disease, may progress to gangrene/amputation
- Neuropathy: slowed conduction in peripheral and autonomic nerves
  - Peripheral neuropathy with numbness, tingling, hyperesthesia, paresthesias, reduced reflexes

- Autonomic neuropathy resulting in orthostatic hypotension, slowed digestion, urinary bladder incontinence or retention, male impotence

Acute Complications

- Type 1:
  - Hypoglycemia (insulin shock) due to excess insulin or lack of food intake
  - Ketoacidosis due to insufficient insulin
- Type 2:
  - HHS with significant hyperglycemia and a plasma osmolarity of 340 mOsm/L or higher

Diagnostic Tests

- Fasting plasma glucose > 126 mg/dL (with manifestations of DM)
- Random plasma glucose > 200 mg/dL (with manifestations of DM)
- Glucose tolerance test > 200 mg/dL during 2-hour testing period
- Urine glucose/ketones positive (none normally present in urine)
- Glycosylated hemoglobin (A1c) > 7% (normal, 4% to 7%) to assess degree of hyperglycemia and compliance over past 2 to 3 months
- Renal function tests (blood urea nitrogen, creatinine, creatinine clearance) and urine protein to detect nephropathy
- Serum cholesterol and triglyceride levels to evaluate risk of CHD

Interdisciplinary Management

- Patients with type 1 DM require a lifelong exogenous source of the insulin hormone to maintain life. Oral hypoglycemic agents may be used to treat patients with type 2 DM.

- The goals of dietary management include restoring normal blood glucose and optimal lipid levels, attaining and maintaining reasonable body weight, staying consistent in timing of meals and snacks, and improving overall health through optimal nutrition. The diet should be high in fiber and low in saturated fat and cholesterol. Nonnutritive sweeteners and fructose, sorbitol, and xylitol may be used. Alcohol may be consumed only in restricted amounts: no more than two drinks at one time and only with a meal.

- Regular exercise reduces glucose levels by increasing the uptake of glucose by muscle cells, potentially reducing the need for insulin. Exercise also reduces cholesterol and triglyceride levels, decreasing the risk of CHD.
- Surgical management of DM involves replacing or transplanting the pancreas, pancreatic cells, or beta cells.

Selected Nursing Diagnoses with Interventions

Risk for Impaired Skin Integrity

- Conduct baseline and ongoing assessments of the feet, as patients with diabetes are at significant risk for lower extremity gangrene due to the effects of peripheral neuropathy and angiopathy.
- Teach foot hygiene.
- Stress the importance of well-fitting shoes and avoiding barefoot walking.
- Wear cotton socks.
- Discuss the importance of not smoking.
- Discuss the importance of maintaining blood glucose levels through prescribed diet, medication, and exercise.

Risk for Infection

- Use and teach meticulous hand hygiene.
- Monitor for clinical manifestations of infection in patients at high risk.
- Discuss the importance of skin care. Keep the skin clean and dry, using lukewarm water and mild soap.
- Teach dental health measures.
- Teach women with diabetes the symptoms of and preventive measures for vaginitis caused by *Candida albicans*.

Risk for Injury

- Assess for the presence of contributing or causative factors that increase the risk of injury, including blurred vision, cataracts, decreased adaptation to dark, decreased tactile sensitivity, hypoglycemia, hyperglycemia, hypovolemia, joint immobility, and unstable gait.
- Reduce environmental hazards in the healthcare facility, and teach the patient about safety in the home.

- Monitor for, and teach the patient with type 1 DM and significant others to recognize and seek care for, the manifestations of diabetic ketoacidosis, including hyperglycemia, thirst, headaches, nausea and vomiting, abdominal pain, increased urine output, ketonuria, dehydration, and decreasing level of consciousness.

- Monitor for, and teach the patient with type 2 DM and significant others to recognize and seek care for, the manifestations of HHS, including extreme hyperglycemia, increased urinary output, thirst, dehydration, hypotension, seizures, and decreasing level of consciousness.

- Monitor for, and teach the patient and significant others to recognize and treat the manifestations of, hypoglycemia, including low blood glucose, anxiety, headache, uncoordinated movements, sweating, rapid pulse, drowsiness, and visual changes.

- Recommend that the patient wear a MedicAlert bracelet or necklace identifying self as a person with diabetes.

Ineffective Coping

- Assess the patient's psychosocial resources.

- Explore with the patient and significant others the effects (actual and perceived) of the diagnosis and treatment on finances, occupation, energy levels, and relationships.

- Teach constructive problem-solving techniques:

  1. Identify the problem.

  2. Find the cause of the problem.

  3. Determine the options.

  4. List the advantages and disadvantages of each option.

  5. Choose an option and make a plan.

- Provide information about support groups and resources, such as suppliers of products, journals, cookbooks, and so on.

Community-Based Care

- Explain the importance of strict compliance with treatment regimens, including diet, exercise, medications, and blood glucose monitoring techniques and injection of insulin.

- Explain the effects of blood glucose levels on long-term health.

- Teach how to perform regular foot care.

- Explain the importance of reading nutritional labels for hidden sugar content.

- Refer to a social worker or home health nurse as appropriate. Consider income level, as money to purchase medications and supplies often must be taken out of a fixed income.

- Provide information on how to purchase supplies, and how to obtain a MedicAlert bracelet or necklace.

- Encourage regular dental and eye examinations.

- Provide a list of community resources such as the American Diabetes Association.

For more information on diabetes mellitus, see Chapter 20 in *Medical-Surgical Nursing*, Fifth Edition, by LeMone, Burke, and Bauldoff.

DIABETIC KETOACIDOSIS

Overview
- Diabetic ketoacidosis (DKA) is a form of metabolic acidosis that results when insulin deficit causes fat stores to break down, releasing fatty acids and ketones.

Causes
- Untreated type 1 diabetes mellitus
- May occur in people with diagnosed type 1 diabetes mellitus when energy requirements increase during stress, causing release of gluconeogenic hormones that stimulate carbohydrate formation from protein or fat
- Lack of insulin, leading to hyperglycemia, hyperosmolarity, and resulting osmotic diuresis
- Ketoacid accumulation, causing metabolic acidosis

Manifestations
- Fatigue, confusion, coma
- Polyuria secondary to high blood glucose
- Poor skin turgor/dry mucous membranes secondary to fluid losses
- Fever secondary to fluid volume deficit
- Hypotension

- Kussmaul's (deep, rapid, labored) respirations
- Anorexia, nausea, vomiting, abdominal pain
- Altered levels of consciousness: confusion, stupor, coma

Diagnostic Tests

- Arterial blood gases show plasma pH < 7.3; plasma bicarbonate (HCO_3) < 15 mEq/L, decreased $PaCO_2$
- Blood glucose levels > 300 mg/dL
- Ketones present in blood and urine; glycosuria

Interdisciplinary Management

- DKA requires immediate medical attention. Fluids are administered for dehydration, and insulin is given to reduce hyperglycemia and acidosis.
- Potassium replacement is begun early in the course of treatment.

Selected Nursing Diagnoses with Interventions

Deficient Knowledge

- Explain "sick day" management.
- Explain manifestations of impending DKA and ways to prevent condition.
- Provide individual diabetes management plan; reinforce teaching where needed.

Deficient Fluid Volume

- Administer fluids, insulin, and potassium as prescribed.
- Monitor blood sugars using the fingerstick method.
- Encourage resumption of diabetic diet, oral fluid intake, and insulin self-administration as soon as possible.

Community-Based Care

- Stress the need for long-term follow-up care with the physician, diabetes nurse educator, and dietitian.
- A referral to a social worker or psychologic counselor for assistance in coping with chronic diabetes may be appropriate.

For more information on diabetic ketoacidosis, see Chapter 20 in *Medical-Surgical Nursing*, Fifth Edition, by LeMone, Burke, and Bauldoff.

Disseminated Intravascular Coagulation

Overview

- Disseminated intravascular coagulation (DIC) is a disruption of hemostasis characterized by widespread intravascular clotting and bleeding.

- It may be acute and life-threatening or relatively mild.

- The sequence of DIC follows:

  1. Endothelial damage, tissue factors, or toxins stimulate the clotting cascade.

  2. Excess thrombin within the circulation overwhelms naturally occurring anticoagulants.

  3. Widespread clotting occurs within the microvasculature.

  4. Thrombi and emboli impair tissue perfusion, leading to ischemia, infarction, and necrosis.

  5. Clotting factors (including platelets) are consumed faster than they can be replaced.

  6. Clotting activates fibrinolytic processes that begin to break down clots.

  7. Fibrin degradation products (potent anticoagulants) are released, contributing to bleeding.

  8. Clotting factors are depleted, the ability to form clots is lost, and hemorrhage occurs.

Causes

DIC always occurs secondarily to another disorder. Precipitating causes may include the following:

- Burns, especially extensive ones

- Embolism: pulmonary, fat

- Infection: especially bacterial septicemia, but possible with any organism

- Hemolysis: transfusion reaction, sickle cell crisis

- Obstetric complications: abortion, abruptio placenta, amniotic fluid embolus, endometritis with sepsis, fetal demise, hemorrhage, toxemia of pregnancy

- Necrotizing disorders: frostbite, gunshot wounds, head injury, trauma, transplant rejection, liver necrosis

- Neoplastic disease, especially leukemias, lymphomas, metastatic carcinoma
- Other: acute respiratory distress syndrome, cardiac arrest, cardiopulmonary bypass, diabetic ketoacidosis, drug reactions, shock, heat stroke, snakebite, cirrhosis

Manifestations

D

- Spontaneous bleeding following a known or suspected precipitating event
- Epistaxis (nosebleed)
- Skin: ecchymosis, hematoma, petechiae, purpura, oozing of blood from surgical incisions or venipuncture sites
- Respiratory: dyspnea, tachypnea, hemoptysis
- Cardiovascular: hypotension, reduced pulse amplitude, chest pain
- Gastrointestinal: nausea, vomiting, abdominal pain, hematemesis, rectal bleeding/melena
- Renal: hematuria, oliguria, flank pain
- Neurologic: decreased level of consciousness, seizures
- Muscle or back pain
- Chronic DIC may be asymptomatic

Diagnostic Tests

- Complete blood cell and platelet counts show reduced hemoglobin, hematocrit, and circulating platelets. Fragmented red blood cells may be noted.
- Coagulation studies include the following:
  1. Prolonged prothrombin time, partial thromboplastin time, and thrombin time.
  2. Low fibrinogen level due to depletion of clotting factors. The fibrinogen level helps predict bleeding in DIC: As it falls, the risk of bleeding increases (Braunwald et al., 2001).
  3. Increased fibrin degradation products or fibrin split products.
  4. Positive D-dimer test.

Interdisciplinary Management

- Fresh frozen plasma and platelet concentrates are given to restore clotting factors and platelets.

- Heparin may be administered, as it interferes with the clotting cascade and may prevent further clotting factor depletion due to uncontrolled thrombosis. It is used when bleeding is not controlled by plasma and platelets, and when manifestations of thrombotic problems such as acrocyanosis and possible gangrene are present.

Selected Nursing Diagnoses with Interventions

Ineffective Tissue Perfusion

- Assess extremity pulses, warmth, and capillary refill. Assess level of consciousness and mental status.
- Promptly report changes in mental status, extremities, gastrointestinal function, and urinary output.
- Carefully turn from side to side at least every 2 hours.
- Discourage the patient from crossing the legs, and do not elevate the knees on the bed.
- Minimize use of adhesive tape on the skin.

Impaired Gas Exchange

- Monitor oxygen saturation and arterial blood gases; report abnormal results to the physician.
- Administer oxygen as prescribed.
- Maintain bed rest in semi- or high Fowler's position.
- Encourage deep breathing and effective coughing; assist with incentive spirometer.

Fear

- Encourage the patient and significant others to verbalize concerns.
- Answer questions truthfully.
- Help identify coping strategies the patient and significant others may be able to use.
- Provide emotional support.
- Maintain a calm environment.
- Respond promptly when the patient calls for help.

Community-Based Care

- Teach the patient and significant others about the disorder, its treatment, and expected outcome.

- Teach the patient and family about specific care needs, such as foot care or dressing changes.

- Provide instruction about continuing medications and follow-up care.

- Patients with chronic DIC may require continuing heparin therapy, using either intermittent subcutaneous injections or a portable infusion pump. Teach how to administer the injection or manage the infusion pump.

- Provide a referral to home health care or a home intravenous management service as needed.

- Discuss manifestations of excessive bleeding or recurrent clotting to report to the physician.

For more information on disseminated intravascular coagulation, see Chapter 33 in *Medical-Surgical Nursing*, Fifth Edition, by LeMone, Burke, and Bauldoff.

DIVERTICULAR DISEASE

Overview

- Diverticular disease is the formation of abnormal herniations, called *diverticula*, of bowel mucosa through the muscle layers of the gastrointestinal tract.

- Diverticula can form in any portion of the gastrointestinal tract, but usually affect the sigmoid colon.

- Diverticula are thought to form due to high intraluminal pressures.

- *Diverticulosis* is the presence of diverticula; most are asymptomatic.

- *Diverticulitis* is an inflamed diverticula. Diverticulitis develops when fecal material becomes trapped in a diverticulum and forms a hard mass (or fecalith). It may lead to obstruction, infection, perforation, hemorrhage, or fistula formation.

- Diverticulosis usually affects adults: In the United States, 5% of people in their 40s and 50% or more of those over 80 have diverticula.

Causes

- Risk factors include a low-fiber diet. Diverticular disease is almost unknown in less developed countries where unrefined (high-fiber) diets are consumed.

- Sedentary lifestyle and postponement of defecation may be contributing factors.

Manifestations

Diverticulosis

- Usually asymptomatic but may cause abdominal cramping, decreased stool caliber, constipation, and occult blood in the stool.

Diverticulitis

- Symptoms may occur in paroxysmal attacks
- Pain: mild to severe left lower quadrant abdominal; crampy; often relieved upon defecation; rebound tenderness
- Nausea, vomiting, anorexia; gas; flatus
- Irregular bowel habits; alternating constipation, diarrhea
- Manifestations of infection: fever, chills, leukocytosis

Diagnostic Tests

- Barium enema is used to illustrate the diverticula.
- Sigmoidoscopy or colonoscopy is used to detect diverticulosis.
- Abdominal x-rays detect presence of gas; bowel obstruction; and air in the abdominal cavity, which may indicate perforation.
- Computed tomography scan can identify diverticula, bowel wall changes, abscesses, and fistulas.
- Guaiac testing of the stool often reveals the presence of occult blood.

Interdisciplinary Management

- Medications include systemic broad-spectrum antibiotics effective against usual bowel flora. Pentazocine may be prescribed for pain relief. A stool softener such as docusate sodium may be prescribed. Laxatives are avoided.
- Bowel rest is prescribed for the patient with acute diverticulitis. A high-residue diet with fiber is recommended following recovery.
- Resection of the affected bowel segment, with anastomosis of the proximal and distal portions, may be performed for acute diverticulitis; temporary colostomy is a possibility.

Selected Nursing Diagnoses with Interventions

Potential Complication: Perforation

- Monitor vital signs including temperature at least every 4 hours.
- Assess abdomen every 4 to 8 hours; more often as indicated.
- Observe for gross blood in the stools, and test stools for occult blood.
- Maintain intravenous fluids, total parenteral nutrition, and accurate intake and output records.

Acute Pain

- Assess pain using a standard pain scale. Document the level of pain; note any changes in the location or character of pain.
- Administer prescribed analgesic, assessing its effectiveness. Avoid morphine administration.
- Maintain bowel rest and total body rest as prescribed.
- Reintroduce oral foods and fluids slowly, providing a soft, low-fiber diet, followed by a high-fiber diet with bulk-forming agents after recovery.

Anxiety

- Assess and document level of anxiety.
- Demonstrate empathy and awareness of the perceived threat to the patient's health.
- Spend as much time as possible with the patient.
- Assess level of understanding about the condition.
- Encourage supportive significant others to remain with the patient as much as possible.
- Assist to identify and use appropriate coping mechanisms.
- Involve the patient and significant others (as appropriate) in care decisions.

Community-Based Care

- Explain all diagnostic and therapeutic procedures. Discuss oral food and fluid limitations, and explain the rationale for a low-residue diet with acute diverticulitis.
- Stress the importance of maintaining a high-fiber diet for life. Discuss ways to increase dietary fiber, and refer to a dietitian as needed.

- Discuss the complications of diverticular diseases and their manifestations.

- Following surgery, provide instructions for home care, including information on where to purchase supplies as indicated.

- Provide information about colostomy management if necessary, as well as referral to the United Ostomy Association.

- A referral to a home health agency may be appropriate.

For more information on diverticular disease, see Chapter 24 in *Medical-Surgical Nursing*, Fifth Edition, by LeMone, Burke, and Bauldoff.

DYSFUNCTIONAL UTERINE BLEEDING

Overview

- Dysfunctional uterine bleeding (DUB) is defined as abnormal uterine bleeding patterns.
- It is due to abnormal hormonal patterns, especially when estrogen is secreted unopposed by progesterone, producing endometrial hyperplasia.

Causes

- Polycystic ovary syndrome
- Anovulatory cycles: perimenopausal
- Obesity
- Immature hypothalamic-pituitary function (adolescents)

Manifestations

- Amenorrhea: absence of menses, or oligomenorrhea, scant menses
- Menorrhagia: excessive bleeding with menses
- Hypermenorrhea: prolonged menstrual periods (> 8 days)
- Polymenorrhea: frequent menstrual periods (< 18 days)
- Metrorrhagia: bleeding in the middle of the cycle
- Postmenopausal bleeding
- Manifestations of anemia

Diagnostic Tests

- Dilation and curettage to obtain endometrial tissue for biopsy.
- Biopsy can reveal endometrial hyperplasia.
- Hemoglobin and hematocrit will be low if anemia is present.

Interdisciplinary Management

- DUB in some patients can be corrected with hormonal agents. Progesterone or medroxyprogesterone may be prescribed. Oral iron supplements may be used to replace iron lost through bleeding.
- Surgical options include therapeutic dilation and curettage, endometrial ablation, and hysterectomy.

Selected Nursing Diagnoses with Interventions

Anxiety

- Discuss the results of tests and examinations with the patient face to face.
- Monitor bleeding pattern, including duration and amount of bleeding.
- Monitor vital signs, hemoglobin, and hematocrit to determine severity of blood loss.
- Involve the patient in developing the treatment plan.
- Assist the patient in identifying personal strengths and coping strategies.
- Encourage the patient to be involved in care activities, demonstrate feelings, express concerns, and request the attention and involvement of significant others.

Sexual Dysfunction

- Offer information about engaging in sexual intercourse during menstruation.
- Provide an opportunity for the patient to express concerns related to alterations in lifestyle and sexual functioning.
- Encourage frequent rest periods.
- Provide information about alternative methods of sexual expression.

- Administer prescribed medications and monitor response to therapy.

Community-Based Care

- Explain the disorder and the therapeutic interventions indicated.
- Describe medication regimen, including oral contraceptives, iron supplements, and other agents, including dosage, effects, and side effects.
- Center nutritional teaching on the need to maintain a balanced diet, increasing iron-rich foods such as beans, liver, beef, and shrimp.
- Encourage the patient to document her menstrual cycles on a calendar to assist in diagnosis and to monitor the effectiveness of treatment.
- Emphasize the need to report recurring episodes of dysfunctional uterine bleeding, particularly in postmenopausal women.

For more information about dysfunctional uterine bleeding, see Chapter 49 in *Medical-Surgical Nursing*, Fifth Edition, by LeMone, Burke, and Bauldoff.

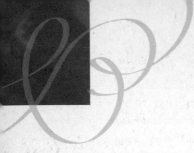

EMPHYSEMA

Overview

- Emphysema is characterized by destruction of the walls of the alveoli and development of abnormal air spaces.

- Alveolar wall destruction causes alveoli and air spaces to enlarge with loss of corresponding portions of the pulmonary capillary bed.

- This reduces the surface area for alveolar-capillary diffusion, affecting gas exchange.

- Loss of elastic recoil and support tissue decreases passive expiration and leads to air trapping.

- Either respiratory bronchioles or alveoli may be the primary tissue involved.

Causes

- Cigarette smoking is a causative factor in most cases.

- Deficiency of alpha$_1$-antitrypsin, an enzyme that normally inhibits the activity of proteolytic enzymes and tissue destruction in the lungs, leads to early-onset emphysema.

Manifestations

- Insidious onset

- Dyspnea, initially with exertion, progressing to at rest

- Minimal cough

- Increased anterior-posterior chest diameter (barrel chest)

- Tachypnea, prolonged expiratory phase of respirations

- Use of accessory muscles of respiration

- Decreased breath sounds, hyperresonant percussion tone

- Anorexia, weight loss

Diagnostic Tests

- Chest x-ray shows hyperinflation with flattened diaphragm, reduced vascular markings, and increased anterior-posterior diameter.

- Pulmonary function tests show increased residual volume and total lung capacity, and reduced expiratory flow rate.

- Ventilation/perfusion scanning demonstrates the extent to which lung tissue is ventilated but not perfused ("dead space").

- Exhaled carbon dioxide ($ETCO_2$) is decreased when pulmonary perfusion is impaired.

- Arterial blood gases show mild hypoxemia and normal or low carbon dioxide tension. Respiratory alkalosis may be present due to an increased respiratory rate.

- Serum alpha$_1$-antitrypsin levels may be low. Normal adult serum alpha$_1$-antitrypsin levels range from 80 to 260 mg/dL.

Interdisciplinary Management

- Medications include antibiotics, bronchodilators, and alpha$_1$-antitrypsin replacement therapy.

- Smoking cessation is vital.

- Pulmonary hygiene measures include hydration, controlled breathing, and cough techniques to prevent airway collapse (e.g., pursed-lip breathing).

- Oxygenation and inspiratory positive-pressure assistance with a face mask or intubation and mechanical ventilation may be necessary for acute exacerbation.

- Lung transplantation may be an option.

Selected Nursing Diagnoses with Interventions

(Also see Chronic Obstructive Pulmonary Disease)

Ineffective Breathing Pattern

- Monitor respiratory status and diagnostic test results. Report significant changes.

- Teach pursed-lip and abdominal breathing techniques.

Ineffective Airway Clearance

- Provide chest physiotherapy and postural drainage every 4 hours or as needed.

- Administer prescribed medications, including inhalers and nebulizers, and monitor response.
- Schedule respiratory treatments at least 1 hour before or after meals.
- Encourage fluid intake of 2 to 3 L per day.

Impaired Gas Exchange
- Monitor arterial blood gases and oxygen saturation.
- Administer oxygen as ordered, observing closely for respiratory depression.

Activity Intolerance
- Provide a calm, quiet environment and encourage frequent rest periods.
- Encourage verbalization of concerns and fears; answer questions honestly.

Community-Based Care
- Explain the importance of smoking cessation.
- Instruct to avoid respiratory irritants such as secondhand smoke, air pollution, and cold, dry air.
- Advise to avoid crowds and people with known infections.
- Teach effective coughing and breathing techniques, chest physiotherapy, and postural drainage as appropriate.
- Review medication regimen, including proper use of inhalers and nebulizers.
- Encourage a high-kilocalorie, protein-rich diet.
- Instruct to report sudden, sharp chest pain that is exacerbated by chest movement, breathing, and coughing.
- Referral to a smoking cessation program may be appropriate.
- Refer to home health care and respiratory therapy services as needed for home oxygen.
- Stress the need for continuing medical care.

For more information on emphysema, see Chapter 37 in *Medical-Surgical Nursing,* Fifth Edition, by LeMone, Burke, and Bauldoff.

Empyema

Overview

- Empyema is accumulation of purulent exudate in the pleural cavity.
- Empyema is a space-occupying lesion that leads to atelectasis (collapse) of lung.

Causes

- Pulmonary infection such as pneumonia or lung abscess
- Thoracic surgery, chest trauma

Manifestations

- Fever, chills, night sweats
- Anorexia, weight loss
- Chest pain
- Dyspnea, cough
- Decreased chest wall movement on affected side
- Decreased breath sounds over affected area, flat percussion tone

Diagnostic Tests

- Chest x-ray may show visible opaque effusion if volume is sufficient.
- Culture and sensitivity of collected fluid.

Interdisciplinary Management

- Thoracentesis is performed to drain the pus from the pleural cavity.
- Antibiotics are the primary pharmacologic treatment.
- An open thoracotomy and surgical debridement of the pleural space may be used in severe cases.

Selected Nursing Diagnoses with Interventions

Impaired Gas Exchange

- Frequently assess respiratory status, including rate and depth, respiratory excursion, and breath sounds.
- Monitor oxygen saturation and arterial blood gases. Report significant changes.
- Prepare for thoracentesis and chest tube insertion.

Risk for Infection

- Use standard precautions. Maintain strict aseptic technique when caring for chest tubes, including on air-occlusive dressing around tube insertion site.

- Administer antibiotics and oxygen as prescribed and monitor responses.

Community-Based Care

- Explain all tests and procedures, medications, and their effects and side effects.

- Discuss home management of the drainage tube, if planned.

- Encourage immunization for pneumonia and annual influenza immunization.

- Refer to a smoking cessation program as appropriate.

- Home health care referral may be required for tube management and oxygen therapy.

- Stress the importance of continued medical follow-up care.

For more information on empyema, see Chapter 36 in *Medical-Surgical Nursing,* Fifth Edition, by LeMone, Burke, and Bauldoff.

ENCEPHALITIS

Overview

- Encephalitis is an inflammation of the brain parenchyma (functional tissue) and meninges (covering membranes).

- It is usually due to viral organisms; however, any organism is possible.

- Viral infections are characterized by infiltration of lymphocytes; bacterial types by polymorphonuclear leukocytes.

- Brain tissues are inflamed; edema formation increases intracranial pressure.

- Cerebral edema can be mild or severe enough to cause brainstem herniation, a medical emergency.

- Brain cells are destroyed; number and type vary with the cause.

- Residual neurologic deficits may follow.

- Prognosis depends on the specific offending organism and the patient's resistance.

Causes

- Viral infections (prognosis varies with type):

  1. Common viruses include arboviruses (epidemic type), enteroviruses, herpes simplex virus-1, and mumps.

  2. Less common viruses are cytomegalovirus, Epstein-Barr virus, human immunodeficiency virus, varicella-zoster virus, and measles.

  3. Rare viruses include Colorado tick-fever virus, lymphocytic choriomeningitis virus, adenoviruses, influenza A, rubella, and rabies.

- Other infections:

  1. Bacteria (*Listeria monocytogenes*, *Mycobacterium tuberculosis*)

  2. Mycoplasma

  3. Fungi (*Cryptococcus*)

  4. Protozoa (*Toxoplasma gondii*)

  5. Rickettsia

- Noninfectious causes include ingested lead, and postvaccination (associated with vaccines for measles, mumps, and rabies).

Manifestations

- Infection: fever, chills, malaise

- Meningeal irritation: nuchal rigidity (stiff neck), neck pain, positive Brudzinski sign, positive Kernig's sign

- Increased intracranial pressure: headache; changes in level of consciousness such as irritability, confusion, drowsiness, stupor, coma, and declining Glasgow coma scale; vital sign changes such as bradycardia, hypertension, widening pulse pressure, and altered respiratory patterns; pupillary changes such as inequality or dilation; brainstem herniation is rapidly fatal

- Focal: vary widely but may include photophobia, aphasia, sensory deficits (blindness, deafness, loss of taste/smell), motor deficits (ataxia), psychosis, or seizures

Diagnostic Tests

- Lumbar puncture and cerebrospinal fluid analysis may reveal elevated cerebrospinal fluid pressure, increased white blood cells, increased protein, but normal glucose; fluid is usually clear.
- Electroencephalogram may show focal or general electric slowing.
- Computed tomography scanning or magnetic resonance imaging can rule out other neurologic conditions or show areas of swelling.
- Brain biopsy collects brain tissue specimens to identify specific virus.

Interdisciplinary Management

- Medications include antiviral drugs (intravenous acyclovir or vidarabine) or antifungal drugs (amphotericin-B, flucytosine, and fluconazole) to treat the infection and osmotic diuretics and corticosteroids to control cerebral edema. Antiepileptic drugs (AEDs) may be given to prevent seizures.

Selected Nursing Diagnoses with Interventions

Ineffective Protection

- Assess for fever, malaise, headache, listlessness, joint pain, nausea, vomiting, change in level of consciousness, hemiparesis, tremors, seizures, stiff neck, aphasia, and cranial nerve dysfunction.
- Maintain a quiet, calm environment and organize care to minimize unnecessary stimulation.
- Maintain the bed in the low position, with side rails up and padded and the head of the bed elevated 30 to 45 degrees.

Risk for Imbalanced Body Temperature

- Assess vital signs frequently and administer analgesics/antipyretics as prescribed to reduce temperature.
- Institute measures to prevent complications resulting from immobility (e.g., turn the patient every 2 hours, use an air mattress to reduce pressure, provide range of motion exercises, and change wet linens promptly).

Risk for Deficient Fluid Volume

- Monitor nutritional and fluid balance status and report any abnormalities.

- Monitor daily weights, skin turgor, BUN:creatinine ratio.
- Administer prescribed medications and fluids
- Assess patient and family support and coping skills and intervene to assist in coping with potential long-term rehabilitation and possible neurologic deficits.

Community-Based Care

- Explain the disease process and its treatments, medications, prognosis, and any necessary restrictions or precautions.
- Review necessary procedures for home care if appropriate. These include techniques for communicating if the patient has aphasia, preventing seizures, and assisting with self-care.
- Refer patient and caregiver to a social worker and/or spiritual counselor if appropriate to assist with developing coping skills and planning for long-term care.
- The patient with permanent neurologic deficits as a result of encephalitis is usually discharged to a rehabilitation setting or long-term care facility.

For more information on encephalitis, see Chapter 43 in *Medical-Surgical Nursing,* Fifth Edition, by LeMone, Burke, and Bauldoff.

ENDOCARDITIS

Overview

- Endocarditis is inflammation of the endocardium.
- Endocarditis is usually infectious, characterized by colonization or invasion of the endocardium and heart valves by a pathogen.
- Lesions develop on deformed valves, on valve prostheses, or in areas of endothelial tissue damage. The left side of the heart and mitral valve are usually affected.
- Endocarditis is classified by its acuity and disease course:
  1. *Acute infective endocarditis* has an abrupt onset and is a rapidly progressive, severe disease. *Staphylococcus aureus* is commonly the infecting organism.
  2. *Subacute infective endocarditis* has a more gradual onset, with predominant systemic manifestations. It usually affects people with preexisting heart disease. *Streptococcus viridans*

and other gram-negative and gram-positive bacteria often cause subacute forms of endocarditis.

3. *Prosthetic valve endocarditis* (PVE) may occur in patients with a mechanical or tissue valve replacement.

- The initial lesion is a sterile platelet-fibrin vegetation formed on damaged endothelium or healthy valve structures.

- Vegetations are colonized by bacteria, and enlarge as platelets and fibrin cover the infecting organism, shielding them from immune defenses.

- Vegetations expand, and are loosely attached to valve edges. Friable vegetations can break off to become emboli that lodge in small vessels, causing hemorrhages, infarcts, or abscesses.

- Valves are scarred and deformed, leading to turbulent blood flow and valvular stenosis or incompetence.

- Infective endocarditis is almost always fatal if untreated.

Causes

- Endocarditis develops secondarily to bacterial invasion of the blood (bacteremia).

- Risk factors for endocarditis are as follows:

  - Previous heart damage

  - Intravenous (IV) drug use

  - Invasive catheters (e.g., a central venous catheter, hemodynamic monitoring, or an indwelling urinary catheter)

  - Dental procedures or poor dental health

  - Recent heart surgery

Manifestations

- Early manifestations often nonspecific:

  - Temperature above 101.5°F (39.4°C)

  - Flulike symptoms

  - Cough, shortness of breath, and joint pain

- Acute staphylococcal endocarditis: a more severe, sudden onset with chills and a high fever

- Heart murmur

- Manifestations of embolic complications: anginal, flank, or abdominal pain—symptoms of transient ischemic attack or stroke

- Splenomegaly
- Peripheral manifestations: petechiae on trunk, conjunctiva, and mucous membranes; splinter hemorrhages; Osler's nodes (small, painful growths on finger and toe pads); Janeway lesions (flat, painless, red to bluish-red spots on hands and feet); and Roth's spots (cotton-wool spots on the retina)
- Possible manifestations of heart failure

Diagnostic Tests

- Blood cultures identify the infecting organism.
- Echocardiography shows vegetations and valve function. Either transthoracic echocardiography or transesophageal echocardiography may be done. When combined with positive blood cultures, echocardiography can be diagnostic.
- Serologic immune testing may show circulating antigens to infective organisms.
- Other diagnostic tests may include complete blood cell count, erythrocyte sedimentation rate, serum creatinine, chest x-ray, and electrocardiogram.

Interdisciplinary Management

- Antibiotic therapy is the mainstay of treatment for infective endocarditis.
- Surgical intervention is used to replace severely damaged valves, remove large vegetations, or remove a valve that is a continuing source of infection.

Selected Nursing Diagnoses with Interventions

Risk for Imbalanced Body Temperature

- Record temperature every 2 to 4 hours. Notify the physician if it rises above 101.5°F (39.4°C). Assess for complaints of discomfort.
- Obtain blood cultures as prescribed before giving the first dose of antibiotics.
- Administer anti-inflammatory or antipyretic agents as ordered.
- Administer antibiotics as ordered; obtain peak and trough drug levels as indicated.

Risk for Ineffective Tissue Perfusion

- Document and report manifestations of decreased organ system perfusion:
  - Central nervous system: decreased level of consciousness, numbness or tingling in extremities, hemiplegia, visual disturbances
  - Renal: oliguria, hematuria, elevated blood urea nitrogen or creatinine
  - Pulmonary: dyspnea, hemoptysis, shortness of breath, diminished breath sounds, restlessness, sudden chest or shoulder pain
  - Cardiovascular: chest pain radiating to jaw or arms, tachycardia, anxiety, tachypnea, hypotension
  - Gastrointestinal: abdominal pain, decreased bowel sounds, abdominal distention
- Assess and document skin color and temperature, quality of peripheral pulses, and capillary refill.

Community-Based Care

- Teach about the disease process, its manifestations, treatment, and prognosis.
- Emphasize the need to continue antibiotic therapy for the entire course of prescribed treatment.
- Instruct to promptly report unusual manifestations such as vision change, sudden pain, or weakness to the physician.
- Discuss future need for prophylactic antibiotics preceding procedures such as dental work or urologic procedures.
- If endocarditis resulted from IV drug abuse, discuss the risks associated with IV injection of drugs and resources for drug treatment.
- Provide educational materials from the American Heart Association.
- Refer to home health services and IV therapy providers as indicated.
- Refer to a substance abuse treatment program or facility as appropriate.

For more information on endocarditis, see Chapter 31 of *Medical-Surgical Nursing,* Fifth Edition, by LeMone, Burke, and Bauldoff.

Endometrial (Uterine) Cancer

Overview

- Endometrial (uterine) cancer is the most common cancer found in the female pelvis, occurring twice as often as cervical cancer.
- It is a fairly slow-growing neoplasm, usually discovered during the postmenopausal period.
- It arises from glandular endometrial tissues to produce an adenocarcinoma.
- Initially cancer affects only the superficial uterine lining; later it invades the cervix and underlying myometrium.
- Cancer eventually invades the vagina, uterine tubes, ovaries, and local lymphatics.
- It metastasizes via both blood and lymph to lungs, liver, bones, and also intra-abdominally.
- The prognosis depends on stage at diagnosis.

Causes

The cause is unknown. Risk factors are as follows:

- Prolonged estrogen stimulation: early menarche/late menopause, anovulatory menstrual cycles
- Nulliparity/infertility
- Estrogen-secreting neoplasms
- Conditions that alter estrogen metabolism (obesity, diabetes mellitus, hypertension, polycystic ovary syndrome)
- Unopposed estrogen replacement therapy (i.e., estrogen without progestin)
- Genetic predisposition: family history of hereditary nonpolyposis colon cancer

Manifestations

- Early: dysfunctional uterine bleeding
- Later: palpable mass on pelvic examination; cramping, pelvic discomfort; postcoital bleeding

Diagnostic Tests

- Aspiration curettage/endometrial biopsy (office procedure) can identify dysplastic or neoplastic cells.

- Dilation and curettage with biopsy (a surgical procedure) collects endometrial cells for biopsy, which can identify neoplastic cells.

- Hysteroscopy visualizes the uterine lining; may show malignant growth areas.

- Metastatic workup includes chest x-ray, intravenous urography, sigmoidoscopy, and computed tomography or magnetic resonance imaging scans.

Interdisciplinary Management

- Surgery includes a total abdominal hysterectomy and bilateral salpingo-oophorectomy.

- Radiation therapy may be used as a preoperative measure, postoperatively to reduce the incidence of recurrence, or as adjuvant treatment in advanced cases.

- Progesterone agents and the antiestrogen tamoxifen are used to treat invasive disease.

Selected Nursing Diagnoses with Interventions

Acute Pain

- Assess the patient's level of pain on a standard pain scale before and after administering medications.

- Administer analgesics as prescribed and monitor for effects and side effects.

- Encourage ambulation.

- Apply heat to the abdomen and recommend that the patient use a heating pad at home.

Disturbed Body Image

- Actively listen to the patient and acknowledge her concerns about the disease prognosis, treatment, and effects.

- Assist the patient in identifying personal strengths; develop with her a plan of care that identifies coping mechanisms and acknowledges limitations.

- Encourage the patient to maintain her usual daily grooming routine as far as possible and to dress in a way that enhances her self-esteem.

- Allow time and the opportunity for the patient to verbalize concerns about body image and to grieve.

Ineffective Sexuality Patterns

- Encourage the patient and her partner to express their feelings about the effect of cancer on their lives and sexual relationship.
- Tell the patient that sexual intercourse may be resumed 3 weeks after a vaginal hysterectomy and 6 weeks after an abdominal hysterectomy.
- Suggest that the couple explore alternative sexual positions and coordinate sexual activity with rest periods and with periods that are relatively free from pain.

Community-Based Care

- Provide information about the specific treatment and prognosis for her cancer.
- Explain the expected side effects of radiation implant therapy, if used.
- Review medications and alternative methods of pain control, including relaxation, guided imagery, and distraction.
- Instruct that it is normal to experience feelings of weakness, fatigue, emotional lability, and depression at this time.
- Instruct to avoid tub baths for 2 to 3 weeks; avoid sitting for prolonged periods; and avoid jogging, fast walking, horseback riding, and douching for several months.
- Teach to avoid heavy lifting and strenuous activity for 6 to 8 weeks.
- Advise patient to report to the physician any signs of bleeding or temperature elevation.
- For patients receiving radiation therapy, emphasize the importance of keeping appointments and, if necessary, help them arrange for transportation to and from the facility.
- Refer to local cancer support group and psychologic counselor if appropriate for assistance with sexual and body image adjustment.
- Home care may be necessary to assist with maintaining activities of daily living.
- Refer patients with terminal cancer to hospice services.

For more information on endometrial (uterine) cancer, see Chapter 49 in *Medical-Surgical Nursing,* Fifth Edition, by LeMone, Burke, and Bauldoff.

ENDOMETRIOSIS

Overview

- Endometriosis is growth of endometrial tissue in ectopic locations such as the fallopian tubes, or on pelvic organs such as the ovaries, external surface of the uterus, bladder, or bowel. Endometrial tissue located within the myometrium is called adenomyosis.

- It is usually diagnosed in women 30 to 40 years old; it is uncommon before age 20.

- Lesions are hormone dependent, and they proliferate and bleed during the menstrual cycle just like uterine tissue. Bleeding in ectopic locations produces inflammation with subsequent formation of fibrous tissue adhesions.

- Endometriosis is a major cause of fallopian tube obstruction, resulting in infertility, ectopic pregnancy, or spontaneous abortion.

- Manifestations worsen during the menstrual years and abate following menopause.

Causes

- No direct cause is known.

- Theorists suggest possible causative factors, such as embryonic epithelial cells that respond to hormonal changes, reflux of endometrial cells through the fallopian tubes, or spread of endometrial tissue via lymph or blood.

- Risk factors are as follows:
  - Early menarche
  - Short menstrual cycles (< 27 days)
  - Long flow (> 7 days)
  - Heavy flow
  - Dysmenorrhea
  - Delayed childbearing

Manifestations

- Acquired dysmenorrhea: constant (i.e., not crampy) vaginal, pelvic, back pain; begins 5 to 7 days prior to menses, lasts until 2 to 3 days after
- Dyspareunia
- Possibly painful urination, defecation
- Infertility

Diagnostic Tests

- Pelvic examination may reveal tenderness at characteristic cycle times, ovarian enlargement, or thickened adnexa.
- Hysterosalpingogram may show obstruction of oviduct; can be therapeutic.
- Laparoscopy allows visualization of pelvic lesions and ablation treatment.

Interdisciplinary Management

- Medications include oral contraceptives for women who do not desire pregnancy, danazol for women who wish to become pregnant, and analgesics to control pain.
- Surgical resection of any visible implants of endometrial tissue is often accomplished during laparoscopy.
- Laser vaporization may be used for all but the deepest implants.
- In advanced cases in which childbearing is not an issue, a hysterectomy may be performed.

Selected Nursing Diagnoses with Interventions

Deficient Knowledge

- Explain the condition, its symptoms, treatment alternatives, and prognosis. Help the patient evaluate treatment options and make choices appropriate for her.
- If medication is begun, review the dosage, schedule, possible side effects, and any warning signs.

Chronic Pain

- Provide comfort measures such as back rubs and position changes to assist with pain relief.

- Assess vital signs, pad count, complete blood cell count, abdominal distention, and abdominal pain for indications of severe bleeding.

Ineffective Sexuality Pattern

- Assess the patient's stage in the grieving process for loss of reproductive ability. Be a nonjudgmental listener: Accept the patient's emotional state, encourage her to discuss her feelings about her potential loss of fertility, and provide support.

- Assess the couple's coping mechanisms and assist them in identifying additional strategies for coping with loss. Provide a private, empathetic environment to allow them to openly discuss their feelings.

- Suggest the patient and her partner try alternative positions to reduce pain associated with sexual intercourse.

Community-Based Care

- Instruct about medications, including drug name, dosage, schedule, purpose, precautions, potential side effects, and warning signs.

- Explain the importance of reporting manifestations of excessive blood loss and, if surgery has been performed, of caring for the wound and reporting indications of infection.

- Discuss the advantages of having children soon and in rapid succession, using oral contraceptives between pregnancies to reduce bleeding.

- Discuss the possible risks and benefits of long-term oral contraceptive therapy for the patient with endometriosis.

- Stress the importance of exercise, smoking cessation, and weight control.

- Emphasize the importance of follow-up visits to the physician for continuing care.

For more information on endometriosis, see Chapter 49 in *Medical-Surgical Nursing,* Fifth Edition, by LeMone, Burke, and Bauldoff.

EPILEPSY (SEIZURE DISORDER)

Overview

- Epilepsy is a chronic, idiopathic condition with recurrent episodes of seizure activity.

- A seizure (convulsion) is an abnormal, excessive electric discharge within the brain.

- It may be primary or secondary to another condition.

- Epilepsy occurs in more than 3 million people of all ages in the United States. Any age may be affected; the prevalence and incidence of epilepsy increases in older adults.

- Large amounts of glucose and oxygen are consumed by neurons during a seizure.

- Status epilepticus is prolonged seizure activity that may result in neuron death due to lack of glucose and/or oxygen; it is usually precipitated by antiepileptic drug (AED) withdrawal or noncompliance, metabolic disturbances, drug toxicity, or central nervous system pathology such as infection, tumor, or injury.

- Epileptic seizures can be classified as generalized or local.

Causes

- Primary: idiopathic, cause not known

- Secondary: fever, infection (meningitis, encephalitis, brain abscess); cerebrovascular disease; head injury, brain tumor, metabolic conditions (electrolyte/blood sugar derangements), and toxins (carbon monoxide, mercury, ethyl alcohol)

Manifestations

- Seizures are classified as partial (focal) or generalized.

- Partial seizures occur within discrete regions of the brain; the patient may remain conscious (simple partial seizures) or consciousness may be impaired (complex partial seizures). In some instances, partial seizures may spread to involve the entire cerebral cortex (partial seizures with generalization).

- Generalized seizures involve both cerebral hemispheres of the brain simultaneously.

Partial (Focal) Seizures

- **Simple partial seizures** cause motor, sensory, autonomic, or psychic manifestations without impaired consciousness. Partial motor seizures cause symptoms such as involuntary movements of a hand or the face; in some cases, the movements may spread from a very restricted focus (such as the fingers) to involve a larger portion of the extremity (Jacksonian march).

Other forms of simple partial seizures may cause changes in sensation (paresthesias), vision, hearing, smell, equilibrium, autonomic function (flushing, sweating, piloerection), or psychic manifestations.

- **Complex partial seizures** are characterized by focal seizure activity with transient alteration in consciousness. The patient is unable to respond to commands and may exhibit involuntary, automatic behaviors such as chewing, lip smacking, swallowing, picking movements, a display of emotion, or running. A period of confusion usually follows the seizure activity.

Generalized Seizures

- **Absence seizures** (petit mal) are characterized by sudden, brief lapses of consciousness without loss of posture; duration typically in seconds. Nearly always begin in childhood or early adolescence; 60% to 70% of affected children will experience spontaneous remission during adolescence.

- Atypical absence seizures usually involve a longer lapse of consciousness and are associated with diffuse or multifocal structural brain abnormalities.

- **Tonic-clonic seizures** (grand mal) usually begin abruptly without warning, although some patients may experience an aura, or abnormal sensation (smell, flashing lights, or vague premonition), prior to the seizure. Seizure sequence: tonic contraction of muscles throughout the body that interferes with breathing and increases heart rate, blood pressure, and pupil size; clonic phase with alternating muscle relaxation and contraction; postictal period, during which patient is unresponsive, with flaccid muscles and excessive salivation that may impair airway and breathing. Bowel and bladder incontinence may occur. Consciousness gradually returns over minutes to hours, with confusion common.

Status Epilepticus

- Continuous seizure activity or repetitive discrete seizures with impaired consciousness between seizures. A medical emergency; cardiorespiratory dysfunction, hyperthermia, and metabolic disruptions can lead to irreversible neuronal injury after approximately 2 hours.

Diagnostic Tests

- Electroencephalogram (EEG) performed during a seizure will reveal excessive electric discharge; may also reveal abnormal patterns of discharge; may be normal during periods between seizures.

- Positron emission tomography (PET) locates areas of neural glucose depletion, indicative of excessive discharge; especially useful in identifying focal disease.

- Magnetic resonance imaging (MRI) and computed tomography (CT) scan are used to rule out space-occupying lesions.

- Lumbar puncture and cerebrospinal fluid analysis can rule out infection or increased intracranial pressure.

- Serum chemistry and electrolytes may reveal electrolyte or metabolic causes.

Interdisciplinary Management

- Most seizure activity can be reduced or controlled through the use of automated external defibrillators (AEDs).

- Status epilepticus is a medical emergency that requires immediate intervention to preserve life. Interventions include establishing and maintaining an airway, intravenous administration of dextrose to prevent hypoglycemia, and intravenous administration of diazepam to stop seizure activity. Phenytoin is also administered intravenously for longer-term control of seizures.

- When all attempts to control the patient's seizures fail, surgical excision of the tissue involved in the seizure activity may be an effective and safe treatment alternative.

Selected Nursing Diagnoses with Interventions

Risk for Ineffective Airway Clearance

- Provide interventions during a seizure to maintain a patent airway:
  - Loosen clothing around neck.
  - Turn the patient on the side.
  - Do not force anything into the mouth.
  - If prescribed and available, administer oxygen by mask.

- Teach significant others how to care for the patient during a seizure.

Risk for Injury

- Obtain information about past seizures, including most recent seizure and precipitating factors.
- Provide interventions during a seizure to reduce the risk of injury:
  - Maintain the bed in low position and keep the side rails up and padded.
  - If the patient is sitting or standing, ease to the floor.
  - Place a folded towel or pillow under the patient's head.
- Teach the patient and significant others measures to prevent injury at home:
  - Avoid smoking when alone or in bed.
  - Avoid alcohol.
  - Avoid becoming excessively tired.
  - Install grab bars in the shower and tub area.
  - Do not lock bedroom or bathroom doors.
  - Avoid excessive caffeine.

Community-Based Care

When teaching the patient with epilepsy, include family and/or caregivers as appropriate.

- Explain seizure management, especially how to maintain a patent airway and prevent injury (see the Selected Nursing Diagnoses with Interventions section).
- Review AEDs, including dosage and side effects. Stress the importance of maintaining dosage as prescribed even when no seizures are experienced. Emphasize the importance of avoiding alcohol and limiting caffeine.
- Discuss factors that may trigger a seizure, such as abrupt withdrawal from medication, constipation, fatigue, excessive stress, fever, menstruation, and sights and sounds such as television, flashing video, and computer screens.
- Provide the name and location of community and national resources such as the Epilepsy Foundation of America.
- Stress the importance of follow-up care and keeping medical appointments.

- Review state and local laws regarding operation of a motor vehicle that apply to people with seizure disorders, as well as employment requirements and hazards.

- Stress the importance of wearing a MedicAlert tag at all times, and provide information on how to obtain one.

For more information about epilepsy, see Chapter 42 in *Medical-Surgical Nursing,* Fifth Edition, by LeMone, Burke, and Bauldoff.

E

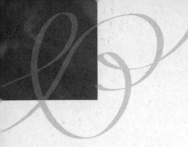

FIBROCYSTIC CHANGES (FIBROCYSTIC BREAST DISEASE)

Overview

- Fibrocystic changes (FCC) is the physiologic nodularity and breast tenderness that increases and decreases with the menstrual cycle

- Cystic change refers to the dilation of ducts in the subareolar, lobular, or lobe areas.

- FCC is found primarily in women age 30 to 50 and is rare in postmenopausal women who are not taking hormone replacement.

- FCC includes fibrosis, epithelial proliferation, and cyst formation in the breasts. Patients with the proliferative form have a higher risk of developing breast cancer, whereas those with nonproliferative fibrocystic changes (the more common form) have no increased risk.

Causes

The exact cause is unknown, but may be related to the following:

- Imbalance of estrogen and progesterone with excessive tissue response

- Increased sensitivity of the glandular epithelium to hormones

- Incomplete resolution of hormonal effect within the glandular epithelium

- Dysplastic cell changes

Manifestations

- Bilateral or unilateral pain or tenderness in the breasts' upper, outer quadrants.

- Patients may report thick and lumpy breasts the week prior to menses; some women report an increase in breast size.

- Nipple discharge and pain may be present.

- Multiple, mobile cysts may form, usually in both breasts.

- Fluid aspirated from these cysts ranges in color from milky white to yellow, brown, or green. If the fluid is tinged with blood, there is reason to suspect malignancy.

Diagnostic Tests

- Diagnosis of FCC is based on complete history, physical examination, and imaging studies.

- A biopsy may be required for diagnosis.

- Analysis of nipple discharge, mammography, and possibly ductography may be used. The affected duct is excised in an open biopsy procedure.

Interdisciplinary Management

- Treatment is usually symptomatic. Cyst aspiration may relieve pain, and also allows examination of fluid to confirm the cystic nature of the disease.

- Hormonal therapy is controversial due to the benign nature of the disease and potential adverse effects of therapy. Danazol, a synthetic androgen, may relieve severe pain.

Selected Nursing Diagnoses with Interventions

Anxiety

- Explain that fibrocystic changes are not a disease but are normal changes, probably influenced by hormonal cycles and aging, that are common in premenopausal women.

- Encourage the patient to verbalize her feelings of discomfort and her fears.

Knowledge Deficit

- Teach breast self-examination (BSE) and encourage monthly BSE, annual clinical breast examination, and mammography as recommended by primary care provider.

- Stress the importance of becoming aware of the normal feeling of breast tissue, and the need to be aware of any changes in the size, consistency, or mobility of lumps.

- Premenopausal women should perform BSE 7 to 10 days from the first day of their menstrual period, because hormonal changes increase breast tenderness and lumpiness prior to menses.

- Postmenopausal women should choose one date of the month (for example, the first day of the month) for BSE.

- If a palpable mass is present, ask how long the lesion has been present, if the patient is experiencing pain, or if she noticed a change in mass size or association to the menstrual cycle.

- Review available prescription and nonprescription medication options, and their effects and side effects.

Community-Based Care

- Eliminate coffee, tea, cola, and chocolate (xanthenes) from the diet, especially right before the menstrual period. Limiting salt premenstrually may also help.

- A well-fitting brassiere that provides good support worn day and night helps relieve discomfort. Aspirin, mild analgesics, and local heat or cold and Vitamin E may help relieve breast pain. Emphasize the benign nature of the disease, and reassure that manifestations are rare after menopause.

- Teach how and when to do monthly BSE.

For more information on fibrocystic breast disease, see Chapter 49 in *Medical-Surgical Nursing*, Fifth Edition, by LeMone, Burke, and Bauldoff.

FIBROMYALGIA

Overview

- Fibromyalgia is a common rheumatic syndrome characterized by musculoskeletal pain, stiffness, and tenderness.

- Fibromyalgia may resolve spontaneously or become chronic and recurrent.

- It primarily affects older women but can develop at any age.

- An estimated 0.5% to 5% of the world's population has fibromyalgia.

- Central findings include disordered pain processing with abnormal cerebrospinal fluid levels of neurotransmitters and abnormal hypothalamic-pituitary-adrenal axis responses.

Causes

- The cause is unknown; genetic and environmental factors are thought to contribute.

- Possible causes include sleep disorders, depression, infections, and an altered perception of normal stimuli.

- Onset is typically associated with physical or emotional trauma.

Manifestations

- Skeletal/muscular: Gradual onset of chronic, achy muscle pain aggravated by exertion. Local tightness or muscle spasm may occur.

- General: fatigue, sleep disruptions, headaches, morning stiffness, painful menstrual periods, and problems with thinking and memory ("fibro fog").

- Pain may be localized or generalized; the neck, spine, shoulders, and hips are often affected.

- Palpation of localized "tender points" produces pain.

Diagnositic Tests

- No laboratory or diagnostic tests are available. Diagnosis is based on history and physical assessment.

- American College of Rheumatology diagnostic criteria for fibromyalgia include the following:

  a. History of widespread pain for at least 3 months

  b. Pain at 11 of the 18 tender points on palpation

Interdisciplinary Management

- Heated pool treatments with or without exercise are beneficial.

- A program of structured aerobic exercise for conditioning, as well as stretching exercises is recommended. Approved medications include duloxetine (Cymbalta), milnacipran (Savella), and pregabalin (Lyrica). Tramadol (Ultram) or an NSAID analgesic may be used for pain relief.

- Tricyclic antidepressants (amitriptyline or doxepin) or SSRIs (fluoxetine and paroxetine) may be ordered to promote better sleep and relieve manifestations.

- Cognitive behavioral therapy, hypnotherapy, biofeedback, and acupuncture have shown mixed results.

Selected Nursing Diagnoses with Interventions

Chronic Pain

- Provide verbal and written instructions about the use of heat, exercise, and stress-reduction techniques.

- Acknowledge patient's symptoms and discuss ways to manage pain and anxiety.

Anxiety

- Emphasize that fibromyalgia is a treatable disease that is not progressive.

- Provide information about Internet resources and support groups.

- Provide teaching about prescribed medications to relieve pain and anxiety.

Community-Based Care

- Provide contact information for national and community resources such as the following:
  - Fibromyalgia Network
  - National Fibromyalgia Research Association
  - American College of Rheumatology
  - National Institute of Arthritis and Musculoskeletal and Skin Diseases

For more information about fibromyalgia, see Chapter 40 in *Medical-Surgical Nursing*, Fifth Edition, by LeMone, Burke, and Bauldoff.

Flail Chest

Overview

- Flail chest is instability of the chest wall caused by fracture of three or more ribs in two or more places.

- The multiple fractures result in a free-floating, or flail, unsupported chest wall segment.

- The flail segment moves inward with negative intrathoracic pressure during inspiration, and bulges outward during expiration (paradoxical chest movement).

- Pulmonary contusion with edema and bleeding into lung tissue is common underlying the flail segment and can further compromise ventilation and gas exchange.

- Atelectasis develops under the flail segment, impairing gas exchange.

- The work of breathing is greatly increased, resulting in fatigue.

- Respiratory failure may result.

Cause

- Blunt trauma (motor vehicle crash, fall) to the chest wall

Manifestations

- Respiratory: Obvious paradoxical chest motion, dyspnea, tachypnea, rales, decreased breath sounds

- Skin/mucous membranes: Cyanosis, palpable crepitus

- General: Severe chest pain, especially with inspiration, grunting

Diagnostic Tests

- Arterial blood gases show the extent of hypoxia, hypercapnia, and acidosis.

- Chest x-rays identify the area and extent of chest wall injury.

Interdisciplinary Management

- The preferred treatment for flail chest is intubation and positive pressure mechanical ventilation. A double lumen endotracheal tube may be used to independently ventilate each lung.

- Intercostal nerve blocks or continuous epidural analgesia may be used to manage pain.

- In some cases, internal fixation of the flail segment may be done. Bronchoscopy may be performed to clear debris from affected pleural segment underlying injury.

Selected Nursing Diagnoses with Interventions

Acute Pain

- Administer prescribed analgesics on a schedule or by patient-controlled analgesia to maintain pain control and facilitate effective ventilation.

- Assess frequently for adequate pain control.

Ineffective Airway Clearance

- Assess frequently for respiratory depression resulting from narcotic analgesia.

- Assess lung sounds and respiratory rate, depth, and effort frequently. Continuously monitor oxygen saturation.

- Assist to cough, deep breathe, and change position every 1 to 2 hours. Encourage use of incentive spirometer. Suction airway as needed.

- Teach how to splint the affected area when coughing.

- Elevate the head of the bed to facilitate lung expansion.

- Promptly report signs of complications to the physician: diminished breath sounds, increasing crackles (rales) or rhonchi, dull or hyperresonant percussion tones, unequal chest movement, hemoptysis, chills or fever, low oxygen saturation, or vital sign changes.

- For severe flail chest with respiratory failure, prepare for intubation and mechanical positive pressure ventilation.

Community-Based Care

- If intubation and mechanical ventilation are required, teach communication strategies. Reassure the patient and significant others that mechanical ventilation is a short-term measure.

- Teach the importance of coughing and deep breathing.

- Demonstrate how to splint the affected area when coughing.

- Explain the reasons for not taping or wrapping the chest continuously.

- Discuss the importance of effective pain management in preventing respiratory complications.

- Discuss manifestations of potential complications to report to the physician: chills and fever, productive cough, purulent or bloody sputum, shortness of breath or difficulty breathing, and increasing chest pain.

- Emphasize the importance of avoiding respiratory irritants such as cigarette smoke and respiratory infection by avoiding large crowds or close contact with obviously ill people.

For more information on flail chest, see Chapter 36 of *Medical-Surgical Nursing,* Fifth Edition, by LeMone, Burke, and Bauldoff.

FLUID VOLUME DEFICIT (DEHYDRATION)

Overview

- Dehydration is excessive water loss from the body.

- The term *dehydration* often is used interchangeably with fluid volume deficit (FVD), a decrease in intravascular, interstitial, and/or intracellular fluid in the body.

- FVD can develop slowly or rapidly.

- Loss of extracellular fluid can lead to hypovolemia, decreased circulating blood volume. Fluid is drawn into the vascular compartment from the interstitial spaces to maintain tissue perfusion, eventually depleting intracellular fluid as well.

- Third spacing is a shift of fluid from the vascular space into an area where it cannot support normal physiologic processes. Fluid may be sequestered in the abdomen, bowel, or soft tissues.

Causes

Fluid Volume Deficit

- Excessive loss of gastrointestinal (GI) fluids from vomiting, diarrhea, GI suctioning, intestinal fistulas, and intestinal drainage
- Insufficient fluid intake
- Excessive renal losses due to diuretic therapy, renal disorders, or endocrine disorders
- Water and sodium losses during sweating
- Hemorrhage
- Chronic abuse of laxatives and/or enemas

Dehydration

- Inadequate fluid intake due to lack of access to fluids, inability to request or to swallow fluids, oral trauma, or altered thirst

Manifestations

- Cardiovascular: tachycardia, decreased blood pressure, postural hypotension, thready pulses, flat veins
- Renal: oliguria, dark urine, increased specific gravity
- Skin/mucous membranes: poor skin turgor; dry, sticky tongue; sunken eyeballs; pallor
- Neurologic: lethargy, confusion, coma
- GI: anorexia, nausea, vomiting, decreased motility and bowel sounds, constipation (unless dehydration is due to diarrhea)
- General: fever, thirst, weakness, dizziness, weight loss

Diagnostic Tests

- Serum electrolytes may show imbalances of sodium and potassium.
- Serum osmolality is high in dehydration (water loss), and may be within normal limits with an isotonic fluid loss.
- The hematocrit often is high due to hemoconcentration.
- Urine specific gravity and osmolality increase as the kidneys conserve water.

- Central venous pressure (CVP) measures the mean pressure in the superior vena cava or right atrium, reflecting fluid volume status. It is low in dehydration and FVD.

Interdisciplinary Management

- Oral or enteral rehydration with a balanced electrolyte solution is preferred.

- Intravenous (IV) fluids are often prescribed to correct FVD:

    1. Isotonic electrolyte solutions (0.9% NaCl or Ringer's solution) are used to expand plasma volume in hypotensive patients or to replace abnormal losses.

    2. Five percent dextrose in water (D5W) or one-half normal saline (0.45% NaCl) are given to treat total body water deficits.

    3. Hypotonic saline solutions (0.45% NaCl with or without added electrolytes) or hypotonic mixed electrolyte solutions 5% dextrose in 0.45% sodium chloride (D_5 1/2 NS) are used as maintenance solutions.

- A fluid challenge may be done to evaluate fluid volume prior to IV fluid therapy.

Selected Nursing Diagnoses with Interventions

Deficient Fluid Volume

- Assess for continuing fluid losses from the GI tract, wounds, or decreased intake.

- Weigh daily using standard conditions; assess intake and output, hourly if indicated. Report urine output of less than 30 mL per hour.

- Measure urine specific gravity.

- Assess vital signs at least every 4 hours, including orthostatic blood pressure, CVP, and peripheral pulse volume. Monitor for fluid overload with IV fluid replacement: dyspnea, tachypnea, tachycardia, increased CVP, jugular vein distention, adventitious lung sounds.

- Assess skin condition and turgor, mucous membranes; presence of edema.

- Administer and monitor oral fluid intake as prescribed.

- Administer IV fluids as prescribed using an electronic infusion pump.
- Monitor laboratory values (electrolytes, serum osmolality, blood urea nitrogen [BUN], and hematocrit).

Ineffective Tissue Perfusion

- Assess for restlessness, anxiety, agitation, excitability, confusion, vertigo, fainting, and weakness; changes in muscle strength.
- Monitor serum creatinine, BUN, and cardiac enzymes and report elevated levels.
- Provide good skin care: Turn at least every 2 hours, keep skin clean and dry, avoid drying soaps.

Risk for Injury

- Institute safety precautions, including keeping the bed in a low position, using side rails, and slowly raising the patient from supine to sitting or sitting to standing position.
- Teach the patient and caregivers to change positions slowly to avoid lightheadedness, use a walker, avoid prolonged standing, rest in a recliner, and use assistive devices to pick up objects from the floor.

Community-Based Care

- Emphasize the importance of maintaining adequate fluid intake, and measures to prevent fluid deficit.
- Discuss early manifestations of FVD and measures to correct it such as using Gatorade or Pedialyte for oral fluid replacement.
- Provide both verbal and written instructions:
  1. Amount and type of fluids to take each day.
  2. Increase fluid intake in hot weather.
  3. Decrease activity during hot weather.
  4. If vomiting, take frequent small amounts of ice chips or clear liquids such as weak tea, flat cola, or ginger ale.
  5. Avoid coffee, tea, alcohol, and large amounts of sugar as they increase urine output and can cause fluid loss.
  6. Replace fluids lost through diarrhea with fruit juices or bouillon, rather than large amounts of tap water.

- Refer to a home health agency as appropriate for continued evaluation and monitoring.

- Refer to social services as appropriate to evaluate home environment, or assess the need for long-term or residential care placement.

For more information on dehydration, see Chapter 10 in *Medical-Surgical Nursing,* Fifth Edition, by LeMone, Burke, and Bauldoff.

FLUID VOLUME EXCESS (HYPERVOLEMIA)

Overview

- Fluid volume excess occurs when both water and sodium are retained in the body. It may be caused by fluid overload or by impaired homeostasis.

- Excess fluid can lead to excess intravascular fluid (hypervolemia) and excess interstitial fluid (edema).

- Water and sodium are gained together; total body sodium increase causes an increase in total body water.

- The serum sodium and osmolality remain normal, and the excess fluid remains in the extracellular space.

Causes

- Conditions causing sodium and water retention: heart failure, cirrhosis, renal failure, adrenal gland disorders, corticosteroid administration, and stress conditions causing antidiuretic hormone and aldosterone release

- Excess intake of high-sodium foods

- Drugs that cause sodium retention

- Administration of excess amounts of intravenous fluids such as 0.9% NaCl or Ringer's solution

Manifestations

- Cardiovascular: full, bounding pulses, tachycardia, increased blood pressure, distended neck and peripheral veins, increased central venous pressure

- Skin/mucous membranes: taut skin turgor
- Respiratory: cough, dyspnea, orthopnea (difficulty breathing when supine), moist crackles (rales), wheezes in the lungs; pulmonary edema if severe
- Renal: decreased or normal urine output, decreased specific gravity
- Neurologic: mental status changes and anxiety
- General: weight gain over a short period, ascites, peripheral dependent edema; if severe, anasarca (severe, generalized edema)

Diagnostic Tests

- Serum electrolytes and serum osmolality often are within normal ranges.
- Hematocrit and hemoglobin are decreased due to plasma dilution.
- Tests of renal and liver function (e.g., serum creatinine, blood urea nitrogen, and liver enzymes) may help determine the cause.

Interdisciplinary Management

- Diuretics are commonly ordered to treat fluid volume excess, primarily loop or thiazide-type diuretics; potassium-sparing diuretics also may be used.
- Fluid intake may be restricted. A sodium-restricted diet often is prescribed. In moderate and severely sodium-restricted diets, salt is avoided altogether, as are all foods containing significant amounts of sodium.

Selected Nursing Diagnoses with Interventions

Excess Fluid Volume

- Assess vital signs, heart sounds, central venous pressure, and volume of peripheral arteries.
- Assess presence and extent of edema, particularly in the lower extremities, the back, sacral, and periorbital areas.
- Weigh daily using consistent conditions.
- Administer oral fluids cautiously, adhering to any prescribed fluid restriction.

- Maintain accurate intake and output records.
- Provide frequent oral hygiene (at least every 2 hours).
- Administer prescribed diuretics as ordered, monitoring response to therapy. Report abnormal changes in serum electrolytes or osmolality.
- Teach patient and caregivers about importance of maintaining a sodium restricted diet.

Risk for Impaired Skin Integrity

- Frequently assess skin, particularly in pressure areas and over bony prominences.
- Reposition at least every 2 hours. Provide skin care with each position change.
- Provide an egg crate mattress or alternating-pressure mattress, foot cradle, heel protectors, and other devices to reduce pressure on tissues.

Risk for Impaired Gas Exchange

- Assess breath sounds for crackles or wheezes, and heart sounds for S_3.
- Place in Fowler's position.
- Monitor oxygen saturation and arterial blood gases ($SaO_2 < 92\%$ to 95%; $PaO_2 < 80$ mmHg). Administer oxygen as indicated.

Community-Based Care

- Explain the underlying cause of fluid volume excess.
- Relate signs and symptoms of excess fluid and when to contact the care provider.
- Explain prescribed medications: when and how to take, intended and adverse effects, what to report to care provider.
- Review recommended or prescribed diet; ways to reduce sodium intake; how to read food labels for salt and sodium content; use of salt substitutes (if allowed).
- If restricted, teach the amount and types of fluids to take each day, and how to balance intake over 24 hours.
- Advise about monitoring weight and changes to report to care provider.

- Discuss ways to decrease dependent edema:
  a. Change positions frequently.
  b. Avoid restrictive clothing.
  c. Avoid crossing the legs when sitting.
  d. Wear support stockings or hose.
  e. Elevate feet and legs when sitting.
- Provide information about protecting edematous skin from injury:
  a. Do not walk barefoot.
  b. Buy well-fitting shoes; shop in the afternoon when feet are more likely to be swollen.
- Suggest using additional pillows or a recliner to sleep to relieve orthopnea.
- Referral to home health services may be appropriate.

For more information about fluid volume excess, see Chapter 10 of *Medical-Surgical Nursing,* Fifth Edition, by LeMone, Burke, and Bauldoff.

FRACTURE

Overview

- A fracture is any break in the continuity of the bone.
- Local soft tissue is always damaged to some extent with a fracture.
- Bone can fracture in an infinite number of ways. Some general categories are the following:
  - **Closed (simple):** fracture line in bone is well opposed; skin intact over fracture; minimal soft-tissue injury.
  - **Open (compound):** skin over fracture site is lacerated; increased possibility of infection.
  - **Complete:** fracture line extends through entire bone.
  - **Incomplete (greenstick):** fracture line through bone is incomplete; occurs more often in children.

- **Oblique:** fracture occurs at an angle to the bone.
- **Spiral:** fracture curves around the bone.
- **Avulsed:** fracture occurs when the fracture pulls bone and other tissues away from the point of attachment.
- **Comminuted:** bone is shattered into multiple fragments at fracture site.
- **Compressed:** the bone is crushed.
- **Impacted:** the broken bone ends are forced into each other.
- **Depressed:** the broken bone is forced inward.
- **Stable (nondisplaced):** fractured bones maintain their anatomic alignment.
- **Unstable (displaced):** fractured ends of bone are widely separated from each other. Immediate intervention is required to prevent further damage to soft tissue, muscle, and bone.
- **Stress or Pathologic:** a fracture of any bone with a preexisting disease that has weakened the bone; only small forces are necessary to induce fracture.

Cause

- Any direct or indirect force to the bone that is greater than the bone can withstand

Manifestations

- Pain, tenderness, or guarding with movement
- Skeletal/muscular: deformity or bulging at fracture site; increase or decrease in limb length; paresthesias (numbness, tingling); crepitus (a grinding noise made when bone edges rub together); muscle spasms or decreased function/paralysis
- Cardiovascular: Decreased distal or peripheral pulses (signal impaired arterial perfusion)
- Skin/mucous membranes: Coolness, pallor, mottling, or cyanosis due to arterial perfusion disruption; swelling and bruising (ecchymosis) due to extravasation or inflammation at fracture site

- Complications: hemorrhagic or hypovolemic shock, fat embolus, aseptic necrosis, renal calculi, permanent deformity or reduced function

Diagnostic Tests

- X-ray reveals fracture line.
- A bone scan may be necessary to determine presence of a fracture.
- Blood chemistry and coagulation studies are performed to assess blood loss, renal function, muscle breakdown, and risk of excessive bleeding or clotting.

Interdisciplinary Management

- Medications include narcotics for pain relief, NSAIDS, and antibiotics. Anticoagulants may be ordered to prevent deep vein thrombosis formation and stool softeners may be given to combat constipation caused by immobility and narcotic use.
- Traction is applied to return or maintain the fractured bones in normal anatomic position. External fixation devices may be applied to maintain bone alignment.
- Casts are applied for relatively stable fractures.
- Electrical bone stimulation, application of electric current at the fracture site, may be used to treat fractures that are not healing properly.
- Surgery (internal reduction and fixation or open reduction internal fixation) is used for fractures that require direct visualization for repair, fractures with long-term complications, and fractures that are severely comminuted and threatening vascular supply.

Selected Nursing Diagnoses with Interventions

Acute Pain

- Monitor baseline vital signs, since some analgesics decrease respiratory effort and blood pressure.
- Ask the patient to rate the pain on a standard pain scale before and after any intervention.
- Splint and support the injured area.

- Apply ice, if ordered.
- Move the fractured area gently and slowly.
- Administer pain medications as prescribed.

Impaired Physical Mobility

- Teach or assist patient with range-of-motion exercises of the unaffected limbs.
- Teach isometric exercises and encourage the patient to perform them every 4 hours.
- Teach and observe use of assistive devices in conjunction with the physical therapist, as appropriate.
- Turn the patient on bed rest every 2 hours. If the patient is in traction, teach to shift weight every hour.

Risk for Peripheral Neurovascular Dysfunction

- Support the injured extremity above and below the fracture site when moving the patient.
- Assess the 5 Ps every 1 to 2 hours (*unrelenting pain, pallor, diminished distal pulses, paresthesias, and paresis*). Report any abnormal findings immediately.
- Elevate the injured extremity above the heart, unless contraindicated. If compartment syndrome develops, elevation may further reduce arterial flow to the extremity.
- If compartment syndrome is suspected, assist the physician in measuring compartment pressure. Normal compartment pressure is 10 to 20 mmHg.
- If casted, assess for tightness. If the cast is tight, prepare to assist with bivalving (splitting the cast down both sides to alleviate pressure on the injured extremity).
- Maintain skeletal traction weight and alignment at all times.
- Administer anticoagulants and apply antiembolism stockings or pneumatic compression boots, if ordered to prevent clot formation.

Community-Based Care

- Show how to use all assistive devices and teach crutch walking, if appropriate.

- Explain measures to prevent complications from immobility.

- Teach care of the cast, splint, brace, external fixator, or wound, as appropriate.

- Discuss how to recognize signs of infection.

- Stress the importance of eating well-balanced meals to promote healing.

- Review medications, including dosage desired and adverse effects.

- Refer to a home health agency and community services as appropriate, especially for the older adult.

- Evaluate living situation for possible hazards to safety and mobility.

- Discuss the importance of follow-up care as needed.

For more information on fracture, see Chapter 39 in *Medical-Surgical Nursing,* Fifth Edition, by LeMone, Burke, and Bauldoff.

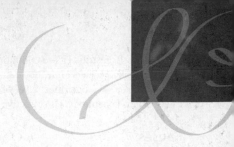

Gastritis

Overview

- Gastritis, inflammation of the stomach lining, results from irritation of the gastric mucosa. It may be either acute or chronic in nature.

- Acute gastritis, the most common form, generally is benign and self-limiting.

  1. It is characterized by disruption of the mucosal barrier by a local irritant (e.g., aspirin or nonsteroidal anti-inflammatory drug use).

  2. This disruption allows hydrochloric acid and pepsin to contact gastric tissue, leading to irritation, inflammation, and superficial erosions.

  3. Gastric mucosa rapidly regenerates; resolution and healing occur within several days.

- Erosive or stress-induced gastritis is a severe form of acute gastritis that may complicate life-threatening conditions such as shock or burns. *Curling's ulcers* may follow a major burn or may follow a head injury.

  1. Sympathetic vasoconstriction causes ischemia of the gastric mucosa, which disrupts the gastric mucosal barrier, allowing tissue injury. Multiple superficial erosions develop.

  2. Maintaining the gastric pH 3.5 and medications to inhibit gastric acid secretion are preventive measures.

- Chronic gastritis is characterized by progressive and irreversible changes in the gastric mucosa. Glands are destroyed and the gastric mucosa thins and atrophies. Chronic gastritis is classified as type A and type B.

  1. Type A or autoimmune gastritis (less common) is an autoimmune disorder causing tissue atrophy and loss of hydrochloric acid and pepsin secretion. Lack of intrinsic factor leads to development of pernicious anemia.

2. Type B gastritis (more common) usually affects older adults. Chronic *H. pylori* infection causes inflammation of the gastric mucosa. The outermost layer of gastric mucosa thins and atrophies, becoming a less effective barrier against gastric juices.

Causes

Acute Gastritis

- Ingestion of gastric irritants such as aspirin, alcohol, caffeine, or foods contaminated with certain bacteria
- Accidental or purposeful ingestion of a corrosive alkali (such as ammonia, lye, Lysol, and other cleaning agents) or acid
- Iatrogenic: radiation therapy and certain chemotherapeutic agents
- Erosive: shock, major trauma or surgery, sepsis, burns, or head injury

Chronic Gastritis

- *H. pylori* infection
- Autoimmune process
- Risk factors: aging, ethnic heritage, chronic alcoholism, cigarette smoking

Manifestations

Acute Gastritis

- Possibly asymptomatic
- Mild heartburn
- Severe gastric distress, vomiting
- Hematemesis (vomiting blood)
- Melena

Chronic Gastritis

- Vague epigastric heaviness after meals
- Anorexia and weight loss
- Gnawing, burning, ulcerlike epigastric pain unrelieved by antacids

Diagnostic Tests

- Gastric analysis may show decreased hydrochloric acid secretion in chronic gastritis.

- Hemoglobin, hematocrit, and red blood cell indices may show evidence of pernicious anemia due to parietal cell destruction, or iron-deficiency anemia because of chronic blood loss.

- Serum vitamin B_{12} levels are reduced in pernicious anemia resulting from chronic gastritis.

- Upper endoscopy is done to identify changes or bleeding sites, obtain tissue for biopsy, and treat bleeding sites.

Interdisciplinary Management

- Sucralfate, a proton pump inhibitor such as lansoprazole or omeprazole, or a histamine H_2- receptor blocker such as cimetidine, ranitidine, or famotidine are used to reduce gastric acid secretion and protect the gastric mucosa.

- Discontinuing alcohol consumption or the offending drug also is an important treatment measure for acute gastritis.

- Type B chronic gastritis may be treated with combination antibiotic therapy and a proton pump inhibitor to eradicate the *H. pylori* infection.

- Vitamin B_{12} injections are necessary when intrinsic factor is no longer produced.

Selected Nursing Diagnoses with Interventions

Nausea

- Monitor subjective complaints of nausea.

- Administer antiemetic medication as ordered, prior to meals and before treatments or procedures known to stimulate nausea.

- Monitor vital signs, intake and output, urine color, amount, and specific gravity. Weigh daily.

- Document skin turgor and condition and status of oral mucous membranes. Provide frequent skin and mouth care.

- Monitor laboratory values for electrolytes and acid–base balance.

- Administer medications and fluids as prescribed.
- Ensure the safety of patients with orthostatic hypotension.

Imbalanced Nutrition: Less than Body Requirements

- Monitor and record food and fluid intake and any abnormal losses (such as vomiting).
- Monitor laboratory values for serum albumin, RBC indices, hemoglobin, and hematocrit.
- Arrange for consultation with dietitian, and consider food preferences.
- Provide nutritional supplements between meals, or frequent small feedings as needed.
- Instruct to consume small quantities of clear fluids and dry foods at separate times.
- Maintain enteral or parenteral nutrition as prescribed.

Community-Based Care

- Help to identify causative factors and ways to avoid future episodes of acute gastritis.
- Emphasize the importance of taking nonsteroidal anti-inflammatory drugs or aspirin with food to decrease the risk of gastritis.
- Teach management of acute symptoms and reintroduction of fluids and solid foods.
- Provide information about manifestations that should be reported to the physician, such as intractable vomiting, or signs of dehydration or electrolyte imbalance.
- For chronic gastritis, provide information on maintaining nutrition, using prescribed medications, and avoiding known irritants such as aspirin, alcohol, and cigarette smoke.
- Discuss treatment plans for *H. pylori* infection and their potential benefit.
- Provide referral to home health nursing services as needed.
- Refer to smoking cessation classes and programs to treat alcohol abuse as indicated.

For more information on gastritis, see Chapter 23 in *Medical-Surgical Nursing,* Fifth Edition, by LeMone, Burke, and Bauldoff.

Gastroenteritis (Enteritis, Food Poisoning, Cholera, Traveler's Diarrhea)

Overview

- Gastroenteritis is inflammation of the stomach and small intestine.

- Bacterial or viral infection of the gastrointestinal (GI) tract produces inflammation, tissue damage, and symptoms by the following mechanisms:

  1. *Exotoxins* excreted by bacteria damage and inflame GI mucosa, impairing intestinal absorption and drawing fluids and electrolytes into the bowel lumen.

  2. Direct invasion and ulceration of bowel mucosa by the organism causes bleeding, fluid exudate formation, and water and electrolyte secretion.

- Manifestations result from distension of the upper GI tract by unabsorbed chyme and excess water; inflammation and fermentation of undigested food; and secretion of excess fluid and electrolytes into the bowel.

- Gastroenteritis can lead to secondary fluid, electrolyte, and acid–base disruptions, and is a major cause of morbidity and mortality in undeveloped countries.

- In the United States, gastroenteritis can be life-threatening in children, older adults, or the immunocompromised.

Causes

- Bacteria: *Staphylococcus, Shigella, Salmonella, Clostridium perfringens, C. botulinum, Escherichia coli,* and *Vibrio cholerae*
- Viruses: rotavirus, Norwalk virus, enteric adenovirus, enteric cytopathic human orphan virus, coxsackieviruses
- Amoebae: especially *Entamoeba histolytica*
- Parasites: *Ascaris, Enterobius, Trichinella spiralis*
- Immune reactions: food allergy, drug reactions

Manifestations

- Diarrhea: copious, foul smelling, watery/mucoid; possibly bloody
- Abdominal pain ranging from mild cramping to severe pain
- Borborygmi (loud, rushing, hyperactive bowel sounds)
- Anorexia, nausea, and vomiting
- Fever and general malaise
- Fluid volume deficit: poor skin turgor, dry mucous membranes, orthostatic hypotension, oliguria
- Possible headache, myalgia

Diagnostic Tests

- Stool culture (requires up to 6 weeks) to reveal ova and parasites, and fecal leukocytes.
- Gram stain of vomitus may reveal staphylococci in staphylococcal food poisoning.
- Serum toxin levels may be ordered if botulism is suspected.
- Serum osmolality and electrolytes, and arterial blood gases to assess fluid, electrolyte, and acid–base balance.
- Sigmoidoscopy may be done to differentiate inflammatory bowel disease from infectious enteritis.

Interdisciplinary Management

- Enteritis often is self-limiting and requires no treatment.
- Antibiotics may be used to treat cholera, salmonellosis, or shigellosis.
- Antidiarrheal drugs may be prescribed to reduce stool frequency and fluid loss associated with diarrhea.
- Botulism antitoxin is administered to patients with suspected botulism. Antidiarrheals are contraindicated for these patients.
- Oral rehydration is preferred. Intravenous fluids may be used with significant vomiting or severe fluid loss.
- Gastric lavage may be ordered to remove unabsorbed toxin from the GI tract. Plasmapheresis may be used to remove circulating toxin in patients with botulism or hemorrhagic colitis caused by *E. coli*.

Selected Nursing Diagnoses with Interventions

Deficient Fluid Volume

- Replace fluids as ordered with oral rehydration solutions such as Resol or intravenous solutions such as Ringer's solution.

- Encourage oral intake of small amounts of clear liquids with electrolytes (e.g., Gatorade).

- Advise to progress slowly to diet as tolerated.

Diarrhea

- Obtain stool culture prior to start of antibiotic therapy.

- Administer antibiotics specific to the organism as prescribed.

- Cautious use of antidiarrheal preparations (can increase risk of complications in certain types).

- Apply repellent cream such as zinc oxide, Desitin, A&D ointment, or moisture barriers to protect skin in the anal area.

Community-Based Care

- Teach proper hand hygiene, especially after toileting, to reduce transmission of bacteria to others.

- Stress the importance of not sharing utensils, glasses, and so on, and of washing soiled garments separately in hot water and detergent.

- Encourage to maintain adequate fluid intake.

- Provide written and oral instructions for medications.

- Provide information about proper food handling, preparation, and storage. Emphasize the importance of following instructions when home-canning foods.

- Encourage patients traveling out of the country to consume only bottled water or to use water purification tablets.

- Instruct to return to the physician for follow-up care if diarrhea, vomiting, or dizziness do not resolve or recur.

For more information on gastroenteritis, see Chapter 24 in *Medical-Surgical Nursing,* Fifth Edition, by LeMone, Burke, and Bauldoff.

Gastroesophageal Reflux Disease (GERD)

Overview

- Gastroesophageal reflux disease (GERD) is a common disorder characterized by the backward flowing of gastric contents into the esophagus.

- Gastroesophageal reflux may result from transient sphincter relaxation, an incompetent lower esophageal sphincter, or increased gastric pressure.

- In GERD, corrosive gastric juices damage and inflame the esophageal mucosa. Esophagitis and superficial ulcers develop. Bleeding may occur.

- Untreated GERD may lead to scaring and esophageal stricture, and may increase the risk for esophageal cancer.

Causes

Although the cause of GERD is unknown, risk factors include the following:

- Obesity
- Hiatal hernia
- Anticholinergic medications
- Gastric outlet obstruction

Manifestations

- Heartburn following meals and when bending over or reclining
- Regurgitation of sour material into the mouth, belching
- Dysphagia (difficult or painful swallowing)
- Atypical chest pain
- Sore throat and hoarseness; chronic cough; laryngitis, pharyngitis

Diagnostic Tests

- Barium swallow may reveal impaired esophageal peristalsis, reflux, stricture, or hiatal hernia.

- Upper endoscopy shows red, ulcerated esophageal tissue. Biopsy may be done.

- Bernstein test (acid solution instilled in esophagus produces heartburn, saline solution does not).

- A 24-hour ambulatory pH monitoring may be used to establish the diagnosis of GERD.

- Esophageal manometry may show reduced esophageal pressure and peristalsis.

Interdisciplinary Management

- Antacids and histamine H_2-receptor blockers effectively relieve GERD symptoms. Proton-pump inhibitors (e.g., omeprazole or pantoprazole) reduce gastric secretions and promote healing of erosive esophagitis. Metoclopramide (Reglan) may improve esophageal clearance and gastric emptying.

- Dietary and lifestyle changes include smoking cessation and eliminating acidic foods, fatty foods, chocolate, peppermint, and alcohol from the diet. The patient is advised to maintain ideal body weight, eat smaller meals, refrain from eating for 3 hours before bedtime, and stay upright for 2 hours after meals. Elevating the head of the bed on 6- to 8-inch blocks is beneficial.

- Laparoscopic surgery to tighten the lower esophageal sphincter or an open surgical procedure known as Nissen fundoplication may be done.

Selected Nursing Diagnoses with Interventions

Chronic Pain

- Provide small, frequent meals. Restrict intake of fat, acidic foods, coffee, and alcohol.

- Administer antacids, H_2 receptor blockers, and proton-pump inhibitors as ordered.

- Discuss the long-term nature of GERD and its management.

Community-Based Care

- Instruct to stop smoking. Refer to a smoking cessation clinic or program as needed.

- Discuss the need for continued gastric acid reduction using antacids, H_2-receptor blockers, or proton-pump inhibitors.

- Teach continuing management strategies, including dietary changes, remaining upright after meals, and avoiding eating for at least 3 hours before bedtime.

- Advise to maintain ideal weight.

- Suggest elevating the head of the bed on 6- to 8-inch wooden blocks placed under the legs.

For more information about gastroesophageal reflux disease, see Chapter 23 of *Medical-Surgical Nursing,* Fifth Edition, by LeMone, Burke, and Bauldoff.

GLAUCOMA

Overview

- Glaucoma is a group of eye disorders characterized by increased intraocular pressure (IOP).

- Increased IOP, left untreated, reduces blood flow to the retina and optic nerve, resulting in degeneration and (if untreated) eventual blindness.

- Glaucoma is the second leading cause of irreversible blindness in the United States, and the most common cause in African Americans.

- It may be congenital, primary, or secondary.

- Congenital glaucoma is the result of abnormal development of the trabecular network.

- Primary glaucoma results from impaired circulation and/or reabsorption of aqueous humor. There are two forms:

  - **Open angle (chronic) glaucoma** is usually due to degeneration of the trabecular network or canal of Schlemm, obstructing aqueous humor outflow.

  - **Closed, or narrow, angle (acute) glaucoma** develops when aqueous humor outflow is blocked due to narrowing of the angle between the iris and the cornea (i.e., the anterior chamber).

Causes

- Congenital glaucoma is an autosomal-dominant trait.

- Primary glaucoma has no identified precipitating cause.
- Secondary glaucoma results from trauma, hemorrhage into the anterior chamber, surgery, infection, tumor, prolonged steroid use, or microvascular effects of diabetes mellitus.

Manifestations

- Probable increased IOP
- Chronic open angle glaucoma is bilateral and develops insidiously; manifestations are late:
  - Mild ache in eyes
  - Peripheral field vision loss
  - Loss of visual acuity
  - Reduced night vision
  - Halos around lights
- Acute closed (narrow) angle glaucoma develops rapidly and unilaterally; it is an ocular emergency:
  - Pressurelike eye pain
  - Nonreactive/dilated pupil, cloudy cornea
  - Blurred vision
  - Halos around lights
  - Nausea, vomiting
  - Photophobia

Diagnostic Tests

- Tonometry measures IOP.
- Slit-lamp ophthalmic examination can show changes in anterior chamber structures.
- Gonioscopy measures the anterior chamber angles, distinguishes open angle from closed angle.
- Perimetry establishes degree of peripheral field loss.
- Ophthalmoscopy reveals changes in the fundus such as cupping, pallor, and/or atrophy of optic disk.
- Serial photographs of the fundus can be used to monitor changes over time.

Interdisciplinary Management

- The primary pharmacologic agents used to treat glaucoma are topical beta-adrenergic blocking agents or carbonic anhydrase inhibitors to decrease aqueous humor production, adrenergics (mydriatics), or prostaglandin analogs to increase aqueous outflow. An oral carbonic anhydrase inhibitor also may be used.

- Surgical intervention is indicated for patients with glaucoma that is not controlled with medications and for patients with acute closed angle glaucoma.

Selected Nursing Diagnoses with Interventions

Disturbed Sensory Perception: Visual

- Address by name and identify yourself with each interaction. Orient to time, place, person, and situation as indicated. Explain the purpose of your visit.

- Provide any visual aids that the patient routinely uses. Keep them in close proximity, making sure that the patient knows where they are and can reach them easily.

- Orient to the environment. Explain the location of the call bell, personal items, and the furniture in the room. If the patient is able to ambulate, provide a walking tour of the room and immediate facilities, including the toilet and sink.

- Provide other tools or items that can help compensate for diminished vision, such as bright, nonglare lighting, large-print books and magazines, books on tape, telephones with oversize pushbuttons, and a clock with large numbers that can be felt.

- Assist with meals by reading menu selections and marking choices, describing the position of foods on the meal tray, placing utensils in or near the patient's hands, and removing lids from containers.

- Assist with mobility and ambulation by having the patient hold your arm or elbow, describing the surroundings as you proceed, and advising the patient to feel the chair, bed, or commode with the hands and the backs of the legs before sitting.

Risk for Injury

- Assess ability to provide for self-care in activities of daily living.

- Provide for a safe environment by removing furniture and other objects from traffic pattern areas. Be sure that frequently used items are readily accessible.

- If hospitalized, notify housekeeping and place a sign on the door to alert all personnel not to change the arrangement of the patient's room.

- Raise the side rails as needed to promote safety.

- Assist to identify changes in the home environment to help maintain independence and prevent falls or other injuries.

Anxiety

- Assess for indicators of anxiety level and for usual coping mechanisms. Repeated expressions of concern or denial that the vision change will affect the patient's life are indicators of anxiety. Nonverbal indicators include tension, difficulty concentrating, restlessness, poor eye contact, rapid speech, voice quivering, tremors, tachycardia, and dilated pupils.

- Encourage verbalization of fears, anger, and feelings of anxiety. Listen actively.

- Discuss the patient's perception of the eye condition and its effects on lifestyle and roles.

- Help identify past successful coping strategies and their adaptation to the present situation.

- Provide diversional activities and relaxation strategies.

- Identify and enlist the patient's support system.

Community-Based Care

- Emphasize to all patients, particularly those over 40, the need for regular eye examinations.

- Explain the prescribed medications, dosage, desired and adverse effects, and the proper way to instill eye drops. Discuss medications that can increase IOP and should be avoided.

- Instruct postoperative patients to avoid bending from the waist, lifting heavy objects, straining with bowel movements, and coughing. Discuss manifestations of complications to be immediately reported, including brow pain, severe eye pain, headache, nausea, and changes in vital signs.

- Provide referral to community, state, and national agencies and resources specializing in information and assistive devices for the visually impaired.

- A referral to home health care may be appropriate.

- Emphasize the importance of lifetime therapy and periodic eye examinations to prevent blindness.

For more information on glaucoma, see Chapter 46 in *Medical-Surgical Nursing*, Fifth Edition, by LeMone, Burke, and Bauldoff.

GLOMERULONEPHRITIS

Acute

Chronic

Overview

- Glomerulonephritis is inflammation of the glomerular capillary membrane. This inflammatory disorder affects the structure and function of the glomerulus, disrupting glomerular filtration.

- Acute poststreptococcal glomerulonephritis is the most common form of acute glomerulonephritis. It primarily affects children but also can affect adults.

  - Circulating antigen-antibody immune complexes formed during the primary infection are trapped in the glomerular membrane, causing an inflammatory response that damages the membrane, increasing its permeability to plasma proteins and blood cells.

- Rapidly progressive glomerulonephritis (RPGN) causes severe glomerular injury. It may be idiopathic or related to a systemic disorder such as systemic lupus erythematosus or Goodpasture's syndrome. Glomerular cells proliferate and form crescent-shaped lesions that obliterate Bowman's space, leading to a rapid, progressive decline in renal function.

- Chronic glomerulonephritis may be the end stage of other glomerular disorders such as RPGN or diabetic nephropathy, or may develop without an identifiable cause. It is characterized by slow, progressive destruction of the glomeruli and a gradual decline in renal function. The kidneys shrink in size as entire nephrons are lost.

- Nephrotic syndrome is characterized by massive proteinuria, hypoalbuminemia, hyperlipidemia, and edema. *Minimal change disease* is the most common cause of nephrotic syndrome in children and also can affect adults. The glomeruli appear normal. *Membranous glomerulonephropathy* is the most common cause of idiopathic nephrotic syndrome in adults. The glomerular basement membrane thickens, although no inflammation is present.

  - In nephrotic syndrome, loss of plasma proteins and resulting hypoalbuminemia cause fluid shifts that, together with salt and water retention, cause edema. Loss of plasma proteins stimulates albumin production and lipoprotein synthesis in the liver, leading to hyperlipidemia. Thromboemboli are a relatively common complication of nephrotic syndrome.

Causes

- Idiopathic
- Immunologic
  1. Post group A beta-hemolytic streptococcal pharyngitis or cutaneous infection
  2. Systemic lupus erythematosus
  3. Goodpasture's syndrome
- Diabetic nephropathy
- Hypertension
- Toxins such as *E. coli* toxin
- Nephrotoxic drugs such as gold, penicillamine, captopril, non-steroidal anti-inflammatory drugs, probenecid, trimethadione, chlormethiazole, mercury
- Malignancy

Manifestations

- Abrupt or gradual onset
- Hematuria, gross or microscopic; cocoa- or coffee-colored urine
- Proteinuria
- Hypertension
- Edema, primarily facial and periorbital, and dependent edema of hands and upper extremities in particular

- Azotemia with elevated serum creatinine and blood urea nitrogen
- Fatigue
- Anorexia, nausea, and vomiting
- Headache

Diagnostic Tests

Tests to identify the cause and type of glomerulonephritis:

- Throat or skin cultures and antistreptolysin O titer to detect group A beta-hemolytic streptococci and exoenzymes that stimulate the immune response.
- A kidney, ureter, bladder abdominal x-ray may show enlarged kidneys in acute glomerulonephritis or bilateral small kidneys in late chronic glomerulonephritis.
- Kidney scan shows delayed uptake and excretion of radioactive material in glomerular diseases.
- Ultrasound of the kidneys may be done to evaluate size.
- Biopsy helps determine the type of glomerulonephritis, the prognosis, and appropriate treatment. Kidney tissue for biopsy is usually obtained percutaneously.

Studies to evaluate kidney function:

- Blood urea nitrogen and serum creatinine are metabolic by-products excreted by the kidneys that provide good indicators of renal function. They are elevated in glomerular disorders.
- eGFR (estimated GFR) 60 mL/min/1.73 m^2 or higher is WNL for adults more than 20 years old.
- Urine creatinine decreases when renal function is impaired.
- Creatinine clearance is used to evaluate the glomerular filtration rate by evaluating the amount of blood cleared of creatinine in 1 minute.
- Serum electrolytes are evaluated.
- Urinalysis often shows red blood cells and abnormal proteins in the urine.

Interdisciplinary Management

- Penicillin or another antibiotic is prescribed to eradicate continuing infection in poststreptococcal glomerulonephritis.

Antihypertensives are ordered to maintain the blood pressure within normal levels. Corticosteroids or an immunosuppressant drug may be used for acute inflammatory glomerulonephritis.

- Plasmapheresis, removal of harmful components in the plasma, may be used to treat RPGN and Goodpasture's syndrome.

- When edema is significant or the patient is hypertensive, sodium intake may be restricted.

- If renal failure develops as a result of a glomerular disorder, dialysis may be required to restore fluid and electrolyte balance and remove waste products from the body.

Selected Nursing Diagnoses with Interventions

Excess Fluid Volume

- Monitor vital signs, oxygen saturation, and breath sounds at least every 4 hours.

- Record intake and output every 4 to 8 hours, weigh daily using standard technique.

- Assess presence, location, and degree of edema.

- Monitor serum electrolytes, hemoglobin and hematocrit, blood urea nitrogen, and creatinine. Report abnormal values or significant changes.

- Maintain fluid restriction as prescribed, offering ice chips in limited and measured amounts and frequent mouth care to relieve thirst.

- Arrange for consultation with a dietitian to plan the diet when sodium is restricted and proteins are restricted or increased.

- Administer prescribed medications, monitoring for desired and adverse effects.

- Provide frequent position changes and good skin care.

Fatigue

- Assess and document energy level.

- Provide for adequate rest and energy conservation through activity and procedure scheduling. Prevent unnecessary fatigue.

- Assist with activities of daily living as needed.

- Discuss the relationship between fatigue and the disease process.

- Reduce energy demands by scheduling more frequent, small meals and short periods of activity. Limit the number of visitors and visit length.

- Provide a diet with complete proteins and adequate calories, iron, and minerals.

- Enhance coping by providing support, understanding, and active listening.

Risk for Infection

- Assess vital signs, including temperature and mental status, every 4 hours.

- Assess frequently for other signs of infection such as purulent wound drainage, productive cough, adventitious breath sounds, and red or inflamed lesions. Monitor for signs of urinary tract infection.

- Monitor the complete blood cell count, paying particular attention to the white blood cell count and differential.

- Use good hand hygiene and protect from cross-infection by providing a private room and limiting ill visitors.

- Avoid or minimize invasive procedures.

- If urinary catheterization is required, use intermittent straight catheterization or maintain a closed drainage system. Prevent reflux of urine from the drainage system to the bladder or the bladder to the kidneys by ensuring a patent, gravity system.

Community-Based Care

- Provide information about the disease process and prognosis; the use, effects, and side effects of medications; activity and diet restrictions; and the risks, manifestations, prevention, and management of complications such as edema and infection.

- Teach the manifestations and implications of improving or declining renal function.

- Stress the importance of long-term follow-up medical care.

- Discuss measures to avoid further glomerular injury such as maintaining hydration and avoiding nephrotoxic drugs.

- Refer to a home health nurse for continued assessment and reinforcement of teaching.

For more information on glomerulonephritis, see Chapter 28 in *Medical-Surgical Nursing,* Fifth Edition, by LeMone, Burke, and Bauldoff.

Gonorrhea

Overview

- Gonorrhea is a sexually transmitted disease caused by *Neisseria gonorrhoeae,* a gram-negative diplococcus.
- Symptoms appear 3 to 10 days after unprotected intercourse with an infected partner.
- In males, the most commonly infected site is the urethra, producing urethritis. The genital tract may also become infected, causing prostatitis, seminal vesicle inflammation, and/or epididymitis.
- In females, the cervix and urethra are the most commonly infected sites. Upper genital tract infections (endometritis, salpingitis, oophoritis, peritonitis, pelvic inflammatory disease) are not as common, but are much more serious.
- A systemic form exists in about 1% of those infected, and sterility is a complication.
- The oral mucous membranes can be infected via oral sex and the rectal mucous membranes via anal sex.

Causes

- Infection with *N. gonorrhoeae* acquired through unprotected intimate sexual contact with an infected partner.
- Neonates may acquire the disease *in utero* or during the birth process.
- Hand-to-eye transmission is possible.

Manifestations

May be asymptomatic, particularly in women.

In the male:

- Dysuria, frequency
- Discharge: penile or anal—profuse yellow-green or scant clear

In the female:

- Dysuria, frequency
- Discharge: vaginal, urethral, or anal—profuse, purulent
- Pruritus of vulva
- Manifestations of pelvic inflammatory disease

In both males and females:

- Anal itching, inflammation, pain, bleeding
- Painful defecation
- Pharyngitis
- Conjunctivitis
- Arthritis, if systemic
- Rash

Diagnostic Tests

- Nucleic acid amplification test (NAAT) of specimens obtained from urine or infected mucous membranes (cervix, urethra, rectum, or throat).
- Culture and sensitivity testing of infectious site (penis, cervix, throat, anus/rectum, conjunctiva) may be necessary for gonorrhea resistant to treatment.

Interdisciplinary Management

- The antibiotic ceftriaxone is recommended for the treatment of gonorrhea.
- Erythromycin or doxycycline is also given to treat any coexisting chlamydial infection.

Selected Nursing Diagnoses with Interventions

Impaired Social Interaction

- Provide privacy, confidentiality, and a safe, nonjudgmental environment.
- Emphasize that gonorrhea is a consequence of sexual behavior, not a "punishment," and that it can be avoided in the future.

Community-Based Care

- Stress the need to take all medications as directed and keep follow-up appointments to be sure no reinfection has occurred. Explain the prevalence of gonorrhea and the potential complications if it is not cured.

- Refer sexual partner(s) for evaluation and treatment.

- Discuss the importance of sexual abstinence until the infection is cured, and safer sex practices such as condom use to prevent reinfection or other sexually transmitted infections.

For more information on gonorrhea, see Chapter 50 in *Medical-Surgical Nursing,* Fifth Edition, by LeMone, Burke, and Bauldoff.

GOUT (GOUTY ARTHRITIS)

Overview

- Gout is a metabolic disorder characterized by elevated serum uric acid levels and deposits of urate crystals in synovial fluid and surrounding tissues.

- Gout occurs most often in men, with incidence peaking in the 40s or 60s.

- It may be due to primary or secondary hyperuricemia.

Causes

- *Primary gout* is caused by one of several X-linked genetic disturbances in purine metabolism. Uric acid production is greater than renal excretion, producing hyperuricemia. The increased uric acid levels set the stage for precipitation of urate crystals in the tissues, especially synovial tissue.

- *Secondary gout* is associated with excess breakdown of nucleic acids, resulting in excess uric acid production. Potential causes include malignancies, leukemia, multiple myeloma, polycythemia, and sickle cell anemia. Chronic renal disease, hypertension, starvation, diabetic ketoacidosis, and some drugs cause hyperuricemia by reducing the amount of uric acid secreted by the kidneys.

Manifestations

Manifestations of acute gout often start at night, and may follow excessive exercise, medications, foods, alcohol, or dieting.

- Arthritis of a single joint, usually the big toe; may affect foot, ankle, heel, knee, elbow, or hand
- Pain, severe in affected joints
- Redness and swelling of affected joints
- After 10 years or more: tophi (hard, large nodules)

Diagnostic Tests

- Analysis of synovial fluid reveals presence of urate crystals.
- Serum uric acid levels are increased.
- Urine uric acid levels are decreased.

Interdisciplinary Management

- Medications include nonsteroidal anti-inflammatory drugs for pain and inflammation. Colchicine may be prescribed, or a corticosteroid may be injected into the affected joint. Drugs that inhibit the formation of uric acid (such as allopurinol) or increase renal excretion of uric acid (such as probenecid and sulfinpyrazone) also may be prescribed for recurrent attacks.

Selected Nursing Diagnoses with Interventions

Deficient Knowledge

- Explain the disease, its causes, treatment, and prevention. Provide information about the primary disease process and its relationship to secondary gout as indicated.
- Advise to avoid alcohol and to drink 3000 mL of fluids per day. Foods high in purine, such as organ meats and shellfish, should be consumed in moderation.

Acute Pain

- Assess pain using a standard scale before and after treatment. Encourage to report activities that increase pain and fatigue.

- Take anti-inflammatory, anti-gout, and analgesics as prescribed. Avoid aspirin.

- Suggest positions to provide comfort, reduce the risk of skin breakdown, promote skin integrity, and promote healing. During an acute attack, even the weight of the bedclothes on the affected joint may cause tremendous pain.

Community-Based Care

- Review the prescribed medication regimen, including dosage, effects, and side effects.

- Stress the importance of avoiding alcohol (which is high in purines and interferes with uric acid excretion) and maintaining a liberal fluid intake to prevent future attacks.

- Emphasize the need for long-term medical management and to continue prescribed medication even when asymptomatic.

For more information on gout, see Chapter 40 in *Medical-Surgical Nursing,* Fifth Edition, by LeMone, Burke, and Bauldoff.

GUILLAIN-BARRÉ SYNDROME

Overview

- Guillain-Barré syndrome (GBS) is an acute polyneuropathy characterized by inflammation and demyelinization.

- It results in areflexic motor paralysis with possible sensory deficits.

- Both sexes are affected equally.

- About 30% of people with GBS require ventilatory support due to respiratory muscle paralysis.

- Recovery is spontaneous and complete in 80% to 90% of affected persons.

- Neurologic deficits such as weakness may persist, especially in the lower extremities.

Causes

- Usually follows a viral infection by about 1 to 3 weeks; most often with Epstein-Barr virus or cytomegalovirus

- May also be triggered by other infectious agents, such as *Campylobacter jejuni* gastroenteritis, immunization, or trauma, including surgery

- Probably is an autoimmune response to the original trigger; exact mechanism is unknown

Manifestations

- Muscle weakness progressing to flaccid paralysis that begins distally and progresses in a proximal pattern; legs usually precede arms or cranial nerves

- Paresthesias and numbness

- Areflexia

- If autonomic nervous system is involved: postural hypotension, dysrhythmias, facial flushing, sweating abnormalities, and urinary retention

Diagnostic Tests

- Cerebrospinal fluid analysis reveals clear fluid with elevated total protein and normal white blood cell count; pressure may be slightly elevated.

- Electromyography often shows repetitive firing of single motor units rather than normal diffuse stimulation.

- Nerve conduction velocities are slower than normal following the onset of symptoms.

Interdisciplinary Management

- There are no medications available for the specific treatment of GBS; however, high-dose immunoglobulin may be given during the acute phase.

- Ventilatory support with endotracheal intubation and mechanical ventilation may be necessary if respiratory muscle paralysis develops.

- Plasma exchange (plasmapheresis) may be beneficial, particularly when performed within the first 2 weeks of the syndrome's development.

- Nutritional support and physical and occupational therapy are important for recovery.

Selected Nursing Diagnoses with Interventions

Impaired Verbal Communication

- Choose alternative methods of communication while the patient is able to participate. With full progression of paralysis, the patient may only be able to click the tongue or blink the eyes. Cognitive abilities, however, are retained throughout the course of the disease.

- Use therapeutic communication techniques even when the patient is unable to respond verbally. Maintain eye contact and talk directly to the patient rather than to others in the room.

- Involve the patient in decisions regarding care and daily routines to reduce the sense of isolation and powerlessness caused by the inability to talk.

- Develop a regular schedule of visits to the patient's room to identify care needs; remember that the patient may be unable to use call devices to signal for help.

Risk for Impaired Skin Integrity

- Inspect bony prominences and provide skin care at least every 2 hours. Reposition the patient and clean, dry, and lubricate the skin as needed.

- Pad bony prominences such as sacral areas, heels, and elbows.

- Use an alternative-pressure mattress or water bed.

- Monitor for incontinence and provide thorough skin care following any episode of incontinence.

Community-Based Care

- Explain the disease process and the long-term effects.
- Review the medication regimen, including dosage, effects, and side effects.
- Review the use of adaptive and assistive devices, especially for ambulating.

- Show how to prevent and assess for skin breakdown.
- Show how and when to do range-of-motion exercises.
- A home care referral may be appropriate for evaluation of needs and hazards in the home environment.
- Referral to a rehabilitation facility may be required.
- The patient and significant others may benefit from referral to social services for help with coping strategies.

For more information on Guillain-Barré syndrome, see Chapter 44 in *Medical-Surgical Nursing,* Fifth Edition, by LeMone, Burke, and Bauldoff.

G

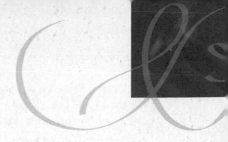

Heart Failure (Congestive Heart Failure)

Overview

- Heart failure is the inability of the heart to pump enough blood to meet the metabolic demands of the body. It may be acute or chronic. It is more common in older adults.

- Decreased tissue perfusion stimulates compensatory mechanisms that lead to vascular congestion and congestive heart failure. These mechanisms are as follows:

  1. The sympathetic nervous system increases heart rate and contractility.

  2. Vasoconstriction increases venous return and ventricular filling, increasing the force of contraction (*Frank-Starling mechanism*).

  3. Renin-angiotensin-aldosterone system activation leads to sodium and water retention.

  4. Ventricular remodeling with dilation and hypertrophy.

- Cardiac reserve (the ability to adjust output to metabolic needs) falls in heart failure, leading to activity intolerance and dyspnea on exertion.

- Classifications of heart failure:

  1. *Systolic failure* occurs when the ventricle cannot contract adequately to eject a sufficient blood volume. *Diastolic failure* results from inadequate ventricular relaxation and impaired filling.

  2. *Left-sided heart failure* usually is caused by coronary heart disease or hypertension. Its manifestations are those of decreased cardiac output and pulmonary congestion. *Right-sided heart failure* typically is caused by left-sided failure or

acute or chronic pulmonary disease. Both ventricles usually are impaired in chronic heart failure.

3. *High-output failure* occurs in hypermetabolic states when increased blood flow cannot meet the oxygen demands of the tissues and compensatory mechanisms are activated.

4. *Acute failure* is the abrupt onset of myocardial injury, decreased cardiac function, and signs of decreased cardiac output. *Chronic failure* is a progressive deterioration of the heart muscle.

Causes

Impaired Myocardial Contraction

- Coronary heart disease
- Myocardial infarction
- Cardiac muscle disorders such as cardiomyopathy, myocarditis, or rheumatic carditis

Excessive Workload

- Hypertension
- Structural cardiac disorders such as valvular disorders, congenital defects, or bacterial endocarditis

Acute Excess Demands

- Fluid volume overload
- Pregnancy, hyperthyroidism
- Fever, infection
- Massive pulmonary embolism

Manifestations

Decreased Cardiac Output

- Weakness, fatigue
- Decreased exercise tolerance
- Dizziness, syncope

Increased Pressure and Congestion behind the Failing Ventricle

- Left ventricle: shortness of breath, dyspnea, tachypnea, orthopnea (difficulty breathing while lying down); cough; inspiratory crackles (rales) and wheezes; S_3 gallop; cyanosis
- Right ventricle: distended neck veins; anorexia and nausea, liver enlargement with right upper quadrant pain; dependent edema

Other Manifestations

- Weight gain
- Nocturia (voiding more than one time at night)
- Paroxysmal nocturnal dyspnea (acute shortness of breath that develops at night)
- Severe heart failure: dyspnea at rest; S_3 and S_4 gallop
- Hepatomegaly, splenomegaly, and ascites
- Dysrhythmias
- Pleural effusion

Diagnostic Tests

- Atrial natriuretic peptide and B-type natriuretic peptide blood levels increase.
- Chest x-ray may show pulmonary vascular congestion and cardiomegaly.
- Electrocardiography may show dysrhythmias and changes related to ventricular enlargement and myocardial ischemia.
- Echocardiography with Doppler flow studies evaluate left ventricular function and measure the velocity of blood flow across valves, within cardiac chambers, and through the great vessels.
- Radionuclide imaging is used to evaluate ventricular function and size.
- Hemodynamic monitoring shows increased central venous pressure with fluid overload or right-sided heart failure. Pulmonary artery pressure and pulmonary artery wedge pressure are elevated in left-sided heart failure. Cardiac output and the cardiac index are low.

Interdisciplinary Management

- The main drug classes used to treat heart failure are the angiotensin-converting enzyme inhibitors, beta blockers, diuretics, inotropic medications (e.g., digitalis, sympathomimetic agents, and phosphodiesterase inhibitors), and direct vasodilators.

- A sodium-restricted diet is recommended. Activity is restricted during acute episodes; otherwise, moderate, progressive activity is prescribed to improve myocardial function.

- In end-stage heart failure, ventricular assist devices may be used. Heart transplant is the only clearly effective surgical treatment for end-stage heart failure.

- End-of-life care for heart failure may necessitate hospice services. Severe dyspnea is common, and may be managed with narcotic analgesics, intravenous diuretics, and continuous infusion of a positive inotropic drug.

Selected Nursing Diagnoses with Interventions

Decreased Cardiac Output

- Monitor vital signs and oxygen saturation as indicated.

- Administer supplemental oxygen as needed.

- Auscultate heart and breath sounds regularly for presence of an S_3 or S_4, respiratory crackles, and wheezes.

- Report manifestations of decreased cardiac output: changes in mentation; decreased urine output; cool, clammy skin; diminished pulses; pallor or cyanosis; dysrhythmias.

- Administer prescribed medications as ordered.

- Maintain a quiet environment; encourage expression of fears and feelings.

Excess Fluid Volume

- Assess respiratory status and auscultate lung sounds at least every 4 hours.

- Immediately notify the physician if the patient develops air hunger, an overwhelming sense of impending doom or panic, tachypnea, severe orthopnea, or a cough productive of large amounts of pink, frothy sputum.

- Monitor intake and output. Notify the physician if urine output is less than 30 mL per hour. Weigh daily.

- Monitor abdominal girth. Note complaints of a loss of appetite, abdominal discomfort, or nausea.

- Monitor and record hemodynamic measurements. Report significant changes and negative trends.

- Restrict fluids as ordered. Allow choices of fluid type and timing. Offer ice chips and frequent mouth care; provide hard candies if allowed.

Activity Intolerance

- Monitor vital signs and cardiac rhythm during and after activities. Instruct to rest if tachycardia, dysrhythmias, dyspnea, blood pressure changes, diaphoresis, pallor, chest pain, excessive fatigue, or palpitations develop.

- Organize care to allow rest periods. Assist with activities of daily living as needed. Encourage independent activities of daily living within prescribed limits.

- Encourage small, frequent meals rather than three heavy meals per day.

- Plan and implement progressive activities. Consult with physical therapist on activity plan.

Community-Based Care

Provide written and verbal information about the following topics:

- The disease process and its effects.

- Warning signals of cardiac decompensation that requires treatment.

- Desired and adverse effects of prescribed drugs; monitoring for effects; importance of compliance with drug regimen.

- Prescribed diet and sodium restriction; practical suggestions for reducing salt intake; American Heart Association materials and recipes.

- Exercise recommendations.

- Consult with dietitian to plan and teach a low-sodium and, if necessary for weight control, low-kilocalorie diet. Provide a list of high-sodium, high-fat, high-cholesterol foods to avoid.

- Stress the importance of keeping scheduled follow-up appointments.

- Provide referrals for home health care and household assistance as indicated. Referrals to community agencies, such as local cardiac rehabilitation programs, heart support groups, or the American Heart Association, may be appropriate.

For more information about heart failure, see Chapter 31 in *Medical-Surgical Nursing*, Fifth Edition, by LeMone, Burke, and Bauldoff.

HEMOPHILIA

Overview

- Hemophilia is a group of hereditary clotting factor disorders that lead to persistent and sometimes severe bleeding.

- Types of hemophilia:

  1. Hemophilia A, the most common, is caused by deficiency or dysfunction of clotting factor VIII. It is an X-linked recessive disorder transmitted from mothers to sons, affecting 1 in 10,000 male births. Hemophilia A may range from mild to severe.

  2. Hemophilia B (Christmas disease) is caused by a deficiency in factor IX. It is clinically identical to hemophilia A and also is transmitted from mother to son as an X-linked recessive disorder.

  3. Von Willebrand's disease is the most common hereditary bleeding disorder. It is caused by insufficient von Willebrand factor, a protein that mediates platelet adhesion. It is transmitted in an autosomal-dominant pattern, affecting men and women equally. Bleeding rarely is severe.

  4. Factor XI deficiency (hemophilia C), a mild bleeding disorder, is inherited in an autosomal-recessive pattern, and usually affects Ashkenazi Jews.

- In hemophilia, formation of a stable fibrin clot is impaired, resulting in prolonged or extensive bleeding. With a severe clotting factor deficit, spontaneous bleeding into joints (*hemarthrosis*), deep tissues, and central nervous system can occur, leading to joint deformity and disability.

Causes

- Hemophilia A and B: These X-linked recessive hereditary diseases almost always affect males. Females with the trait have a 50% chance of passing the gene to each child; male children develop the disease, while female children are carriers.

- Von Willebrand's disease is inherited in an autosomal-dominant pattern; each child of a parent with the trait has a 50% chance of developing the disease.

- Hemophilia C is inherited in an autosomal-recessive pattern; the trait must be inherited from both parents to develop the disorder.

Manifestations

- Hemarthrosis
- Easy bruising, cutaneous hematomas, and prolonged bleeding with minor trauma
- Bleeding gums
- Gastrointestinal bleeding: hematemesis (vomiting blood), occult blood in the stools, gastric or abdominal pain
- Spontaneous hematuria or epistaxis (nosebleed)
- Pain or paralysis
- Manifestations of intracranial hemorrhage

Diagnostic Tests

- Factor assays reveal decreased factor VIII in hemophilia A and von Willebrand's disease, and decreased factor IX in hemophilia B.
- Activated partial thromboplastin time is prolonged.
- Thrombocyte count, function, bleeding time, and prothrombin time are all normal.
- Amniocentesis or chorionic villus sampling may identify the genetic defect when there is a known family history of the disease.

Interdisciplinary Management

- Deficient clotting factors are replaced regularly as a prophylactic measure before surgery and dental procedures and to control bleeding. Clotting factors may be given as fresh-frozen plasma, cryoprecipitates, or concentrates. Factor levels are measured on a regular basis to determine whether the treatment is adequate.

Selected Nursing Diagnoses with Interventions

Ineffective Protection

- Monitor for signs of bleeding, including hematomas, ecchymoses, and purpura. Check emesis and stool for occult blood. Notify the physician of any apparent bleeding.

- Avoid intramuscular injections, rectal temperatures, and enemas.

- Use safety measures such as an electric razor in personal care.

- If bleeding occurs, control blood loss using gentle pressure, ice, or a topical hemostatic agent.

Risk for Ineffective Health Maintenance

- Assess knowledge of disorder and the related treatments.

- Provide emotional support, expressing confidence in self-care abilities.

- Provide supervised learning and practice opportunities for administering clotting factors and topical hemostatic agents.

Community-Based Care

- Instruct to immediately report manifestations of internal bleeding, including pallor, weakness, restlessness, headache, disorientation, pain, and swelling.

- Teach to apply cold packs and immobilize the joint for 24 to 48 hours if hemarthrosis occurs.

- Stress the need to avoid taking aspirin. Instruct to request a prescription analgesic if pain is severe.

- Stress the importance of good dental hygiene to decrease potential tooth decay and extractions. Instruct to discuss prophylactic clotting factor administration with dentist and physician if dental procedures are necessary.

- Teach how to prepare and administer IV medications.

- Instruct to avoid activities associated with a risk of trauma, including contact sports and jobs requiring physical exertion, and to eliminate safety hazards in the home.

- Encourage maintenance of a safe home environment; for example, pad sharp edges of furniture, leave a light on at night, avoid using scatter rugs, and wear protective gloves when working in the house or yard.

- Provide information about obtaining and wearing a MedicAlert tag.

- Referral to a home health nurse may be appropriate to evaluate the home environment and review administration of intravenous medications.

For more information on hemophilia, see Chapter 33 in *Medical-Surgical Nursing*, Fifth Edition, by LeMone, Burke, and Bauldoff.

HEMORRHOIDS

Overview

- Hemorrhoids are dilated, torturous veins of the superior or inferior hemorrhoidal plexus.

- Internal hemorrhoids develop above the mucocutaneous junction of the anus. They rarely cause pain, usually presenting with bright bleeding.

- External hemorrhoids develop below the mucocutaneous junction. They rarely bleed, but may cause anal irritation and discomfort.

- Hemorrhoids can prolapse (protrude through the anus) or become thrombosed. Thrombosed hemorrhoids are extremely painful.

- They are very common, affecting nearly all adults in the United States.

Causes

- Impaired venous return from anal canal and increased venous pressure. Risk factors are as follows:
  1. Straining to defecate in sitting or squatting position
  2. Pregnancy, labor
  3. Prolonged sitting
  4. Obesity
  5. Chronic constipation

6. Low-fiber diet
7. Liver disease with portal hypertension

Manifestations

- Often asymptomatic
- External hemorrhoids possibly protruding from the rectum
- Anal discomfort and itching, mild to severe
- Bright red bleeding unmixed with stool
- Sensation of incomplete evacuation

Diagnostic Tests

- Rectal examination confirms presence of distended veins.
- Proctoscopy confirms diagnosis and rules out polyps or other neoplasms.
- Additional tests include testing of stool for occult blood, barium enema, and sigmoidoscopy to rule out colorectal cancer or diverticular disease.

Interdisciplinary Management

- A high-fiber diet and increased water intake are recommended to prevent constipation.
- Stool softeners or laxatives may be prescribed to relieve constipation.
- Anesthetic suppositories and creams may reduce discomfort.
- Sclerotherapy, rubber band ligation, hemorrhoidectomy, or cryosurgery may be used for hemorrhoids that are permanently prolapsed, thrombosed, or produce significant symptoms.

Selected Nursing Diagnoses with Interventions

The following nursing diagnoses and interventions are appropriate for the patient who has undergone a hemorrhoidectomy.

Acute or Chronic Pain

- Maintain side-lying position or position of comfort.
- Apply ice packs over the dressing.

- Assist with a sitz bath three to four times in the first 12 hours postoperatively.

- Administer narcotic analgesic prior to first bowel movement as ordered.

Constipation

- Ensure adequate cleaning, usually with a sitz bath, following defecation postoperatively.

- Stress the importance of drinking plenty of fluids, avoiding caffeine, and eating a high-fiber diet.

- Administer stool softeners as prescribed.

- Assess for urinary retention.

Community-Based Care

- Instruct to respond to the urge to defecate, rather than delaying defecation.

- Discuss proper use of over-the-counter stool softeners, laxatives, and hemorrhoidal suppositories and creams.

- If necessary, teach how to reduce prolapsed hemorrhoids digitally.

- Review the signs of possible complications such as chronic bleeding, prolapse, and thrombosis.

- Discuss the similarity of the manifestations of hemorrhoids and colorectal cancer. Stress the need to seek medical evaluation if symptoms persist.

- For patients who have had surgery, stress the importance of returning to the physician for postoperative care.

For more information on hemorrhoids, see Chapter 24 in *Medical-Surgical Nursing,* Fifth Edition, by LeMone, Burke, and Bauldoff.

HEPATITIS

Overview

- Hepatitis is inflammation of the liver. It may be acute or chronic in nature. Cirrhosis is a potential consequence of severe hepatocellular damage.

- Hepatitis disrupts liver function, including the metabolism and elimination of bilirubin; carbohydrate, protein, and fat metabolism; drug metabolism; and detoxification of alcohol and toxins.

- Viral hepatitis is the most common type, caused by one of five different viruses. These viruses replicate in the liver, damaging liver cells (hepatocytes). They provoke an immune response that causes inflammation and necrosis of hepatocytes.

- Viral hepatitis follows a predictable pattern: the prodromal phase with flulike manifestations, and the convalescent phase with gradual improvement of symptoms and falling liver enzyme levels.

- Other types of hepatitis include the following:

  1. Chronic hepatitis (chronic infection of the liver), the primary cause of liver damage leading to cirrhosis, liver cancer, and liver transplantation. Three known hepatitis viruses can cause chronic hepatitis: hepatitis B virus, hepatitis C virus, and hepatitis D virus.

  2. Toxic hepatitis, caused by direct damage to liver cells by toxins such as alcohol.

  3. Hepatobiliary hepatitis, due to interruption of normal bile flow with resulting inflammation of liver tissue.

Causes

Viral Hepatitis

- Table 25-2 summarizes the mode of transmission, incubation, and features of various types of viral hepatitis.

- Hepatitis A risk factors include international travel, male homosexuality, drug abuse, household contacts, and occupational risks such as working in child care.

- Hepatitis B risk factors include working in the healthcare field, heterosexual or homosexual contact, drug abuse, and household contacts.

Alcoholic Hepatitis

- Chronic alcohol abuse or an acute toxic reaction to alcohol.

Toxic Hepatitis

- Acetaminophen overdose, ingestion of benzene, carbon tetrachloride, halothane, chloroform, poisonous mushrooms, or other agents.

Hepatobiliary Hepatitis

- Cholelithiasis or cholestasis related to use of oral contraceptives and allopurinol.

Manifestations

Preicteric Phase

- General malaise
- Fatigue, body and muscle aching
- Anorexia
- Nausea, vomiting, diarrhea, or constipation
- Mild right upper quadrant abdominal pain
- Chills, fever

Icteric Phase (1 to 2 weeks)

- Jaundice of sclera, skin, mucous membranes
- Pruritus
- Clay-colored stools, dark urine
- Improved appetite and sense of well-being

Posticteric/Convalescent Phase (2 to 12 weeks or longer)

- Gradual improvement in symptoms
- Improving appetite and activity level

Diagnostic Tests

- Liver function tests, including enzymes commonly released with liver cell damage, are elevated. These include alanine aminotransferase (ALT), aspartate aminotransferase (AST), and alkaline phosphatase (ALP).
- Serum bilirubin levels, both conjugated and unconjugated, are elevated.

- Laboratory tests for viral antigens and their specific antibodies may be done to identify the infecting virus and its state of activity. These tests are summarized in Table 25-4.
- A liver biopsy may be done to detect and evaluate chronic hepatitis.

Interdisciplinary Management

- Pre-exposure prophylaxis with hepatitis A vaccine or immunoglobulin and hepatitis B vaccine is recommended for people at risk for hepatitis A and B, such as travelers and healthcare workers.
- Postexposure prophylaxis with immunoglobulin is recommended for people exposed to hepatitis A virus and hepatitis B virus.
- Vitamin supplementation may be indicated during hepatitis.

Selected Nursing Diagnoses with Interventions

Risk for Infection (Transmission)

- Use standard precautions and meticulous hand hygiene.
- Use contact isolation precautions in addition to standard precautions for patients with hepatitis A who are diapered or have fecal incontinence.

Fatigue

- Facilitate self-direction of activities as determined by fatigue level.
- Encourage gradual resumption of activities.
- Promote rest; incorporate safety and fall prevention techniques.

Imbalanced Nutrition: Less than Body Requirements

- Help patients with acute viral hepatitis select a diet that provides a high-kilocalorie intake.
- Because many patients with hepatitis are nauseated later in the day, encourage consumption of the majority of kilocalories in the morning.
- Encourage a low-fat diet.
- Encourage small, frequent meals.

Community-Based Care

- Teach how the disease is transmitted and ways to prevent spreading it to others. For instance, instruct not to share towels or eating utensils. Explain that until serologic indicators return to normal, sexual and close personal contact with others should be avoided.

- Instruct to avoid hepatotoxins, such as alcohol and acetaminophen.

- Encourage patients in high-risk groups to obtain hepatitis A and/or hepatitis B immunizations.

- Emphasize the importance of childhood immunizations.

- Stress the need for follow-up care with the physician.

- Refer patients with alcoholic hepatitis to alcohol treatment and support groups such as Alcoholics Anonymous as appropriate. Stress the importance of continued abstinence.

- Teach safer sex practices to patients with hepatitis, and discuss other important measures such as avoiding sharing needles, syringes, and razors.

- Referral to a home health nurse may be appropriate for some patients.

For more information on hepatitis, see Chapter 25 in *Medical-Surgical Nursing,* Fifth Edition, by LeMone, Burke, and Bauldoff.

HERNIA

Inguinal

Ventral

Overview

- A hernia is a defect in the abdominal wall that allows abdominal contents to protrude from the abdominal cavity.

- Inguinal hernia, prolapse of the small or large intestine into the inguinal canal, is the most common type.

- Hernias may be reducible, incarcerated, or strangulated.

  1. The contents of a reducible hernia can be returned manually to the abdominal cavity through the defect.

  2. The contents of an incarcerated hernia are trapped and do not move back through the defect into the abdominal cavity.

3. In a strangulated hernia, the blood supply to the contents in the hernia is compromised, owing to twisting or edema. Necrosis and obstruction result.

Causes

- Weakness of the abdominal muscles due to congenital malformation, surgery, trauma, or aging
- Increased intra-abdominal pressure due to lifting, pregnancy, coughing, straining, or obesity

Manifestations

- Lump in inguinal area or abdomen upon sitting or standing that disappears when recumbent
- Pain in groin; steady but decreases with hernia reduction
- Severe pain: strangulation

Diagnostic Tests

- Diagnosis is made primarily by physical examination.
- X-ray may show bowel obstruction.
- White blood cell count may be elevated if there is bowel obstruction.

Interdisciplinary Management

- Herniorrhaphy—surgical repair of a hernia—usually involves suturing or using wire mesh over the defect that allowed herniation.
- If incarceration has occurred or strangulation is suspected, any infarcted bowel is resected.
- Heavy lifting and heavy manual labor are restricted for 3 weeks after surgery.

Selected Nursing Diagnosis with Interventions

Risk for Ineffective Gastrointestinal Perfusion

- Assess comfort; report an acute increase in abdominal, groin, perineal, or scrotal pain, which may indicate strangulation.

- Assess bowel sounds and abdominal distention at least every 8 hours.

- Notify the physician if the hernia becomes painful or tender, as this may indicate incarceration and increased risk for strangulation.

- If strangulation occurs, position supine with the hips elevated and the knees slightly bent.

- Withhold food and fluids, and begin preparations for surgery.

Community-Based Care

- Reassure that the risks associated with hernia surgery are lower than not repairing the hernia.

- Reinforce teaching about pain management and activity restrictions.

- Teach wound care and identifying signs of infection.

- Schedule an appointment for the patient to return to the surgeon for follow-up after discharge.

For more information on hernias, see Chapter 24 in *Medical-Surgical Nursing,* Fifth Edition, by LeMone, Burke, and Bauldoff.

HERNIATED INTERVERTEBRAL DISK

Overview

- A herniated disk is the rupture of the soft, internal portion (nucleus pulposus) of a vertebral disk through the tough outer portion (annulus fibrosis).

- The extruded disk material impinges upon spinal nerve roots and/or the spinal cord.

- Most occur in the lumbar vertebrae; cervical vertebrae are the second most common site; thoracic, the least common.

- They are more common in males 30 to 50 years of age.

Causes

- Severe trauma or lumbar strain
- Improper body mechanics, especially with lifting
- Disk degeneration, especially in older adults

Manifestations

- Pain: severe, unilateral, exacerbated by movement
- Lumbar disk: pain radiates in sciatic pattern (buttock, leg, foot)
- Paresthesias such as numbness or tingling
- Possible motor deficits/muscle wasting

Diagnostic Tests

- X-rays are taken of vertebrae to rule out other causes (e.g., fracture); not diagnostic for herniated intervertebral disk.
- Myelography reveals spinal canal compression.
- Computed tomography scan and magnetic resonance imaging reveal spinal cord compression.

Interdisciplinary Management

- Pain is managed with nonsteroidal anti-inflammatory drugs. Muscle spasms are treated with muscle relaxants.
- Transcutaneous electrical nerve stimulation may be used for pain relief.
- Surgery is indicated for patients who do not respond to conservative management.

Selected Nursing Diagnoses with Interventions

Acute Pain

- Encourage discussion of pain. Assess degree of pain and identify contributing and relieving factors.
- Maintain activities as prescribed.
- Use a firm mattress or place a board under the mattress.
- Teach to avoid turning or twisting the spinal column and to assume positions that decrease stress on the vertebral column.
- Encourage analgesic medications on a regular basis around the clock.

Chronic Pain

- Treat reports of pain with respect.

240

- Do not refer to the patient as being addicted to pain medication. Tolerance to medications does not imply addiction.

- Monitor carefully for any changes in condition.

- Ensure understanding of the reason for the pain experienced.

- Do not withdraw pain medications abruptly. Suggest a gradual withdrawal for patients who have been taking narcotic or sedative medications for longer than 3 weeks.

- Follow recommended guidelines for administering pain medications.

- Teach alternative methods of pain management.

- Identify patient support systems and encourage their use.

Constipation

- Reduced mobility, bed rest, and pain medications increase the risk for constipation.

- Assess usual bowel routine, including diet, fluid intake, and the use of laxatives or enemas.

- Encourage a fluid intake of 2,500 to 3,000 mL per day, unless contraindicated by renal or cardiac disease.

- Increase fiber and bulk in the diet. Consult with the physician about the use of stool softeners or bulk-forming agents.

Community-Based Care

- Review methods of pain control including: medications, positioning, use of proper body mechanics, and nonpharmacologic methods of pain management, including relaxation, guided imagery, distraction, hypnosis, and music.

- Explain scheduling of analgesics. Although many people believe that the use of analgesic medications causes addiction, it is now widely accepted that providing medications on a routine schedule is the preferred administration method.

- Encourage to remain physically active and maintain weight within the desired range.

- Make appropriate referrals to a support group or counselor to help the patient cope with chronic pain.

- Refer to a physical therapist for an exercise program if appropriate.

For more information on herniated intervertebral disk, see Chapter 43 in *Medical-Surgical Nursing,* Fifth Edition, by LeMone, Burke, and Bauldoff.

HERPES SIMPLEX VIRUS—HERPES LABIALIS, HERPES GENITALIS, HERPETIC WHITLOW, HERPES SIMPLEX VIRUS KERATITIS

Overview

- Infection occurs with herpes simplex virus I (HSV-I) and/or HSV-II.

- Each strain is highly contagious.

- HSV-I usually affects mucous membranes of the lips (cold sore or fever blister), oral mucosa, and/or facial skin.

- HSV-II usually affects mucous membranes and skin of the genital/rectal area; it is considered a sexually transmitted infection.

- Cross-infection is possible.

- Herpetic whitlow is an HSV infection of the fingers with either strain of the virus.

- HSV keratitis is a corneal infection and is the most common cause of corneal blindness in the United States.

- Infection in early pregnancy may result in spontaneous abortion.

- In immunocompromised patients, including infected neonates, HSV disseminates widely to skin, central nervous system, and viscera.

- During the primary, or initial, infection, peripheral sensory or autonomic nerves are colonized by the herpes virus. Following the primary infection, the virus moves by axonal transport to the cell body of the neurons contained in ganglia.

- Secondary infection (reinfection) of peripheral mucous membranes/skin occurs episodically.

- Secondary attacks may be precipitated by other infections, stress, sunlight, menses, fever, or exposure to excess heat or cold.

Causes

- Herpes virus hominis; strain HSV-I or HSV-II; enveloped DNA viruses
- Acquired through intimate contact: kissing, oral intercourse, sexual intercourse; maternal-to-fetal spread by transplacental or vaginal routes
- Autoinoculation following poor hand hygiene
- Spreads to contiguous area upon reactivation

Manifestations

- Vesicles develop in clusters and initially are small, inflamed, and fluid filled; later, vesicle rupture produces ulceration, oozing, and the formation of a crust.
- Pain, burning in nature, is characteristic of early and late lesions.
- Itch may precede or accompany pain.
- A prodrome of itching or tingling may signal an impending secondary attack.
- Lymphadenopathy may be present with primary infection.

Diagnostic Tests

- Viral culture of lesions reveals HSV-I or HSV-II.
- Biopsy also confirms presence of herpes virus infection.
- A general rise in immunoglobulin titers and white blood cell count supports the diagnosis.

Interdisciplinary Management

There is no cure for herpes infections; the treatment is symptomatic.

- Suppressive therapy using an antiviral (acyclovir, valacyclovir, or famciclovir) for recurrent genital herpes reduces the frequency of outbreaks and transmission to uninfected partners.
- Aspirin and other nonprescription analgesics may reduce the pain of herpes lesions.
- Patients with acquired immunodeficiency syndrome may require prophylactic treatment.

Selected Nursing Diagnoses with Interventions

Acute Pain

- Teach to keep herpes blisters clean and dry. A solution of warm water, soap, and hydrogen peroxide can be used to cleanse the lesions two or three times daily. Loose cotton clothing that will not trap moisture should be worn.

- For dysuria, suggest pouring water over the genitals while urinating, or urinating in the tub or shower. Drinking additional fluids helps dilute the acidity of the urine. Fluids that increase acidity, such as cranberry juice, should be avoided.

- Nonpharmacologic measures to reduce pain include application of heat or cold and sitz baths.

Sexual Dysfunction

- Provide a supportive, nonjudgmental environment to discuss feelings and ask questions about implications for future sexual relationships.

- Provide information about suppressive therapy for patients in mutually monogamous heterosexual relationships.

- Discuss the disease process and factors that may contribute to recurrent infections.

- Offer information about support groups and other resources for people with herpes such as the National Herpes Information Hotline.

Anxiety

Advise about the need for regular Pap smears, as appropriate. Pap smears every 6 months may be recommended for women with genital herpes.

Discuss cesarean delivery to prevent transmission of infection to the neonate with women of childbearing age. In women without manifestations of recurrence, vaginal delivery is possible.

Community-Based Care

- Review the disease process and factors that affect it. Teach to recognize prodromal symptoms and factors that may trigger recurrences (such as emotional stress, acidic food, sun exposure).

- Explain the importance of very careful hand hygiene to prevent the spread of secondary HSV infections.

- For genital herpes infections:

  - Abstain from sexual contact from the onset of prodromal symptoms until 10 days after all lesions have healed.

  - Stress the importance of using latex condoms and careful hygiene practices (such as not sharing towels) even during latency periods.

  - Practice strategies for discussing the condition with current or future sexual partners.

- Stress the need for lifelong follow-up care to manage recurrences.

- Refer the patient to local support groups and information services such as the National Herpes Information Hotline.

For more information on herpes simplex virus, see Chapters 12 and 50 in *Medical-Surgical Nursing,* Fifth Edition, by LeMone, Burke, and Bauldoff.

Hiatal Hernia

Overview

- A hiatal or diaphragmatic hernia is a defect in the esophageal hiatus of the diaphragm that allows part of the stomach to protrude into the chest cavity.

- In a sliding hiatal hernia, the gastroesophageal junction and the fundus of the stomach slide upward through the esophageal hiatus.

- The gastroesophageal junction remains below the diaphragm in a paraesophageal hiatal hernia, while a part of the stomach herniates through the esophageal hiatus.

- A paraesophageal hernia can become incarcerated, leading to tissue ischemia and necrosis.

- Hiatal hernias are relatively common, and their incidence increases with age.

Causes

- Congenital defect in the diaphragm

- Trauma
- Increased intra-abdominal pressure (e.g., obesity, pregnancy, ascites)

Manifestations

- Often asymptomatic
- Heartburn, substernal discomfort or pain
- Gastroesophageal reflux
- Dysphagia
- Indigestion or feeling of fullness
- Belching
- Bleeding, usually occult
- Severe pain and possible hemorrhage with an incarcerated hernia

Diagnostic Tests

- Barium swallow reveals the herniation.
- Endoscopy is used to rule out varices and neoplasms.

Interdisciplinary Management

- Treatment is symptomatic and includes measures to treat gastro-intestinal reflux disease (see Gastroesophageal Reflux Disease). Medications may include antacids, proton-pump inhibitors, histamine H_2 receptor blockers, or sucralfate.
- Surgery may be required, and usually involves a Nissen fundo-plication to prevent the gastroesophageal junction from slipping into the thoracic cavity.

Selected Nursing Diagnoses with Interventions

Imbalanced Nutrition: Less than Body Requirements

- Encourage to eat several small meals throughout the day rather than three large meals, and to avoid bedtime snacks.
- Encourage weight reduction and smoking cessation as appropriate.

Pain

- Elevate the head of the bed 8 to 12 inches.
- Position upright or sitting for at least 2 hours after eating.
- Administer medications as prescribed.

Risk for Injury

- Postoperatively, assess for and report complications of surgery.
- Elevate the head of the bed 30 degrees.
- Supervise initial oral food or fluid intake.
- Teach to support the incision when turning, coughing, and deep breathing.
- Encourage frequent position changes and early ambulation.

Community-Based Care

- Instruct to remain upright for 2 hours after eating and to elevate the head of the bed on 6- to 8-inch blocks.
- Encourage a low-fat diet and avoidance of caffeine, alcohol, acidic foods, carbonated beverages, and gas-producing foods such as cabbage, bananas, and nuts.
- Encourage small meals throughout the day rather than three large meals.
- Teach about use of prescribed or recommended over-the-counter medications.
- Refer to smoking cessation and/or weight reduction programs as necessary.
- Instruct the patient who has had surgery to avoid straining at stools, heavy lifting or manual labor, and climbing stairs for 3 weeks or until approved by physician.
- Stress the importance of follow-up care. Instruct to report immediately any signs of infection such as elevated temperature.

For more information on hiatal hernia, see Chapter 23 in *Medical-Surgical Nursing,* Fifth Edition, by LeMone, Burke, and Bauldoff.

Hodgkin's Disease

Overview

- Hodgkin's disease is a malignant lymphoma that usually affects people between the ages of 15 and 35 or over age 50.

- It is somewhat more common in men than women.

- Hodgkin's disease is curable when diagnosed early and treated appropriately.

- It develops in a single lymph node or chain of nodes. Involved nodes contain Reed-Sternberg cells (malignant cells) that may invade almost any tissue in the body.

- The spleen often is involved; with disease progression, the liver, lungs, digestive tract, and central nervous system may be affected.

- Rapid proliferation of abnormal lymphocytes impairs the immune response, especially cell-mediated immune responses. Infections are common.

Causes

- Exact cause unknown

- Possible risk factors: Epstein-Barr virus infection, genetic predisposition

Manifestations

- One or more painlessly enlarged lymph nodes, usually in the cervical or subclavicular region

- Systemic manifestations: persistent fever, night sweats, fatigue, and weight loss

- Late symptoms: malaise, pruritus, and anemia

- Splenomegaly

Diagnostic Tests

- Complete blood cell count often shows a mild anemia, leukocytosis with high neutrophil and eosinophil counts, and an elevated sedimentation rate.

- Chest x-ray may show enlarged mediastinal lymph nodes and pulmonary involvement.

- Chest or abdominal computed tomography scan may identify abnormal or enlarged nodes.

- Bipedal lymphangiography identifies the extent of iliac, para-aortic, and abdominal lymph node involvement.

- Lymph node biopsy reveals the presence of Reed-Sternberg cells to confirm the diagnosis.

Interdisciplinary Management

- Radiation therapy to the involved lymph node region is the primary treatment for early stage Hodgkin's. Total nodal irradiation may be done for advanced disease.

- Combination chemotherapy often is used in conjunction with radiation therapy. More than 75% of patients who do not have systemic symptoms achieve complete remission with treatment.

- Autologous peripheral blood stem cell transplant is used for patients experiencing remission of malignant lymphoma to restore bone marrow function after chemotherapy or radiation.

- Adverse effects of treatment may include permanent sterility, bone marrow suppression, and long-term risk for secondary cancers and cardiac injury.

Selected Nursing Diagnoses with Interventions

Fatigue

- Inquire about malaise (a vague feeling of body weakness or discomfort) and fatigue (a pervasive, drained feeling that cannot be eliminated).

- Encourage verbalization of feelings about the impact of the disease and fatigue on lifestyle.

- Encourage to establish priorities and include rest periods or naps when scheduling daily activities.

- Encourage a diet high in carbohydrates and fluids.

Nausea

- Provide ordered antiemetics before chemotherapy is started.
- Provide small feedings of high-kilocalorie, high-protein foods and fluids.
- Assist with oral care, general hygiene, and environmental control of temperature, appearance, and odors.

Disturbed Body Image

- Assess perception of body image through subjective information:
  a. Current understanding of health and limitations imposed by illness or treatment
  b. Feelings about the illness and its effect on self-perception as well as perception of others
- Discuss the risk for and measures to cope with alopecia. Suggest wearing wigs, scarves, hats, or caps. Teach proper scalp care using baby shampoo or mild soap, a soft brush, sunscreen, and mineral oil to reduce itching. If eyelashes and eyebrows are lost, teach eye protection, such as wearing eyeglasses and caps with wide brims.
- Discuss available resources for financial assistance with purchase of wigs.

Sexual Dysfunction

- Encourage discussion of actual or potential sexual dysfunction or sterility with the patient and significant other.
- Discuss realistic measures for coping, for example, sperm banking before chemotherapy or radiation therapy.
- Refer for counseling as indicated.

Risk for Impaired Skin Integrity

- Frequently assess skin, especially in areas undergoing radiation.
- Provide and teach measures to promote comfort: Use cool water and a mild soap to bathe; blot (rather than rub) dry skin; use plain cornstarch or nonperfumed lotion or powder unless

contraindicated; use lightweight blankets and clothing; maintain adequate humidity and a cool room temperature; wash bedding and clothes in mild detergent using a second rinse cycle.

Community-Based Care

- Teach about the disease process, prognosis, treatment, and side effects of treatments.

- Discuss the importance of proper skin care and avoiding scratching.

- Advise to plan activities of daily living to ensure adequate rest and exercise, and to eat a well-balanced diet.

- Teach measures to prevent or relieve nausea and vomiting:

  a. Eat soda crackers and suck on hard candy.

  b. Eat soft, bland foods that are cold or at room temperature.

  c. Avoid unpleasant odors, and get fresh air.

  d. Eat before but not immediately before chemotherapy.

  e. Use distraction or progressive muscle relaxation when nauseated.

  f. If vomiting occurs, gradually resume oral intake with frequent sips of clear liquids or ice, progressing to bland foods.

- Teach about the side effects of radiation and chemotherapy, including their management and manifestations that should be reported to the physician.

- Discuss the importance of avoiding exposure to people with contagious diseases.

- Emphasize the need for long-term follow-up care with the oncologist.

- Refer to the local chapter of the American Cancer Society for information, financial assistance, and counseling.

- A home care referral may be appropriate.

For more information on Hodgkin's disease, see Chapter 33 in *Medical-Surgical Nursing,* Fifth Edition, by LeMone, Burke, and Bauldoff.

HUMAN IMMUNODEFICIENCY VIRUS INFECTION

Acquired Immunodeficiency Syndrome

Overview

- Human immunodeficiency virus (HIV) infections range from no symptoms to acquired immunodeficiency syndrome (AIDS) with multiple opportunistic infections and cancers.

- HIV is a retrovirus that contains an RNA genome and reverse transcriptase enzyme that converts RNA to DNA.

- It primarily infects helper T cells of the immune system with CD4 cell-surface receptors.

- HIV is slow growing; the median time from initial infection to the appearance of manifestations of AIDS is 8 to 10 years.

- Generally, HIV infection has a specific course.

Acute Retroviral Syndrome (Primary HIV Infection)

- Begins 2 weeks after infection and lasts about 12 weeks, during which an acute viremia with widespread lymphatic seeding occurs.

- Virus titers peak at about the eighth week, as CD4 counts fall to approximately 500 cells/μL (50% normal).

- During the primary infection 50% to 70% of patients show an acute HIV syndrome, which resembles an acute bout of mononucleosis.

- By the end of this stage, the CD4 count has rebounded to about 700 cells/μL.

- During this phase, antibodies cannot be detected for 6 weeks to 6 months but the infected patient is highly contagious.

- Detectable antibodies are usually found by the end of this stage (seroconversion); however, some patients may not display adequate measurement levels for a year.

Asymptomatic Infection (Latency)

- Three to fifteen years, depending upon availability and adherence to treatment.

- Follows the primary infection and is characterized by the following:
  - Presence of detectable HIV antibodies
  - Reduced viremia
  - Lymphoid sequestration of virus
  - Steady decline in the CD4 count from about 700 to 200 cells/μL over the next 8 to 10 years
- Some patients may display persistent generalized lymphadenopathy, oral lesions, shingles, or other minor opportunistic diseases.

AIDS: HIV-Associated Neoplasms and Opportunistic Infections

- The development of AIDS is heralded when the CD4 count reaches about 200 cells/μL.
- The patient may develop constitutional manifestations or may present with an opportunistic infection or neoplasm.
- Neurologic disease, such as AIDS dementia complex, aseptic meningitis, HIV encephalopathy, and peripheral neuropathies, is common.
- Death usually occurs as the result of overwhelming infection or cancer.

Causes

- HIV is acquired from an infected individual via the following:
  - Sexual intercourse, especially anal sex
  - Blood transfusion
  - Sharing of contaminated needles
  - Perinatal transmission from mother to fetus
- Risk factors include a history of the following:
  - Unprotected sex between men, with multiple partners, or with an infected partner
  - Injection drug use or unprotected sex with an injection drug user
  - Presence of a sexually transmitted infection
  - Transfusion with blood or pooled blood products, especially before 1985

- Pre/perinatal exposure to an HIV-infected mother
- Postnatal exposure, via breast milk, to an infected mother
- Occupational accidents such as needle sticks, cuts, puncture wounds during surgery, or human bites

Manifestations

ARS/Primary Stage

- Fever, lymphadenopathy
- Malaise, fatigue
- Arthralgia, myalgia
- Headache, pharyngitis
- Rash, urticaria
- Abdominal cramps, diarrhea

Asymptomatic/Latent Stage

- May last for many years
- Persistent generalized lymphadenopathy
- Persistent fever, night sweats
- Chronic diarrhea, weight loss
- Fatigue
- Candidiasis of mouth (thrush)

AIDS/HIV-associated Neoplasms and Opportunistic Infections

- AIDS dementia complex and neurologic effects
- Candidiasis of bronchi/lung
- Candidiasis of esophagus
- Coccidioidomycosis, extrapulmonary
- Cryptococcosis, extrapulmonary
- Cryptosporidiosis, intestinal > 1 month
- Cytomegalovirus
- Cytomegalovirus retinitis with loss of vision
- HIV encephalopathy/dementia

- Herpes simplex virus > 1 month
- Herpes simplex virus, disseminated
- Invasive cancer of the cervix
- Isosporiasis with diarrhea > 1 month
- Kaposi's sarcoma
- Lymphoma: immunoblastic, Burkitt's
- *Mycobacterium avium*, or any species
- Tuberculosis (*M. tuberculosis*), any site
- *Pneumocystis carinii* pneumonia
- Pneumonia, any species/recurrent
- Progressive leukoencephalopathy
- Salmonella septicemia, recurrent
- Toxoplasmosis of brain
- HIV wasting syndrome

Diagnostic Tests

End of Primary Stage(Category 1)

- HIV rapid antibody tests; confirmed with positive enzyme-linked immunosorbent assay (ELISA) and Western blot antibody test; negative ELISA and Western blot until end of stage
- CD4 > 500 cells/µL

Latent Stage (Category 2)

- Positive ELISA and Western blot (HIV antibody tests)
- CD4 = 200 to 499 cells/µL
- Decreased red blood cells, hemoglobin, hematocrit, white blood cells, lymphocytes, and platelets

Clinically Apparent Stage (Category 3)

- Positive ELISA and Western blot (HIV antibody tests)
- CD4 < 200 cells/µL and HIV viral load tests to measure disease progression and response to antiretroviral medications.
- Decreased red blood cells, hemoglobin, hematocrit, and white blood cells

- Lymphocytes < 14%
- Blood chemistry abnormalities

Interdisciplinary Management

There is no cure for HIV/AIDS.

- Treatment for HIV infection includes combination of three or more antiretroviral therapy to suppress the HIV infection, prophylaxis and treatment for opportunistic infections and malignancies, and hematopoietic stimulating factors. Highly active antiretroviral therapy (HAART) medications work to interrupt viral replication at a different point. Six classes of drugs used in antiretroviral treatment include nucleoside reverse transcriptase inhibitors (NRTIs), nonnucleoside reverse transcriptase inhibitors (NNRTIs), protease inhibitors (PIs), and three types of entry inhibitors. HAART does not eradicate HIV infection.

Selected Nursing Diagnoses with Interventions

Ineffective Coping

- Assess social support network.
- Promote interaction between the patient, significant others, and family.
- Encourage patient to obtain information and make care decisions.
- Support positive coping behaviors, patient decisions, actions, and achievements.
- Provide referrals to counselors, support groups, and agencies.

Impaired Skin Integrity

- Assess skin frequently.
- Monitor lesions.
- Turn at least every 2 hours, if bedfast.
- Use pressure-relieving devices.
- Keep skin clean and dry.
- Massage around but not over affected pressure sites.
- Caution against scratching.

Imbalanced Nutrition: Less than Body Requirements

- Monitor nutritional status.
- Assess for oral or esophageal lesions, fever, nausea, or diarrhea.
- Administer medications as prescribed.
- Provide a diet high in protein and kilocalories.
- Offer soft foods and serve small portions.
- Provide food preferences, and encourage significant others to bring favorite foods from home (if hospitalized).
- Assist with eating as needed.
- Provide supplementary vitamins and enteral feedings, with products such as Ensure.
- Provide or assist with frequent oral hygiene.

Ineffective Sexuality Patterns

- Examine own feelings about sexuality.
- Establish a trusting, therapeutic relationship with the patient.
- Provide factual information about HIV infection.
- Discuss safer sex practices.
- Encourage the patient and significant others to discuss fears and concerns.
- Refer to local support groups.

Community-Based Care

- Provide information about transmission of HIV and any coexisting infections, and teach how to avoid transmission of HIV through safer sex practices and avoidance of sharing injection drug paraphernalia.
- Explain the need to inform any sexual partners of HIV status.
- Explain the importance of maintaining optimal health through proper nutrition, exercise, smoking cessation, stress reduction, rest, regular check-ups, Mantoux testing, and avoidance of illegal drugs.
- Provide information about HAART medications, effects, and side effects. Stress the importance of precisely following the prescribed medication regimen.

- Show proper care of central or peripheral intravenous lines and venous access devices.

- Stress the importance of regular self-assessment for early signs of opportunistic infections, and to report any signs of infection or any changes in neurologic status.

- Ensure access to follow-up care.

- Provide the names, locations, and phone numbers of local support groups, including local visiting nurses associations, home health agencies, and Meals on Wheels, as well as national information resources such as the National AIDS Information Clearinghouse.

- Discuss assessment of safety of the home environment.

- Discuss the availability of hospice care as appropriate.

For more information on HIV/AIDS, see Chapter 13 in *Medical-Surgical Nursing,* Fifth Edition, by LeMone, Burke, and Bauldoff.

HYPERGLYCEMIA

Overview

- Hyperglycemia is defined as a rise in blood glucose levels to > 120 mg/dL, usually due to diabetes mellitus (DM).

- It results when glucose cannot enter insulin-dependent cells (skeletal muscle and adipose tissue) or when glucose is released from hepatic stores (glycogenolysis and gluconeogenesis).

- It may be attributable to an absolute lack of insulin, as in type 1 DM, or to insulin resistance, as in type 2 DM.

- Secondary hyperglycemia is associated with disorders of insulin target tissue and with pancreatic disorders.

- Hyperglycemia represents a hyperosmolar state that causes cellular dehydration.

- When blood glucose rises to > 180 mg/dL, glucose spills into the urine, producing an osmotic diuresis.

- In type 1 DM, severe hyperglycemia may cause diabetic ketoacidosis possibly progressing to diabetic coma.

- In type 2 DM, severe, profound hyperglycemia causes hyperosmotic hyperglycemic state.

Causes

- DM: type 1 or 2
- Endocrine disorders causing excess production of growth hormone, glucocorticoids, catecholamines, glucagon, or somatostatin
- Medications such as thiazide diuretics, phenytoin, niacin, and high-dose corticosteroids
- Chronic pancreatitis
- Cirrhosis
- Stress

Manifestations

- Polyuria (if blood sugar > 180 mg/dL), due to osmotic diuresis
- Polydipsia, secondary to increased blood osmolarity and dehydration
- Abdominal pain
- Warm, dry, flushed skin
- Poor skin/eye turgor
- Hypotension, tachycardia
- Altered level of consciousness, confusion, stuporous to coma

Diagnostic Tests

- Serum glucose is > 120 mg/dL.
- Serum osmolality is elevated in proportion to blood glucose level.
- Serum sodium and potassium levels vary.
- Blood urea nitrogen and creatinine levels may be elevated.
- Glycosuria when blood glucose exceeds 180 mg/dL.

Interdisciplinary Management

- Insulin replacement therapy as indicated by underlying cause
- Fluid and electrolyte replacement therapy

Selected Nursing Diagnoses with Interventions

Imbalanced Nutrition: More than Body Requirements

- Administer insulin as prescribed.
- Monitor blood glucose levels.
- Encourage fluid intake.
- Encourage adherence to prescribed diet.

Risk for Injury

- Following insulin treatment, monitor for signs of hypoglycemia: change in mental status, diaphoresis, cool and clammy skin. If observed, provide a source of glucose (orange juice, hard candy, glucagon, or 50% glucose).
- Assess for signs of skin breakdown and for decreased urine output.
- Encourage the patient to have baseline ophthalmic examination and regular follow-up care.

Community-Based Care

- Teach diet, exercise, and medication management.
- Show how to self-monitor blood glucose and prevent hyperglycemia and hypoglycemia.
- Review self-administration of insulin, if needed.
- Discuss wound care, if necessary.
- Stress the need for medical management and self-care of the underlying condition.
- Refer to a dietitian for long-term nutritional support and follow-up.
- If appropriate, refer to social services or a psychologic counselor for stress management techniques and coping mechanisms for managing a chronic illness.
- Refer the patient to the American Diabetes Association if indicated.

For more information about hyperglycemia, see Chapter 20 in *Medical-Surgical Nursing,* Fifth Edition, by LeMone, Burke, and Bauldoff.

Hyperosmolar Hyperglycemic State

Overview

- Hyperosmolar hyperglycemic state is a metabolic problem characterized by significantly elevated plasma osmolarity and blood glucose levels, and altered level of consciousness.
- It affects people with type 2 diabetes mellitus, especially the older adult.
- The condition develops insidiously.
- High blood glucose pulls water into the vascular system from body cells; fluid is lost via the urine, resulting in dehydration.
- As water is lost, glucose and sodium increase plasma osmolarity.
- Cellular dehydration primarily affects cells of the central nervous system.

Causes

- Increased insulin resistance
- Excess carbohydrate intake
- Risk factors:
  - Drugs such as glucocorticoids, diuretics, beta-adrenergic blockers, immunosuppressants, chlorpromazine, and diazoxide
  - Acute illness
  - Therapeutic procedures such as dialysis, hyperalimentation (oral or parenteral), surgery
  - Chronic illness such as renal or cardiac disease, hypertension, previous stroke, and alcoholism

Manifestations

- Flushed, warm, dry skin
- Extreme thirst
- Fatigue, malaise
- Nausea, vomiting; abdominal pain

- Hypotension, tachycardia
- Polyuria
- Lethargy progressing to coma; possible seizures

Diagnostic Tests

- Serum glucose > 600 mg/dL
- Serum osmolarity > 340 mOsm/L
- Serum ketones normal
- Serum sodium usually normal to slightly elevated
- Blood urea nitrogen and creatinine elevated

Interdisciplinary Management

Hyperosmolar hyperglycemic state is a life-threatening medical emergency.

- Treatment is immediate, and is directed toward correcting fluid and electrolyte imbalances, lowering blood glucose levels with insulin, and treating underlying conditions.

Selected Nursing Diagnoses with Interventions

Deficient Fluid Volume

- Administer intravenous fluids and insulin as prescribed.
- Monitor response to fluids and insulin.
- Encourage fluid intake (if alert).

Ineffective Tissue Perfusion: Renal

- Monitor fluid status through intake and output, skin turgor, vital signs, and central venous pressure.
- Monitor level of consciousness.
- Monitor blood glucose levels.
- Monitor cardiac activity.

Deficient Knowledge

- Assess knowledge of diabetes management.

- Review diet, medications, and signs and symptoms of hyperglycemia and hypoglycemia and their management.

Community-Based Care

- Stress the need for ongoing follow-up care for management of diabetes.

- A home healthcare referral may be appropriate for continued teaching and monitoring of self-care activities.

For more information on hyperosmolar hyperglycemic state, see Chapter 20 in *Medical-Surgical Nursing,* Fifth Edition, by LeMone, Burke, and Bauldoff.

HYPERPARATHYROIDISM

Overview

- Hyperparathyroidism is overactivity of the parathyroid glands with secretion of excess parathyroid hormone (PTH). Occurs more often in older adults and women.

- There are three types of hyperparathyroidism:

  - *Primary hyperparathyroidism* results from hyperplasia or an adenoma of a parathyroid gland, causing excess PTH secretion.

  - *Secondary hyperparathyroidism* is a compensatory response to chronic hypocalcemia.

  - *Tertiary hyperparathyroidism* is seen most often in chronic renal failure, and results from parathyroid gland hyperplasia and loss of response to serum calcium levels.

- Excess PTH affects the kidneys and bones, resulting in the following:

  - Increased resorption of calcium and excretion of phosphorus by the kidneys

  - Increased bicarbonate excretion and decreased acid excretion by the kidneys

  - Increased calcium and phosphorus release from the bones

  - Soft-tissue deposits of calcium and renal stone formation

Cause

- Primary hyperparathyroidism is caused by intrinsic pathology of the parathyroid glands, including benign adenoma (the most common), hyperplasia, and carcinoma.

Manifestations

Most patients are asymptomatic. Manifestations may include the following:

- Renal: polyuria, polydipsia, renal calculi
- Musculoskeletal: backache, arthralgia, deformity, pathologic fracture, muscle weakness, atrophy
- Central nervous system: paresthesias, fatigue, depression, psychosis, coma
- Gastrointestinal tract: nausea, anorexia, constipation, epigastric pain, peptic ulcers
- Cardiovascular: dysrhythmias, hypertension
- Metabolic: acidosis, weight loss
- Skin: subcutaneous calcification with necrosis

Diagnostic Tests

- Serum calcium is increased in primary and tertiary hyperparathyroidism and decreased in the secondary form.
- Serum phosphorus is decreased in primary hyperparathyroidism and increased in the secondary form.
- Serum PTH is increased.
- Alkaline phosphatase is increased.
- X-rays reveal diffuse demineralization.

Interdisciplinary Management

- Saline fluids are administered intravenously.
- Diuretics are administered to increase renal excretion of calcium.
- Oral or intravenous phosphates and intravenous calcitonin, which reduce calcium levels more rapidly, may be appropriate. Bisphosphonates are prescribed to facilitate movement of calcium into bone and to reduce its release.

- Calcimimetics increase sensitivity of calcium-sensing receptors to serum calcium, thereby decreasing the secretion of PTH, resulting in reduced serum calcium and phosphorous levels.

- The treatment of primary hyperparathyroidism is surgical removal of the parathyroid gland(s) affected by hyperplasia or adenoma.

Selected Nursing Diagnoses with Interventions

Risk for Excess Fluid Volume

- Monitor intake and output carefully.

- Monitor serum calcium levels.

- Monitor vital signs and mental status, and assess for signs of heart failure.

- Administer medications as prescribed.

Risk for Injury

- Provide postoperative care for a patient having parathyroid surgery:

  - Monitor vital signs and serum calcium frequently.

  - Check neck dressing front and back for excessive drainage and bleeding.

  - Assess for respiratory distress caused by hemorrhage or tissue swelling. Keep an emergency tracheostomy tray, oxygen, and suction equipment at bedside.

  - Monitor for signs of hypocalcemia, such as tingling and twitching of the face, and for Trousseau's and Chvostek's signs.

  - Administer calcium and vitamin D as prescribed.

Community-Based Care

- Explain manifestations of hypercalcemia and hypocalcemia.

- Preoperatively, review neck positioning and movement to prevent stress on suture line and to diminish pain.

- Show how to do wound care.

- Stress the need for long-term follow-up medical care.

- Assess the home environment for safety if significant bone demineralization has occurred.

H

- The patient with impaired physical mobility may require a referral to a home health nurse.

For more information on hyperparathyroidism, see Chapter 19 in *Medical-Surgical Nursing,* Fifth Edition, by LeMone, Burke, and Bauldoff.

HYPERSENSITIVITY

Overview

- Hypersensitivity is a harmful altered immune response to an antigen.
- Four different mechanisms may cause hypersensitivity disorders:
  - Type I (immunoglobulin E [IgE]-mediated hypersensitivity)
  - Type II (cytotoxic hypersensitivity)
  - Type III (immune complex-mediated hypersensitivity)
  - Type IV (delayed hypersensitivity)
- IgE-mediated hypersensitivity causes a local or systemic response to a previously encountered antigen to which IgE has been formed and attached to mast cells. The antigen binds to IgE on mast cells, which then release histamine and other chemical mediators, complement, acetylcholine, kinins, and chemotactic factors.
  - Anaphylaxis is an acute systemic type I response that can occur following exposure to the antigen, usually by injection. Histamine and other mediators cause vasodilation and increased capillary permeability, smooth-muscle contraction, and bronchial constriction, which can lead to impaired tissue perfusion and hypotension (anaphylactic shock).
- Cytotoxic hypersensitivity occurs when an antibody attaches to antigens on body cells. This binding leads to phagocytosis, killer cell activity, or complement-mediated lysis of the cell.
- Immune complex-mediated hypersensitivity results when antigen, antibody, and complement proteins interact to form huge complexes that are deposited in tissues. Polymorphonuclear leukocytes are attracted to the area, congregate, and cause local damage.

- Delayed (cell-mediated) hypersensitivity responses are antibody-independent responses of T lymphocytes. Antigen stimulates T cells to secrete lymphokines which then induce inflammation and attract macrophages that release additional inflammatory mediators.
- Latex allergy is a type IV cell-mediated response that can progress to a type I systemic (anaphylactic) response without warning.

Causes

Type I

- Allergens: pollen, dust, molds, dander, insect venom
- Foods: eggs, seafood, nuts, grains, beans, chocolate, sulfite additives
- Antibiotics: penicillin, cephalosporins, sulfonamides, amphotericin B, nitrofurantoin
- Salicylates: acetylsalicylic acid (aspirin)
- Local anesthetics: lidocaine, Xylocaine
- Hormones: exogenous insulin, parathyroid hormone, vasopressin
- Enzymes: chymotrypsin, trypsin, penicillinase
- Diagnostic agents: sodium dehydrocholate, sulfobromophthalein
- Venoms: bee, yellow jacket, wasp, hornet, ant
- Vaccines/serums: antilymphocyte globulin

Type II

- Foreign tissue or cells (e.g., transfusion reaction)
- Drug reaction (e.g., chlorpromazine)
- Endogenous antigens leading to autoimmune disorders such as Goodpasture's syndrome, Hashimoto's thyroiditis, and autoimmune hemolytic anemia

Type III

- Drugs such as penicillin and sulfonamides
- Streptococcal infection
- Inhaled antigens such as dust from moldy hay or pigeon feces
- Systemic lupus erythematosus

Type IV

- Contact dermatitis (e.g., poison ivy)
- Tuberculin reaction
- Foreign tissue grafts such as bone marrow or organ transplants

Latex Allergy

- Persistent exposure to latex: latex gloves, inhalation of corn-starch used to powder latex gloves
- Latex-containing products: balloons, condoms, rubber bands, latex paint

H Manifestations

Type I

- Localized responses: asthma, allergic rhinitis (runny nose; itchy, watery eyes), conjunctivitis, diarrhea or vomiting, atopic dermatitis
- Generalized responses: urticaria (hives); sense of foreboding or uneasiness; lightheadedness; itching palms and scalp; swelling of eyelids, lips, tongue, hands, feet, and genitals; laryngeal edema; bronchial constriction with stridor, wheezing, air hunger, and cough; hypotension and possible shock

Type II

- Type II manifestations relate to specific tissues involved.
- For hemolytic disorders (transfusion reaction): fever, chills, dyspnea, chest pain, urticaria, rash, tachycardia/hypotension, back pain, hematuria, headache.

Type III

- Type III manifestations relate to a specific disorder.
- Serum sickness: urticaria, rash, edema (face, neck, joints), fever.
- Glomerulonephritis: decreased glomerular filtration rate, azotemia, hypertension, coffee-colored urine, oliguria/anuria.
- Systemic lupus erythematosus: multiple (see Systemic Lupus Erythematosus).
- Farmers' lung: fever, chills, malaise, cough, dyspnea.

Type IV

- Contact dermatitis (e.g., poison ivy): itching, erythema, vesicular lesions
- Tuberculin reaction: induration at injection site
- Graft-versus-host disease: fever, rash, nausea, vomiting, diarrhea, bleeding disorders, coma

Latex

- Contact dermatitis (see Type IV manifestations)
- Generalized (systemic) Type I response (see Type I manifestations)

Diagnostic Tests

- Diagnosis mainly depends on history and physical findings.
- White blood cell count with differential is performed to detect possible high levels of circulating eosinophils.
- Radioallergosorbent test may be performed to measure the amount of IgE directed toward specific allergens.
- Blood type and crossmatch are ordered before any anticipated infusions.
- Indirect and direct Coombs' tests are used to detect the presence of antibodies.
- Immune complex assays may be performed to detect the presence of circulating immune complexes. Complement assay also is useful in detecting immune complex disorders.
- A variety of skin tests (patch, prick, intradermal) may be used to determine the causes of hypersensitivity reactions. Food allergy tests are conducted if the patient is suspected of having a food allergy but the implicated food item has not been clearly identified.

Interdisciplinary Management

- Immunotherapy, injections of an extract of the allergen(s) in gradually increasing doses, is used for allergic rhinitis, asthma, and reactions to insect venom.
- Other drugs include antihistamines, cromolyn sodium, and glucocorticoids. Parenteral epinephrine is used for immediate treatment of anaphylaxis.

- Endotracheal intubation or emergency tracheostomy may be required to maintain airway patency in severe laryngospasm.

- Plasmapheresis, removal of harmful components in the plasma, may be used to treat immune complex responses.

Selected Nursing Diagnoses with Interventions

Ineffective Airway Clearance

- Place in Fowler's to high Fowler's position.

- Administer oxygen per nasal cannula at a rate of 2 to 4 L per minute.

- Assess airway: Observe for respiratory rate and pattern, level of consciousness and anxiety, nasal flaring, use of accessory muscles of respiration, chest wall movement, audible stridor; palpate respiratory excursion; auscultate lung sounds and any adventitious sounds, such as wheezes.

- Insert a nasopharyngeal or oropharyngeal airway, and arrange for immediate intubation as indicated.

- Administer parenteral epinephrine (subcutaneous or intramuscular 1:1,000, or intravenous [IV] 1:100,000), as ordered. Repeat in 20 to 30 minutes if necessary. Administer parenteral diphenhydramine as prescribed.

- Provide calm reassurance, as anxiety can increase the respiratory rate, making breathing less effective.

Decreased Cardiac Output

- Monitor vital signs frequently, assessing for changes such as a fall in blood pressure, decreasing pulse pressure, tachycardia, and tachypnea.

- Assess skin color, temperature, capillary refill, edema, and other indicators of peripheral perfusion.

- Monitor level of consciousness.

- Insert one or more large-bore IV catheters.

- Administer warmed IV solutions, such as lactated Ringer's or normal saline, as prescribed.

- Insert an indwelling catheter, and monitor urinary output frequently.

- Place a tourniquet above the site of injected venom and infiltrate the site with epinephrine as prescribed.

- Once airway and breathing are established, place patient flat with legs elevated.

- As status begins to improve, assess for shortness of breath and crackles in the lungs.

High Risk for Injury

- The risk for adverse immunologic response and injury is significant during a blood transfusion, a transplant of living tissue.

- Obtain and record a thorough history of previous blood transfusions and any reactions experienced, no matter how mild.

- Check for a signed informed consent to administer blood or blood products.

- Using two licensed healthcare professionals double-check the type, Rh factor, crossmatch, and expiration date for all blood and blood components received from the blood bank with the patient's data.

- Administer blood within 30 minutes of its delivery from the blood bank.

- Take and record vital signs within 15 minutes before initiating the blood transfusion.

- Using an 18-gauge catheter or larger, infuse blood into a site separate from other IV infusions.

- Administer 50 mL of blood during the first 15 minutes of the transfusion.

- During transfusion, assess for complaints of back or chest pain, temperature increase of more than 1.8°F, chills, tachycardia, tachypnea, wheezing, hypotension, hives, rashes, or cyanosis.

- Stop transfusion immediately if a reaction occurs, no matter how mild. Keep IV line open with normal saline. Notify the physician and the blood bank.

- If a reaction is suspected, send the blood and administration set to the laboratory along with a freshly drawn blood sample and urine sample from the patient.

- If no adverse reaction occurs, administer the transfusion within a 4-hour period.

Community-Based Care

- Explain how to identify possible offending allergens. Discuss possible strategies to avoid these allergens. Refer patients with food allergies to a dietitian.

- Review use of prescription and nonprescription antihistamines and decongestants for symptom relief.

- For patients anticipating surgery, discuss the advantages of autologous blood transfusion and "banking" their own blood prior to surgery.

- Encourage the patient who experiences an anaphylactic reaction to wear a MedicAlert bracelet or necklace at all times identifying the substance(s) that provoke the response.

- Encourage to carry an anaphylaxis kit, and teach the patient and significant others how to inject the medication and use the inhaler.

- Teach patients who have undergone an organ transplant to be alert for and to promptly report signs and symptoms of rejection.

For more information about hypersensitivity, see Chapter 13 in *Medical-Surgical Nursing,* Fifth Edition, by LeMone, Burke, and Bauldoff.

HYPERTENSION

Overview

- Hypertension is a persistently elevated systemic blood pressure. It affects 1 in 3 (over 73 million) people in the United States.

- Primary hypertension, which has no identified cause, is the most common type (> 90%). Secondary hypertension, elevated blood pressure resulting from an identifiable disease process, accounts for only 5% to 10% of identified cases.

- Hypertension usually develops in middle-aged and older adults. Its prevalence is significantly higher in Blacks than in Whites and Hispanics.

- Hypertension is defined as systolic blood pressure of 140 mmHg or higher, or diastolic pressure of 90 mmHg or higher, based on the average of three or more readings taken on separate occasions.

- Factors regulating cardiac output and systemic vascular resistance that are thought to contribute to hypertension include the following:
  1. Sympathetic nervous system overactivity
  2. Renin-angiotensin-aldosterone system overactivity
  3. Chemical mediators of vasomotor tone and blood volume
  4. Interaction between insulin resistance and endothelial function
- Sustained hypertension accelerates atherosclerosis development, increases left ventricular work, and can lead to nephrosclerosis and renal insufficiency.
- *Malignant hypertension* is a medical emergency, marked by a diastolic pressure greater than 120 mmHg. Unless promptly treated, malignant hypertension damages walls of the arterioles and renal blood vessels, and may lead to intravascular coagulation and acute renal failure.

Causes

Primary Hypertension

Although the cause is unknown, a number of risk factors have been identified:

- Family history
- Age: middle-aged and older adults
- Race: highest incidence and severity in Blacks
- High-sodium intake, and low potassium, calcium, and magnesium intakes
- Obesity: central obesity is a greater risk factor than body mass index
- Insulin resistance and hyperinsulinemia
- Excess alcohol consumption
- Stress: physical and emotional

Secondary Hypertension

- Kidney disease
- Coarctation of the aorta
- Endocrine disorders

- Neurologic disorders
- Drugs such as estrogen and oral contraceptives, cocaine, and methamphetamines
- Pregnancy

Manifestations

- Prehypertension: systolic 120 to 139 or diastolic 80 to 89
- Stage 1: systolic 140 to 159 or diastolic 90 to 99
- Stage 2: systolic $\geq$ 160 or diastolic $\geq$ 100
- Asymptomatic in early stages
- Headache (back of the head and neck) on awakening
- Nocturia
- Confusion and visual disturbances
- Narrowed arterioles, hemorrhages, exudates, and papilledema of retina

Diagnostic Tests

- Urinalysis, complete blood cell count, blood chemistry including electrolytes, blood urea nitrogen, and creatinine, glucose, and cholesterol are done to establish baseline values and rule out secondary causes.
- Electrocardiogram and chest x-ray may be done to evaluate possible effects of hypertension.

Interdisciplinary Management

- Hypertension treatment is based on the stage of the disease and risk factors for long-term consequences of elevated blood pressure.
- Lifestyle modifications are recommended for all persons with hypertension, including weight loss; limited alcohol intake; aerobic exercise for 30 to 45 minutes five or more days/week; low-sodium, low-saturated fat, and low-cholesterol diet with adequate calcium and potassium; smoking cessation; stress management.
- Current pharmacologic treatment of hypertension includes use of one or more of the following categories of drugs: diuretics,

beta-adrenergic blockers, angiotensin-converting enzyme inhibitors, angiotensin receptor blockers, centrally acting sympatholytics, vasodilators, and calcium channel blockers.

Selected Nursing Diagnoses with Interventions

Ineffective Health Maintenance

- Assist to identify current behaviors that contribute to hypertension.
- Assist in developing a realistic health maintenance plan.

Risk for Noncompliance

- Inquire about reasons for noncompliance with recommended treatment plan. Listen openly and without judging.
- Evaluate knowledge of hypertension, its long-term effects, and treatment. Provide additional information and reinforce teaching as needed.
- Assess factors contributing to noncompliance, such as adverse drug effects. Suggest measures to manage adverse effects or, if indicated, contact the primary care provider about possible alternative drugs.
- Assist to develop realistic short-term goals for lifestyle changes.

Imbalanced Nutrition: More than Body Requirements

- Assess usual daily food intake, and discuss possible contributing factors to excess weight, such as sedentary lifestyle, or using food as a reward or stress reliever. Inquire about exercise patterns and previous weight-reduction efforts.
- Mutually determine a realistic target weight (e.g., loss of 10% of current body weight over a 6-month period). Regularly monitor weight. Encourage a system of nonfood rewards for achieving small, incremental goals.
- Refer to a dietitian for information about low-fat, low-kilocalorie foods and eating plans. Focus on changing eating habits as opposed to "following a diet."
- Recommend participating in an approved weight-loss program such as Weight Watchers, Overeaters Anonymous, or Take Off Pounds Sensibly (also called TOPS).

Excess Fluid Volume

- Monitor blood pressure and other vital signs as indicated: every 1 to 2 hours or more frequently during acute hypertensive states; once a week or more frequently during initial treatment in the community.

- Monitor intake and output, and weigh daily or weekly.

- Monitor for peripheral edema.

- Monitor laboratory values, such as blood urea nitrogen, urine specific gravity, creatinine, electrolytes, and hematocrit and hemoglobin.

- Refer to a dietitian for teaching about a restricted sodium diet.

Community-Based Care

- Stress the importance of adhering to prescribed medication regimen and recommended diet, limiting alcohol intake, avoiding smoking, and exercising regularly.

- Teach stress-reduction methods such as meditation, relaxation, and deep breathing.

- Encourage frequent follow-up visits.

- Review self-monitoring of blood pressure and suggest the patient keep a daily log.

- Advise to report adverse effects of medications to the physician. Instruct not to discontinue taking the medication unless instructed to do so by the physician.

- A referral to a smoking cessation program, weight-loss program, or cardiovascular fitness program may be appropriate.

For more information on hypertension, see Chapter 32 in *Medical-Surgical Nursing,* Fifth Edition, by LeMone, Burke, and Bauldoff.

HYPERTHYROIDISM (THYROTOXICOSIS)

Overview

- Hyperthyroidism is an endocrine disorder resulting from excess thyroid hormone (TH).

- Increased TH levels increase protein, carbohydrate, and fat metabolism in most body tissues and heighten sympathetic nervous system response to stimulation.

- Heart rate and stroke volume increase.
- The hypermetabolic effects of excess TH result in caloric and nutritional deficiencies.
- The hypermetabolic state increases heat production, mainly by skeletal muscles.
- The most common cause of hyperthyroidism is Graves' disease.
- Thyroid crisis (also called thyroid storm) is an acute and profound rise in TH that is life threatening.

Causes

- Graves' disease: an autoimmune disorder in which antibodies (thyroid-stimulating immunoglobulin) act on the thyroid-stimulating hormone (TSH) receptor, stimulating it; normal feedback regulation is lost.
- Toxic nodular goiter: small discrete, independently functioning nodules within the thyroid gland secrete TH.
- Secondary hyperthyroidism: caused by excess TSH secretion from the pituitary gland.
- Iatrogenic hyperthyroidism: the result of excess exogenous thyroid medication given for hypothyroidism; may be unintentional or intentional.

Manifestations

Hyperthyroidism

- Hyperpyrexia, sweating, heat intolerance
- Nervousness, tremors, irritability
- Increased appetite with weight loss
- Tachycardia, palpitations, dysrhythmias
- Hypertension, bounding pulse
- Warm, flushed skin
- Friable nails, onycholysis
- Muscle fatigue, weakness
- Cardiomegaly, high-output heart failure

Graves' Disease

- Manifestations of hyperthyroidism
- Goiter: smooth, symmetric
- Exophthalmos

Diagnostic Tests

- T_3/T_4 levels are elevated.
- Radioactive iodine (^{131}I) uptake test (thyroid scan) reveals increased ^{131}I uptake.
- TSH level is decreased with primary types of hyperthyroidism; increased with hyperpituitarism.
- TSI autoantibodies are positive.

Interdisciplinary Management

- Antithyroid medications (methimazole, carbimazole, propyl-thiouracil) reduce TH production.
- Radioactive iodine (^{131}I) damages or destroys thyroid tissue so that it produces less TH.
- Iodine (Lugol's solution, potassium iodide) inhibits synthesis and release of TH.
- A subtotal thyroidectomy is performed on patients with breathing or swallowing problems caused by an enlarged thyroid (goiter).

Selected Nursing Diagnoses with Interventions

Risk for Decreased Cardiac Output

- Monitor blood pressure, pulse rate and rhythm, respiratory rate, and breath sounds. Assess for peripheral edema, jugular vein distention, and increased activity intolerance.
- Provide an environment that is cool and as free of distraction as possible. Decrease stress by explaining interventions and teaching relaxation procedures.
- Balance activity with rest periods.

Disturbed Sensory Perception: Visual

- Monitor visual acuity, photophobia, integrity of the cornea, and lid closure if exophthalmos.

- Teach the patient measures for protecting the eye from injury and maintaining visual acuity.

Risk for Imbalanced Nutrition: Less than Body Requirements

- Weigh at the same time.

- Encourage a diet high in carbohydrates and protein.

- Monitor nutritional status through laboratory data.

Disturbed Body Image

- Encourage the patient to verbalize feelings about self and to ask questions about the illness and treatment.

- Provide reliable information and clarify misconceptions.

- Encourage significant others to ask questions about changes they have noticed. Explain the effects of the illness on the patient's physical and emotional status.

Community-Based Care

- Explain the need for lifelong treatment if taking oral medications. Also review medication regimen, effects, and side effects.

- Relate the necessity to consume a diet high in carbohydrates and protein, including between-meal snacks. Caloric intake may need to be increased to 4,000 kcal per day if weight loss exceeds 10% to 20% for height and frame.

- Review the manifestations of hyperthyroidism and hypothyroidism.

- Discuss the risks and benefits of surgery versus radioactive iodine therapy.

- Tell the postoperative patient to inspect the wound for redness, tenderness, swelling, and drainage, and to report temperature elevation, sore throat, or other symptoms of infection.

- Stress the importance of follow-up visits with the physician.

- Arrange for a dietary consultation.

- Depending on the age of the patient and the support systems available, referral to a home health agency may be necessary.

For more information on hyperthyroidism, see Chapter 19 in *Medical-Surgical Nursing,* Fifth Edition, by LeMone, Burke, and Bauldoff.

HYPOGLYCEMIA

Overview

- Hypoglycemia is a blood glucose level of less than 60 mg/dL.
- The brain normally uses glucose as its major fuel; if blood glucose remains low, serious and permanent damage to neurons may occur.
- Damage to neurons may affect cognitive (memory, learning) or motor function.
- A prolonged state of severe hypoglycemia may be fatal.

Causes

In people with diabetes mellitus:

- Excess insulin (insulin reaction/shock)
- Excess oral hypoglycemic agent
- Insufficient food for the dose of insulin or hypoglycemic agent that has been taken
- Vomiting
- Excessive exercise

Other:

- Endogenous insulin secreted out of phase
- Dumping syndrome: status post-gastrectomy
- Drug ingestion (pentamidine)
- Pancreatic tumor
- Hepatitis
- Renal disease
- Idiopathic

Manifestations

- Headache

- Hunger
- Tachycardia
- Skin changes: diaphoresis (cold sweat), pallor
- Motor changes: weakness, tremors, ataxia, "drunk" appearance, slurred speech, hemiplegia
- Behavior changes: irritability, apprehension, combativeness, confusion
- Coma

Diagnostic Tests

- Plasma glucose < 60 mg/dL.
- Plasma insulin levels may define degree of hypoglycemic episode.
- Five-hour glucose tolerance test is used to define phase of insulin secretion.

Interdisciplinary Management

- Treat primary underlying disorder (e.g., administer intravenous glucose to patients with diabetes).
- For pancreatic tumors, surgical resection or treatment with diazoxide and octreotide may be necessary.

Selected Nursing Diagnoses with Interventions

Imbalanced Nutrition: Less than Body Requirements

- Monitor for signs of hypoglycemia: change in mental status, diaphoresis, and cool, clammy skin.
- Provide quiet, darkened environment conducive to rest.
- Provide a source of glucose: orange juice, candy, glucagon, 50% glucose.
- Provide small, frequent meals.

Ineffective Management of Therapeutic Regimen

- Monitor blood glucose levels carefully.
- Teach the signs and symptoms of hyperglycemia and hypoglycemia.

- Explain self-management of medications, insulin, diet, and exercise and the correlations between these factors.

Community-Based Care

- Review glucose self-monitoring.
- Referral to a dietitian for long-term nutritional support and follow-up may be appropriate.
- The patient may require referral to social services or a psychological counselor for coping mechanisms for managing a chronic illness.
- Provide information on obtaining a MedicAlert tag.
- Provide information about the American Diabetes Association, if appropriate.

For more information on hypoglycemia, see Chapter 20 in *Medical-Surgical Nursing,* Fifth Edition, by LeMone, Burke, and Bauldoff.

Hypoparathyroidism

Overview

- Hypoparathyroidism is a deficit of parathyroid hormone that results in impaired renal regulation of calcium and phosphate and produces hypocalcemia.
- Hypocalcemia may induce neuromuscular symptoms such as paresthesias, or result in life-threatening tetany.

Causes

- Damage to or inadvertent removal of all the parathyroid glands during thyroidectomy
- Congenital lack of parathyroid gland development
- Radiation to the neck
- Ischemia
- Hypercalcemia
- Hypomagnesemia

Manifestations

- Neuromuscular irritability/increased deep tendon reflexes
- Tetany/carpopedal spasms/abdominal pain
- Cardiac dysrhythmias
- Dysphagia
- Positive Chvostek's sign, Trousseau's sign
- Seizures
- Psychoses
- Dry skin/hair/alopecia
- Brittle/ridged nails
- Weak tooth enamel/dental caries

Diagnostic Tests

- Parathyroid hormone level is reduced.
- Serum calcium level is reduced.
- Serum phosphorus level is increased.
- Electrocardiogram shows increased Q-T interval and ST segment.

Interdisciplinary Management

- Intravenous calcium is given immediately to treat tetany.
- Long-term therapy includes supplemental calcium, increased dietary calcium, and vitamin D therapy.

Selected Nursing Diagnoses with Interventions

Ineffective Protection

- Assess for tetany, muscle cramping, carpopedal spasms, mental changes, Chvostek's sign, and Trousseau's sign.
- Encourage dietary intake of foods high in calcium and low in phosphorus.

Risk for Injury

- Institute seizure precautions.
- Administer medications as prescribed.

Community-Based Care

- Dietary modifications and other aspects of care must be maintained permanently to prevent recurrence.

- Encourage the patient to wear a MedicAlert tag.

- Referral to a home health nurse may be appropriate.

For more information on hypoparathyroidism, see Chapter 19 in *Medical-Surgical Nursing,* Fifth Edition, by LeMone, Burke, and Bauldoff.

HYPOTHYROIDISM

Overview

- Hypothyroidism is an endocrine disorder resulting from thyroid hormone deficit.

- Primary and secondary forms exist.

- Primary (more common): due to congenital defect, treatment of hyperthyroidism, surgery, thyroiditis, or iodine deficiency.

- Secondary form: results from pituitary thyroid-stimulating hormone (TSH) deficiency or peripheral resistance to thyroid hormones.

- Hashimoto's thyroiditis (chronic autoimmune thyroiditis) is the most common form of primary hypothyroidism, in which antibodies develop that destroy thyroid tissue.

- The incidence of hypothyroidism is higher in women and increases after age 50.

- Myxedema is a serious lack of thyroid hormones that produces multiple symptoms.

- Myxedema coma due to profound lack of thyroid hormones is a life-threatening condition.

- Other complications of untreated hypothyroidism include adrenal insufficiency and cardiovascular disorders.

Causes

- Hashimoto's thyroiditis: autoimmune destruction of thyroid follicular cells

- Infection
- Thyroidectomy
- Radiation therapy to the neck
- Antithyroid medication for the treatment of hyperthyroidism
- Reduced TSH from the pituitary gland
- Reduced thyroid-releasing hormone from the hypothalamus
- Iodine deficiency (necessary for TH synthesis and secretion)
- Interferon α or β therapy for chronic Hepatitis C

Manifestations

Hypothyroidism/Myxedema

- Reduced temperature, cool skin, cold intolerance
- Slow pulse and respiratory rate
- Nonpitting generalized edema, puffy face, periorbital edema, enlarged tongue
- Anorexia with weight gain and constipation
- Dry, loose skin; thick, brittle nails; dry, coarse hair; loss of lateral eyebrows
- Forgetfulness, mental dullness, emotional instability

Hashimoto's Thyroiditis

- Manifestations of hypothyroidism/myxedema
- Goiter: diffuse, tender

Myxedema Coma

- Progressive reduction in level of consciousness to coma
- Hypothermia
- Bradycardia, hypoventilation, hypotension
- Hypoglycemia
- Hyponatremia

Diagnostic Tests

- T_3/T_4 levels are decreased.

- TSH is increased if due to primary thyroid malfunction; decreased if due to pituitary malfunction.

Interdisciplinary Management

- Hypothyroidism is treated with medications that replace thyroid hormone.
- If the patient has a goiter large enough to cause respiratory difficulties or dysphagia, a subtotal thyroidectomy may be performed.

Selected Nursing Diagnoses with Interventions

Decreased Cardiac Output

- Assess blood pressure, rate and rhythm of apical and peripheral pulses, respiratory rate, and breath sounds.
- Prevent chilling; increase room temperature, use additional bed covers, avoid drafts.
- Alternate activity with rest periods. Ask the patient to report any breathing difficulties, chest pain, heart palpitations, or dizziness.

Constipation

- Encourage fluids up to 2,000 mL per day. If kilocalorie intake is restricted, ensure that liquids have no kilocalories or are low in kilocalories.
- Encourage activity as tolerated.

Risk for Impaired Skin Integrity

- Monitor skin for redness or lesions, especially if activity is greatly reduced.
- Turn, reposition, and use pillows, pads, or cushions to prevent tissue ischemia.
- Teach and implement a schedule of range-of-motion exercises.
- Use alcohol-free skin oils and lotions, and use gentle motions when washing and drying skin.

Community-Based Care

- Explain the importance of maintaining a high-fiber diet.

- Teach to assess skin for lesions, use warm (not hot) water when cleansing, and take showers rather than baths.

- Review medication regimen, including effects and side effects, and ask physician before taking any nonprescription drug.

- Stress the importance of lifelong monitoring and care.

- Provide information on obtaining a MedicAlert tag.

- Refer to social services or home health services as appropriate.

For more information on hypothyroidism, see Chapter 19 in *Medical-Surgical Nursing,* Fifth Edition, by LeMone, Burke, and Bauldoff.

H

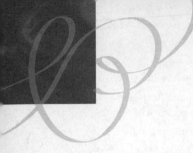

INCREASED INTRACRANIAL PRESSURE

Overview

- Increased intracranial pressure (IICP) (or intracranial hypertension) is sustained elevated pressure (10 mmHg or higher) within the cranial cavity.

- The cranium is a closed vault with a constant volume and pressure; increased volume for any reason results in increased pressure.

- When pressure within the cranium rises above normal, it exerts a damaging force on central nervous system neurons and their blood vessels. IICP of great magnitude and/or duration is a life-threatening condition.

- Initially, pressure forces move cerebrospinal fluid (CSF) into the spinal canal or arachnoid veins. As this adaptive mechanism fails, cranial perfusion is reduced, causing brain hypoxia, ischemia, and necrosis.

- Reduced blood flow stimulates an excitatory response (Cushing's reaction) of the central nervous system cardioregulatory center, significantly increasing the blood pressure.

- Unrelieved IICP eventually causes the brainstem to herniate through the foramen magnum, a fatal complication.

Causes

- Bleeding/hemorrhage/hematoma: intracranial, subarachnoid, subdural, epidural

- Neoplasms: benign or malignant

- Abscess/cyst formation

- Cerebral edema: infection, trauma, surgery

- Hydrocephalus: obstructed CSF flow

Manifestations

- Neurologic: Decreasing level of consciousness: drowsiness to coma (use Glasgow coma scale), seizures
- Pupil/vision changes: unequal/sluggish pupillary responses, diplopia, papilledema
- Motor changes: hemiparesis, ataxia, slurred speech, aphasia, decorticate or decerebrate posturing
- Cardiovascular: bradycardia; hypertension with increased/widened pulse pressure; dysrhythmias; increased mean arterial pressure (MAP)
- Respiratory: altered rate, depth, pattern; labored effort
- General: headache, projectile vomiting, restlessness, irritability, combativeness

Diagnostic Tests

- Skull x-ray can show fracture and/or tissue shifting.
- Computed tomography scan or magnetic resonance imaging may show ischemia/necrosis or subdural, epidural, or intracranial hematomas.
- Cerebral angiogram may reveal abnormal vascular anatomy.

Interdisciplinary Management

- Osmotic diuretics and mannitol are commonly used to reduce intracranial pressure (ICP).
- Other medications include barbiturates to induce coma and anticonvulsants to manage seizures.
- Various intracranial surgical procedures (Burr holes, craniotomy) may be used to relieve pressure and treat the underlying cause.
- ICP monitoring facilitates continual assessment of ICP.

Selected Nursing Diagnoses with Interventions

Ineffective Tissue Perfusion: Cerebral

- Assess for and report indicators of IICP every 1 to 2 hours and as necessary, including level of consciousness, behavior, motor/sensory functions, pupillary size and reaction to light, and vital signs.
- Elevate the head of the bed 30 degrees (or as prescribed). Maintain the head and neck in the neutral plane, and avoid

hyperextension or exaggerated neck flexion. Avoid the prone position. Avoid extreme hip flexion.

- Assess for bladder distention and bowel constipation. Administer stool softeners and use manual techniques or catheterization as needed to prevent urinary retention.

- Provide assistance to prevent Valsalva when turning, moving in bed, or defecating.

- Space nursing care activities. Provide rest periods between procedures.

- Provide a quiet, calm environment. Caution visitors to avoid unpleasant conversations or those that may be emotionally stimulating to the patient.

- Maintain fluid restrictions if prescribed.

- For the patient on mechanical ventilation, maintain airway patency, preoxygenate and hyperventilate with 100% oxygen before suctioning, and limit suctioning to 10 seconds.

- Monitor arterial blood gases; report negative trends.

Risk for Infection

- Keep dressings over the ICP catheter dry, and change dressings per protocol.

- Monitor insertion site for CSF leakage, drainage, or infection.

- Monitor for manifestations of infection, including vital sign changes, chills, increased white blood cell count, and positive cultures of drainage.

- Use strict aseptic technique when caring for or using the device, and check drainage system for loose connections.

Community-Based Care

Provide instructions on the following for the patient and significant others:

- The disease process, treatment, and rehabilitation.

- Avoid coughing, blowing the nose, straining to have a bowel movement, pushing against the bed rails, or performing isometric exercises.

- Maintain head and neck alignment when resting in bed.

- Frequent rest periods.

- Avoid conversations that may be upsetting to the patient.
- Refer to social services, counseling, pastoral services, or a home health nursing service as appropriate.

For more information on increased intracranial pressure, see Chapter 42 in *Medical-Surgical Nursing,* Fifth Edition, by LeMone, Burke, and Bauldoff.

INFLUENZA

Overview

- Influenza, or *flu,* is a highly contagious viral respiratory disease that usually occurs in epidemics or pandemics (global epidemics).
- The virus is transmitted by airborne droplet and direct contact. Its incubation period is 18 to 72 hours.
- The virus infects the respiratory epithelium. Inflammation leads to necrosis and shedding of respiratory epithelial cells.
- Respiratory epithelial necrosis increases the risk for secondary bacterial infections such as sinusitis, otitis media, and pneumonia.
- Influenza pneumonia is a rare but serious complication that progresses rapidly and can cause hypoxemia and death within a few days. Bacterial pneumonia is more likely to occur in older adults and people with chronic disease.
- Reye's syndrome is a rare but potentially fatal complication of influenza usually associated with influenza B virus.

Causes

- The three major strains are influenza A virus, influenza B virus, and influenza C virus. Influenza A causes most infections and severe outbreaks, primarily because it can mutate to avoid existing immune defenses to the virus.

Manifestations

- Abrupt onset of chills and fever, malaise, muscle aches, and headache
- Respiratory: dry, nonproductive cough that may persist for days to weeks, sore throat, substernal burning, coryza (runny nose)

- May develop manifestations of lower respiratory infection (see Pneumonia)

Diagnostic Tests

- Diagnosis is based on history, clinical findings, and presence of influenza in the community.
- Chest x-ray and white blood cell (WBC) count may be done to rule out complications such as pneumonia. The WBC count is commonly decreased in influenza; bacterial infections usually cause an increase in WBC.

Interdisciplinary Management

- Yearly immunization with influenza vaccine is the single most important measure to prevent or minimize manifestations of influenza.
- Amantadine or rimantadine may be used for prophylaxis in unvaccinated people who are exposed to the virus.
- Amantadine, rimantadine, and the antiviral drugs zanamivir, oseltamivir, and ribavirin also may be used to reduce the duration and severity of flu symptoms. Analgesics such as aspirin and acetaminophen provide symptomatic relief of fever and muscle aches.
- Antibiotics are not indicated unless secondary bacterial infection occurs.

Selected Nursing Diagnoses with Interventions

Ineffective Breathing Pattern

- Monitor respiratory rate, pattern, and other vital signs such as pulse rate and temperature.
- Pace activities to provide for periods of rest.
- Elevate the head of the bed.

Ineffective Airway Clearance

- Monitor cough effectiveness and ability to clear airway secretions.
- Maintain adequate hydration. Assess mucous membranes and skin turgor for evidence of dehydration.
- Increase the humidity of inspired air with a bedside humidifier.
- Teach effective cough techniques.

Disturbed Sleep Pattern

- Assess sleep patterns using subjective and objective information.
- Place in semi-Fowler's or Fowler's position for sleep.
- Provide antipyretic and analgesic medications at or shortly before bedtime.
- If necessary, request a cough suppressant medication for night-time use.

Community-Based Care

- Stress the importance of yearly influenza vaccination for patients in high-risk groups and their significant others.
- Teach how the disease is spread, and measures to reduce the risk of contracting influenza, such as avoiding crowds and persons who are ill.
- Encourage appropriate self-care, including hand hygiene and covering mouth when coughing, importance of adequate rest, and use of nonprescription medications.
- Teach about the possible complications of influenza and their manifestations. Tell patients to report complications promptly to the physician.

For more information on influenza, see Chapter 35 in *Medical-Surgical Nursing*, Fifth Edition, by LeMone, Burke, and Bauldoff.

INTESTINAL OBSTRUCTION

Overview

- Intestinal obstruction is failure of intestinal contents to move through the bowel lumen.
- Although either the large or small bowel may be affected, about 85% of bowel obstructions occur in the small intestine.
- Intestinal obstructions may be either mechanical or functional.
  1. Mechanical obstructions may be partial or complete, caused by problems outside or within the intestine. In some mechanical obstructions (e.g., strangulated hernia), blood supply to the bowel is impaired, leading to necrosis and bacterial peritonitis.

2. Functional obstruction occurs when peristalsis fails to propel intestinal contents. Adynamic ileus (paralytic ileus or simple ileus) is the most common functional obstruction.

- When obstruction occurs, gas and fluid accumulate proximal to and within the obstructed segment, distending the bowel.
- Significant bowel distention, vomiting, and third spacing of fluids in the bowel and peritoneal cavity can lead to massive loss of fluids and electrolytes.
- Hypovolemia and hypovolemic shock with multiple organ dysfunction is a significant, potentially fatal, complication of bowel obstruction.

Causes

Mechanical

- Adhesions (bands of scar tissue)
- Hernias
- Tumors
- Intussusception, volvulus, stricture
- Fecal impaction
- Inflammatory bowel disease

Functional

- Gastrointestinal surgery
- Hemorrhage or bowel ischemia
- Peritonitis
- Organ perforation
- Renal colic, spinal cord injuries, uremia, and electrolyte imbalances
- Drugs such as some narcotics, anticholinergic drugs, and antidiarrheal medications

Manifestations

Small Bowel Obstruction

- Cramping, colicky abdominal pain
- Vomiting, may be feculent (smelling of feces)
- Early mechanical: borborygmi, high-pitched tinkling bowel sounds
- Visible peristaltic waves

- Significantly diminished or absent bowel sounds
- Abdominal distention, tenderness
- Tachycardia, tachypnea, hypotension, and possible fever
- Oliguria

Large Bowel Obstruction

- Constipation
- Deep, cramping abdominal pain
- Distended abdomen
- Possible palpable mass

Diagnostic Tests

- White blood cell count often shows leukocytosis.
- Serum osmolality and urine specific gravity increase with fluid loss; hypokalemia and hypochloremia develop due to vomiting.
- Arterial blood gases may show metabolic alkalosis due to loss of hydrochloric acid from the stomach.
- Abdominal x-ray often shows distended loops of intestine or a distended colon.
- Computed tomography scan can confirm mechanical obstruction.

Interdisciplinary Management

- Ninety percent of partial small bowel obstructions are successfully treated with gastrointestinal decompression using a nasogastric tube.
- Surgical intervention is required for complete mechanical obstructions as well as for strangulated or incarcerate obstructions of the small intestine.

Selected Nursing Diagnoses with Interventions

Deficient Fluid Volume

- Monitor vital signs, pulmonary artery pressures, cardiac output, and central venous pressure hourly.
- Record urinary output hourly and nasogastric suction volume every 2 to 4 hours. Report urine output of less than 30 mL/hour.
- Maintain intravenous fluids and blood volume replacement as prescribed. The amount of fluid administered is calculated to replace losses and meet current fluid needs.

- Measure abdominal girth every 4 to 8 hours. Mark level of measurement on the abdomen.
- Notify the physician of changes in status.

Ineffective Gastrointestinal Perfusion

- Assess skin color, temperature, and capillary refill. Assess bowel sounds every 4 hours.
- Monitor temperature at least every 4 hours, reporting elevation > 100°F.
- Frequently assess pain, reporting significant or abrupt increases or pain unrelieved by prescribed analgesia.
- Maintain nothing-by-mouth status until peristalsis is restored.

Ineffective Breathing Pattern

- Assess respiratory rate, pattern, and lung sounds every 2 to 4 hours.
- Elevate the head of the bed.
- Maintain patency of nasogastric or intestinal suction.
- Assist to use incentive spirometry and with effective cough techniques.
- Provide a pillow or folded bath blanket for use in splinting the abdomen while coughing postoperatively.
- Contact respiratory therapy as indicated.
- Provide good oral care every 2 to 4 hours.

Community-Based Care

- Teach health-promotion activities, such as increasing intake of dietary fiber and fluids, and exercising daily.
- For the patient with recurrent obstructions, discuss their cause, early manifestations, and possible preventive measures.
- Provide routine and specific preoperative teaching as indicated.
- If a temporary colostomy has been created, teach care techniques and discuss planned reanastomoses.
- Teach about wound care.
- Discuss activity level after discharge, return to work, and any other restrictions.
- Discuss dietary measures to prevent future episodes of bowel obstruction if appropriate.

- Provide a list of resources for colostomy and wound care supplies as needed.

- Refer to home nursing care services as appropriate.

For more information on intestinal obstruction, see Chapter 24 in *Medical-Surgical Nursing*, Fifth Edition, by LeMone, Burke, and Bauldoff.

IRRITABLE BOWEL SYNDROME (SPASTIC BOWEL)

Overview

- Irritable bowel syndrome (IBS or spastic bowel or mucous colitis) is a chronic motility disorder of the GI tract characterized by abdominal pain with constipation, diarrhea, or both.

- Central nervous system regulation of the motor and sensory functions of the bowel is altered in IBS.

- Stimuli such as food intake, hormonal influences, and physiologic or psychologic stress lead to increased motor reactivity of the small bowel and colon in IBS.

- Sensory responses from the gut are exaggerated as well, and hypersecretion of colonic mucus is common.

Causes

- Although the cause is unknown, a history of emotional, physical, and sexual abuse correlate with IBS.

Manifestations

- Gastrointestinal: Abdominal pain and/or tenderness over the sigmoid colon, excess gas, and bloating relieved by defecation

- Change in bowel habits:

  1. Diarrhea or constipation

  2. Hard or lumpy, loose or watery stools

  3. Straining, urgency, or a sensation of incomplete evacuation with defecation

  4. Mucus passage

- General: Nausea, vomiting, anorexia, fatigue, headache, depression, or anxiety

Diagnostic Tests

- Stool examination may reveal the presence of mucus, but is negative for blood, ova, and parasites.

- Complete blood cell count is done to rule out infectious or other causes of altered bowel elimination (e.g., tumor).

- Sigmoidoscopy or colonoscopy shows normal bowel mucosa, with increased mucus, marked spasm, and possible hyperemia (increased redness). Intraluminal pressures are often increased.

- A small bowel series and barium enema may show increased motility of the entire gastrointestinal tract.

Interdisciplinary Management

- Bulk-forming laxatives are given to reduce bowel spasm and normalize the number and form of bowel movements. An anticholinergic drug may be ordered to inhibit bowel motility and relieve postprandial abdominal pain. Loperamide or diphenoxylate may be used to prevent diarrhea in selected situations.

- Antidepressant drugs (tricyclics and selective serotonin reuptake inhibitors) may help relieve abdominal pain and diarrhea.

- Dietary measures include additional dietary fiber intake. Limiting intake of the following foods may benefit some patients: milk and milk products; gas-forming foods such as cabbage, bananas, and nuts; foods containing fructose; alcohol; and caffeinated drinks.

Selected Nursing Diagnoses with Interventions

Constipation or Diarrhea

- Assist the patient to identify and reduce or eliminate factors that lead to symptoms.

Ineffective Coping

- Encourage regular exercise to promote bowel elimination and to reduce stress.

Community-Based Care

- Discuss the nature of the disorder and the reality of the symptoms, and discuss the relationship between IBS and stress and anxiety.

- Teach stress- and anxiety-reduction techniques, such as meditation, visualization, exercise, time out, and progressive relaxation.

- Discuss foods that may contribute to IBS and suggest dietary changes, such as additional fiber and water intake.

- Instruct about the use and role of prescribed medications, their adverse effects, and when to contact the physician.

- Discuss the importance of routine follow-up appointments and of notifying the primary care provider if manifestations change.

- Refer to a dietitian for nutritional support and teaching as needed.

- Refer to a counselor or other mental health professional for assistance in dealing with psychologic factors as appropriate.

For more information on irritable bowel syndrome, see Chapter 24 in *Medical-Surgical Nursing,* Fifth Edition, by LeMone, Burke, and Bauldoff.

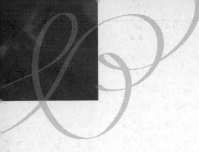

Kaposi's Sarcoma

Overview

- Kaposi's sarcoma (KS) is a malignant neoplasm of blood vessels.
- This opportunistic cancer occurs in people who are immunosuppressed and is the most common cancer associated with AIDS.
- Histologically, an overgrowth of endothelial cells and spindle-shaped cells cause narrowing of vascular lumens and increase the number of blood vessels. Lesions can form anywhere including skin, mucous membranes, and visceral organs; the gastrointestinal tract, lungs, and lymph nodes are most common. Common sites for skin lesions include the palate, toe webs, and the face, especially the tip of the nose and pinnae of the ears.
- KS is locally destructive and rarely invasive or metastatic.

Causes

- KS is caused by the Kaposi sarcoma–associated herpes virus, also known as human herpes virus 8. This virus is readily transmitted by heterosexual and homosexual activities, and via the maternal–infant route.
- People with immunosuppression due to an organ transplant or taking immunosuppressive medications are also at risk of developing KS.

Manifestations

- Skin: early, tiny (1 mm) red to violet macules; painless, non-itchy; progression to larger raised plaques/or nodules; may be edematous or ulcerate, becoming painful. In people with dark skin, lesions appear brown toned.
- Mucous membranes: lesions similar to those on skin; frequently bleed.
- Lymphatic: swollen lymph nodes.

- GI: gastrointestinal bleeding with possible hemorrhage, anemia, and/or obstruction. Gallbladder involvement may result in biliary obstruction/and jaundice.
- Respiratory: Shortness of breath secondary to pulmonary effusion or hemorrhage.

Diagnostic Tests
- Biopsy of lesions is diagnostic.

Interdisciplinaryinter Management
- Rapidly progressing KS is treated with chemotherapy (systemic or intralesional); milder forms may improve with the initiation of highly active antiretroviral therapy (HAART) therapy (a combination of three or more antiretroviral drugs).
- Paclitaxel acts during the G_2 phase to prevent cell division.

Selected Nursing Diagnoses with Interventions

Impaired Skin Integrity
- Assess and monitor progression of lesions. Monitor lesions for signs of infection or impaired healing.
- Institute measures to relieve pressure, such as an air or water mattress, egg-crate mattress, or sheepskin pads. Turn at least every 2 hours, or more frequently if necessary.
- Keep skin clean and dry using mild, nondrying soaps or oils for cleansing. Avoid the use of heat or occlusive dressings.

Fear
- Encourage the patient and significant others to discuss fears and concerns with each other.
- Prepare as appropriate for chemotherapy or radiation treatments.
- Teach patients beginning the HAART protocol regarding the benefits, risks, costs, and effects on leading a normal life.
- Monitor for adherence to HAART therapy; discontinuation or interruption of HAART is considered dangerous.
- Monitor for toxicities associated with Paclitaxel including alopecia, bone marrow depression, and severe hypersensitivity reactions (e.g., hypotension, dyspnea, and urticaria).
- Administer prescribed analgesics for pain.

K

Disturbed Risk for Situational Low Self-Esteem

- Assess negative self-evaluation and statements of self-worth.
- Encourage the patient to express feelings about appearance.
- Monitor for depression, substance abuse, and metabolic syndrome associated with HAART therapy.
- Assist in identifying ways of dressing to cover KS lesions.

Community-Based Care

- Explain the importance of standard precautions, skin care, and wound care if applicable.
- Provide the patient and significant others with information about KS and its transmission. Discuss safer sex practices and use of latex condoms and spermicidal lubricant.
- Explore measures to maintain optimal health, including diet, rest, exercise, and stress reduction.
- Emphasize the importance of long-term follow-up care with the primary physician.
- Refer the patient and significant others to local support groups for persons, partners, and families and friends of persons with HIV as appropriate.
- Provide addresses and phone numbers for local and national information resources and hotlines.
- Refer to social services for help with financial assistance, if needed, for expensive HAART therapy.

For more information on Kaposi's sarcoma, see Chapter 14 in *Medical-Surgical Nursing,* Fifth Edition, by LeMone, Burke, and Bauldoff.

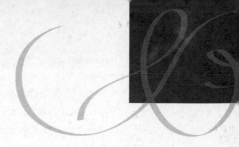

LEGIONNAIRES' DISEASE

Overview

- Legionnaires' disease is a form of bronchopneumonia that occurs sporadically and in outbreaks.

- Consolidation of lung tissue is patchy or lobar.

- The mortality rate is up to 25% without treatment in otherwise healthy people and up to 50% in people who are immunocompromised.

Causes

- *Legionella pneumophila,* a gram-negative bacterium widely found in water, particularly warm standing water.

- Contaminated water-cooled air-conditioning systems and other water sources may spread the disease.

- Risk factors: smoking, increased age, and chronic disease or impaired immune defenses.

Manifestations

- Gradual onset
- Dry cough
- Dyspnea
- General malaise, chills, and fever
- Headache, confusion
- Anorexia and diarrhea
- Muscle and joint pain

Diagnostic Tests

- White blood cell count is significantly increased and increased immature white blood cells are present.

- Sputum Gram stain and culture and sensitivity tests are used to identify the causative organism.
- Arterial blood gases (ABGs) are measured to evaluate gas exchange.
- X-ray shows infiltrates and effusions.
- Direct fluorescent antibody specimen staining is positive.
- Serum indirect fluorescent antibody can detect antibody formed against *Legionella pneumophila.*

Interdisciplinary Management

- Bronchoscopy may be done to obtain a sputum specimen or remove secretions from the bronchial tree.
- Combination antibiotic therapy with erythromycin and rifampin, or a fluoroquinolone antibiotic, is used to treat Legionnaires' disease.
- Bronchodilators are used to relieve bronchospasm. Mucolytic agents and expectorants also may be prescribed.
- Oxygen therapy is indicated if oxygen saturation is low or ABGs reveal hypoxemia.

Selected Nursing Diagnoses with Interventions

Ineffective Airway Clearance

- Assess respiratory status, including vital signs, breath sounds, and skin color, at least every 4 hours.
- Assess cough and sputum.
- Assist to Fowler's position, and to cough, deep breathe, and use assistive devices. Encourage use of incentive spirometry.
- Encourage a fluid intake of at least 2,500 to 3,000 mL per day. Monitor intake and output.
- Administer medications as prescribed and monitor their effects.

Impaired Gas Exchange

- Monitor oxygen saturation and ABGs, reporting abnormal results.
- Administer oxygen therapy as prescribed.

Activity Intolerance

- Encourage to avoid climbing stairs and activities that may increase dyspnea and fatigue.
- Encourage frequent rest periods.

Community-Based Care

- Teach about the disease and its management, including use of medications and the need for rest.

- Teach to avoid crowds, people with colds or flu, and respiratory irritants such as smoke.

- Explain that the course and symptoms of the disease can be prolonged.

- Stress the importance of notifying the physician if chills, fever, persistent cough, dyspnea, hemoptysis, chest pain, or fatigue recur or do not improve.

- Encourage an annual influenza vaccine and a pneumococcal vaccine.

- Refer patients who smoke to a smoking cessation program.

- Provide information about local resources such as the American Lung Association.

For more information on Legionnaires' disease, see Chapter 36 in *Medical-Surgical Nursing,* Fifth Edition, by LeMone, Burke, and Bauldoff.

LEUKEMIA

Acute lymphocytic leukemia (ALL)

Chronic lymphocytic leukemia (CLL)

Acute myeloid leukemia (AML)

Chronic myeloid leukemia (CML)

Overview

- Leukemia is a group of chronic malignant disorders of white blood cells (WBCs) and their cell precursors.

- Leukemias are characterized by replacement of bone marrow by malignant immature WBCs, abnormal immature circulating WBCs, and infiltration of these cells into the liver, spleen, and lymph nodes throughout the body. The usual ratio of red to WBCs is reversed.

- Leukemias are classified by acuity and the predominant cell type involved.

  1. *Acute* leukemias have an acute onset, rapid disease progression, and immature blast cells. *Chronic* leukemias have

a gradual onset, prolonged course, and abnormal mature-appearing cells.

2. *Lymphocytic* (*lymphoblastic*) leukemias involve lymphocytes and their precursor cells. *Myeloid* (*myeloblastic, myelogenous*) leukemias involve myeloid stem cells and interfere with the maturation of all types of blood cells.

- Leukemic cells compete with normal cells in bone marrow, leading to anemia, splenomegaly, bleeding tendencies, and increased risk for infection.

- They infiltrate body tissues such as the central nervous system, testes, skin, gastrointestinal tract, and the lymph nodes, liver, and spleen.

1. AML is characterized by uncontrolled proliferation of myeloblasts. It is the most common adult leukemia. Remission occurs with treatment in 70% of patients; only about 25% achieve cure.

2. CML is characterized by abnormal proliferation of all bone marrow elements. It usually is associated with the Philadelphia chromosome, a translocation of chromosome 22 to chromosome 9. CML causes about 20% of adult leukemias, usually affecting older adults. The disease evolves to acute leukemia in its final stage.

3. ALL is the most common childhood leukemia. It causes abnormal proliferation of lymphoblasts in the bone marrow, lymph nodes, and spleen. Combination chemotherapy produces complete remission in 80% to 90% of adults with ALL.

4. CLL is characterized by proliferation and accumulation of small, abnormal, mature lymphocytes in bone marrow, peripheral blood, and body tissues. It usually affects older adults. It has a slowly progressive course with an average survival of about 7 years.

Causes

- Some leukemias are caused by a retrovirus, human T-cell leukemia/lymphoma virus-1.

- The cause of most leukemias is unknown. Risk factors include the following:

  - Down syndrome and certain other genetic disorders

- Exposure to ionizing radiation and chemicals such as benzene
- Treatment for other cancers

Manifestations

- Pallor, anemia
- Fatigue
- Fever, increased incidence of infection (e.g., herpes zoster)
- Abnormal bleeding (e.g., gingival, epistaxis, petechiae, ecchymosis)
- Weight loss
- Lymphadenopathy
- Hepatomegaly/splenomegaly

Diagnostic Tests

- Complete blood cell count with differential shows low red blood cells, hemoglobin, hematocrit, and platelets, and elevated WBC with an abnormal differential and cells.
- Bone marrow examination shows the presence of leukemic cells.

Interdisciplinary Management

- Single agent or combination chemotherapy is used to eradicate leukemic cells and produce remission in most types of leukemia. Colony stimulating factors often are given to "rescue" the bone marrow following induction chemotherapy.
- Radiation therapy also may be used to prevent the proliferation of leukemic cells.
- Bone marrow transplant (BMT) may be the treatment of choice, used in conjunction with or following chemotherapy or radiation. In *allogenic BMT,* the bone marrow of a healthy donor is infused into the patient; in *autologous BMT,* the patient's own bone marrow is infused.
- Allogeneic stem cell transplant results in complete and sustained replacement of the patient's blood cell lines with cells derived from donor stem cells.
- Biologic therapy with cytokines such as interferons and interleukins may be used to treat some leukemias. These agents modify the response to cancer cells and may be cytotoxic.

Selected Nursing Diagnoses with Interventions

Risk for Infection

- Promptly report fever, chills, throat pain, cough, chest pain, burning on urination, purulent drainage, and other manifestations of infection.

- Institute infection protection measures:

  a. Maintain protective isolation as indicated.

  b. Ensure meticulous hand hygiene among all people in contact with the patient.

  c. Restrict visitors with colds, flu, or infections.

  d. Avoid invasive procedures when possible; when necessary, use strict aseptic technique.

- Monitor vital signs including temperature and oxygen saturation every 4 hours. Report temperature spikes with chilling, tachypnea, tachycardia, restlessness, change in PaO_2, and hypotension.

- Monitor neutrophil levels (measured in mm^3) for relative risk for infection: 2,000 to 2,500, no risk; 1,000 to 2,000, minimal risk; 500 to 1,000, moderate risk; < 500, severe risk.

- Explain infection precautions and restrictions and the temporary nature of these measures.

Impaired Oral Mucous Membrane

- Inspect buccal region, gums, sublingual area, and throat daily for swelling or lesions. Ask about oral pain or burning.

- Culture any oral lesions.

- Assist with mouth care and oral rinses with saline or a solution of hydrogen peroxide and water every 2 to 4 hours. Apply petroleum jelly to the lips to prevent dryness and cracking.

- Encourage use of soft-bristle toothbrush or sponge to clean teeth and gums.

- Administer medications as ordered to treat infection or relieve pain.

- Instruct to avoid alcohol-based mouthwashes, citrus fruit juices, spicy foods, foods that are either very hot or very cold, alcohol, and crusty foods. Suggest bland, cool foods and cool liquids at least every 2 hours.

Ineffective Protection

- Assess for and report bleeding:
  a. Skin and mucous membranes for petechiae, ecchymoses, and purpura
  b. Gums, nasal membranes, and conjunctiva for bleeding
  c. Vomitus, stool, and urine for visible or occult blood
  d. Vaginal bleeding
  e. Prolonged bleeding from puncture sites
  f. Neurologic changes such as headache, visual changes, altered mentation, decreased level of consciousness, seizures
  g. Abdomen for complaints of epigastric pain, diminished bowel sounds, increasing abdominal girth, rigidity or guarding
- Avoid diagnostic procedures such as biopsy or lumbar puncture if the platelet count is less than 50,000.
- Apply pressure to injection sites for 3 to 5 minutes, and to arterial punctures for 15 to 20 minutes.
- Instruct to avoid forcefully blowing or picking the nose, forceful coughing or sneezing, and straining to have a bowel movement.

Anticipatory Grieving

- Assess coping strategies and their effectiveness. Help identify sources of strength and support.
- Discuss changing roles resulting from leukemia diagnosis, and its effect on spiritual, social, economic status, and usual lifestyle.
- Evaluate cultural or ethnic factors that affect grief reactions.
- Use therapeutic communication skills to facilitate open discussion of losses and provide permission to grieve.
- Provide information about agencies that may help in resolving grief, and make referrals as indicated. Consider self-help groups, cancer support groups, and bereavement groups.

Community-Based Care

- Explain the nature of the leukemia and its usual course, the function of bone marrow, and potential complications.
- Discuss treatment options and management of their side effects. Discuss pain control, including nonpharmacologic measures, and provide teaching as appropriate.

- Encourage meticulous personal hygiene, including daily showering or bathing, using a soft-bristle toothbrush for oral care, and inspecting the skin and mucous membranes for bleeding.

- Encourage a balance of activity with rest.

- Teach measures to prevent infection, such as avoiding people who are ill; eating fruits and vegetables cooked, not raw; avoiding immunizations; and using an electric razor rather than razor blades.

- Encourage to report signs of infection or injury to the physician immediately.

- Promote nutrition by encouraging the patient to eat several small meals a day, increase fiber in the diet, drink several glasses of water each day, and report continued weight loss to the physician. A referral to a dietitian may be appropriate.

- Provide referrals to the American Cancer Society, hospice services, and support groups as appropriate.

For more information on leukemia, see Chapter 33 in *Medical-Surgical Nursing,* Fifth Edition, by LeMone, Burke, and Bauldoff.

LYME DISEASE

Overview

- Lyme disease is a systemic inflammatory disorder caused by *Borrelia burgdorferi,* a spirochete bacterium transmitted primarily by deer or mice ticks.

- It manifests as a skin rash, arthritis, and neurologic symptoms. The inflammatory joint changes closely resemble those of rheumatoid arthritis.

- It is common along the Northeast and Middle Atlantic states, upper Midwest, and Pacific Northwest regions; also present in other parts of the world.

- The three stages of infection are as follows:

  Stage 1 occurs when the spirochete enters and infects the skin at the puncture site.

  Stage 2 begins when the organism infects the blood.

  Stage 3 occurs when the organism spreads via the blood to the central nervous system, joints, and possibly the heart, colonizing these tissues.

Cause

- Infection by the spirochete bacterium *B. burgdorferi*

Manifestations

Stage 1 (Local Infection)

- Rash develops:
  - A small red macule forms at bite site.
  - Red macule expands to a red ring surrounding a central area ("bull's eye" lesion).
  - Central area usually remains clear, but may turn red or blue, ulcerate, or become necrotic.
  - Lesions are usually painless.

Stage 2 (Disseminated Infection)

- Skin lesions similar to above form in a disseminated pattern.
- Fever/chills; profound malaise/fatigue.
- Severe headache and mild stiff neck.
- Migratory arthralgia and myalgia.
- Less common: conjunctivitis/iritis, hepatitis, splenomegaly, sore throat, cough, meningitis, cranial neuritis, carditis, cardiomyopathy, and first-degree heart block.

Stage 3 (Persistent Infection)

- Recurrent attacks of arthritis of large or small joints
- Chronic skin lesions
- Chronic neurologic impairment develops; including facial nerve palsy and meningitis

Diagnostic Test

- Enzyme-linked immunosorbent assay will be positive for *B. burgdorferi* antibodies approximately 4 weeks after the initial lesion.

Interdisciplinary Management

- Medications include antibiotics and aspirin or other nonsteroidal anti-inflammatory drugs for symptom relief.
- The joint may be splinted.

Selected Nursing Diagnoses with Interventions

Nursing interventions vary, depending on the stage of the disease.

Chronic Pain

- Emphasize the importance of completing the full course of prescribed antibiotic.

- Advise to take nonsteroidal anti-inflammatory drugs on a regular schedule rather than as needed for pain.

Fatigue

- Teach the manifestations of Lyme disease, including neurologic and cardiac symptoms; instruct to notify the physician if these occur.

- Provide opportunities for adequate rest until energy returns. Reassure that fatigue is temporary.

Community-Based Care

- Explain how to avoid contact with the tick that spreads Lyme disease and what to do if a tick bite occurs:

  - Avoid tick-infested areas, including tall grasses and dense brush. Wear protective clothing and use an insect repellant.

  - After being outdoors, inspect skin and clothing for ticks. Remove any ticks immediately with tweezers and wash the area thoroughly with soap and water. Apply an antiseptic.

  - Notify the physician if a "bull's eye" rash develops around a tick bite.

For more information on Lyme disease, see Chapter 40 in *Medical-Surgical Nursing,* Fifth Edition, by LeMone, Burke, and Bauldoff.

LYMPHOMA, NON-HODGKIN'S

Overview

- Lymphomas are lymphoid tissue malignancies, including non-Hodgkin's lymphoma and Hodgkin's lymphoma.

- Lymphomas are characterized by proliferation of lymphocytes, resident monocytes, macrophages, and their precursors or derivatives. They are closely related to lymphocytic leukemias.

- Non-Hodgkin's lymphoma is more common than Hodgkin's, affecting an estimated 56,000 people annually.

- Non-Hodgkin's lymphomas tend to spread early to other lymphoid tissues and organs such as the nasopharynx, gastrointestinal tract, bone, central nervous system, thyroid, testes, and soft tissue.

- The prognosis ranges from excellent to poor, depending on cell type and grade of differentiation at the time of diagnosis.

Causes

The cause of lymphoma is unknown; identified risk factors are as follows:

- Immunosuppression due to drug therapy following organ transplant or to human immunodeficiency virus disease

- Human T-cell leukemia/lymphoma virus-1 and the Epstein-Barr virus

- Genetic factors

Manifestations

- Early: painless lymphadenopathy, localized or widespread.

- Fever, night sweats, fatigue, and weight loss.

- Abdominal pain, nausea, and vomiting.

- Headaches, peripheral or cranial nerve symptoms, altered mental status, or seizures may signal central nervous system involvement.

Diagnostic Tests

- Chest x-ray may show enlarged mediastinal lymph nodes and pulmonary involvement.

- *Computed tomography scans* of the chest, abdomen, and pelvis can identify abnormal or enlarged nodes.

- *Positron emission tomography or gallium scans* may be used to diagnose the disease and evaluate the effectiveness of treatment.

- Biopsy of the largest, most central enlarged lymph node establishes the diagnosis.

Interdisciplinary Management

- Combination chemotherapy is used to treat non-Hodgkin's lymphoma. It often is followed by radiation therapy to involved lymph node regions.

- The involved lymph node region is treated with radiation therapy; if the disease is advanced, total nodal irradiation may be done.

Selected Nursing Diagnoses with Interventions

Fatigue

- Inquire about feelings of malaise and fatigue.

- Encourage enjoyable but quiet activities, such as reading, listening to music, or hobbies.

- Encourage to establish priorities and include rest periods or naps when scheduling daily activities.

- Encourage delegation of some responsibilities to family members.

Nausea

- Assess precipitating factors for nausea and/or vomiting, the frequency of vomiting, and relief measures used by the patient.

- Provide ordered antiemetics before chemotherapy is started.

- Teach measures to prevent or relieve nausea and vomiting:

  a. Eat soda crackers and suck on hard candy.

  b. Eat soft, bland foods that are cold or at room temperature.

  c. Avoid unpleasant odors, and get fresh air.

  d. Eat before but not immediately before chemotherapy.

  e. Use distraction or progressive muscle relaxation when nauseated.

  f. If vomiting occurs, gradually resume oral intake with frequent sips of clear liquids or ice, progressing to bland foods.

- Provide small feedings of high-kilocalorie, high-protein foods and fluids.

- Assist with oral care, general hygiene, and environmental control of temperature, appearance, and odors.

- Identify and provide preferred foods.

- Assist to a sitting position during and immediately after meals.

Disturbed Body Image

- Assess perception of body image through subjective information:

  a. What the patient likes most and least about his or her body

  b. Pre-illness perception of people who are sick or disabled

  c. Current understanding of health and limitations imposed by illness or treatment

  d. Feelings about the illness and its effect on self-perception as well as perception of others

- Discuss the risk for and measures to cope with alopecia. Suggest wearing wigs, scarves, hats, or caps. Teach proper scalp care using baby shampoo or mild soap, a soft brush, sunscreen, and mineral oil to reduce itching. If eyelashes and eyebrows are lost, teach eye protection, such as wearing eyeglasses and caps with wide brims.

- Discuss available resources for financial assistance with purchase of wigs, including local American Cancer Society chapters and insurance plans.

Sexual Dysfunction

- Encourage discussion of actual or potential sexual dysfunction or sterility with the patient and significant other.

- Assess knowledge, provide information, and clarify misconceptions. Discuss realistic measures for coping, for example, sperm banking before chemotherapy or radiation therapy.

- Refer for counseling as indicated.

Risk for Impaired Skin Integrity

- Frequently assess skin, especially in areas undergoing radiation.

- Provide and teach measures to promote comfort and relieve itching: Use cool water and a mild soap to bathe; blot (rather than rub) dry skin; apply plain cornstarch or nonperfumed lotion or powder to the skin unless contraindicated; use lightweight blankets and clothing; maintain adequate humidity and a cool room temperature; wash bedding and clothes in mild detergent, and put them through second rinse cycle.

Community-Based Care

- Teach about the disease process, treatment options, and prognosis.
- Teach strategies for self-care as described in the previous section, including skin care, rest, and nutrition.

Home Care

- Emphasize the importance of continuing medical care.
- Encourage the patient to contact a support group, local chapter of the American Cancer Society, Leukemia Society of America, or other community service for information, financial assistance, and counseling.

For more information on non-Hodgkin's lymphoma, see Chapter 33 in *Medical-Surgical Nursing,* Fifth Edition, by LeMone, Burke, and Bauldoff.

L

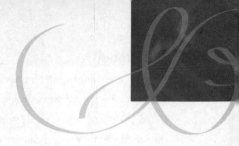

Macular Degeneration

Overview

- Age-related macular degeneration (AMD) is the leading cause of legal blindness and impaired vision in people over the age of 65.

- The risk for AMD is significantly higher in Whites than in Blacks, Hispanics, or people of Asian ancestry. It affects males and females equally.

- The macula, consisting primarily of cone receptors, is the area of the retina that provides sharp central vision.

- Two forms of AMD are identified:

  - *Nonexudative*, or dry, *macular degeneration*, the more common form, is characterized by deposits (*drusen*) beneath the pigment epithelium of the retina. The deposits slowly enlarge and become more numerous. Pigment epithelium detaches and atrophies, impairing central vision. Vision loss typically is not significant. The disorder may progress to an exudative stage of the disease.

  - *Exudative macular degeneration*, is characterized by the formation of new, weak blood vessels between the choroid and the retina. These new vessels are prone to leak, raising the retina from the choroid and distorting vision. Although the process usually is gradual, bleeding can lead to acute vision loss. With significant or repeated bleeding episodes, scar tissue forms, and central vision is permanently lost.

Cause

- The cause of AMD is unknown; however, it usually is associated with aging.

- Risk factors include aging, female gender, smoking, race, genetic factors, and inflammation.

Manifestations

- Blurring and distortion of central vision, may initially be unilateral.
- Straight lines appear wavy or distorted.
- Intact peripheral vision remains intact.
- Impaired ability to engage in activities that require close central vision, such as reading and sewing.

Diagnosis

- Vision and retinal examination reveal distorted central vision.
- The Amsler grid identifies distortion of central vision.
- A fluorescein angiogram may be done to detect leaking vessels in exudative AMD.

Interdisciplinary Management

- High-dose antioxidants (vitamins C, E, and A), zinc, and copper may be used in the early or intermediate stages to slow the progress of dry AMD.
- Wet AMD is treated with laser surgery or photodynamic therapy to slow the rate of vision loss.
- Large-print books and magazines, use of a magnifying glass, and high-intensity lighting can help the patient to cope with the reduced vision of AMD.

Selected Nursing Diagnoses with Interventions

Disturbed Sensory Perception: Visual

- Monitor vision of older adults in home, residential, and long-term care settings for complaints of difficulty reading, engaging in close activities, or driving.
- Refer patients with new or rapid onset of AMD manifestations for ophthalmologic examination.
- Helping the patient and family members adapt to the gradual decline in vision by recommending visual aids and other coping strategies.

Community-Based Care

- Encourage older adults to have annual vision examinations.

- Promptly refer patients with new or rapid onset of AMD manifestations to an ophthalmologist.

- Provide information about visual aids and resources for people with significant vision impairment.

- Refer to home health, social, and other services as appropriate to help the patient maintain independence.

For more information about age-related macular degeneration, see Chapter 46 in *Medical-Surgical Nursing*, Fifth Edition, by LeMone, Burke, and Bauldoff.

MAGNESIUM IMBALANCE

Hypermagnesemia

Hypomagnesemia

Overview

- Most magnesium (Mg^{++}) is found in cells and bone; 1% of total body magnesium is in the extracellular fluid. It is the second most abundant ion in intracellular fluid.

- Magnesium is vital to intracellular processes such as enzyme reactions and protein and nucleic acid synthesis.

- Magnesium has a sedative effect on the neuromuscular junction; it is essential for neuromuscular transmission and cardiovascular function.

- The concentration of magnesium is regulated by gastrointestinal absorption and renal excretion.

- The normal serum magnesium level is 1.6 to 2.6 mg/dL (1.3 to 2.1 mEq/L).

Hypomagnesemia (Serum Magnesium < 1.6 mg/dL)

- Usually occurs along with hypokalemia and hypocalcemia.

- Causes increased neuromuscular excitability, with muscle weakness and tremors, and a risk for seizures and mental status changes.

- Increases the risk of cardiac dysrhythmias, sudden death, and digitalis toxicity.

- Chronic hypomagnesemia may contribute to hypertension.

Hypermagnesemia (Serum Magnesium > 2.6 mg/dL)

- Interferes with neuromuscular transmission, depresses the central nervous system (CNS), and impairs cardiovascular function.

- Relaxes vascular smooth muscle.

Causes

Hypomagnesemia

- Loss of gastrointestinal (GI) fluids (diarrhea, ileostomy drainage, or intestinal fistula)

- Impaired intestinal absorption

- Chronic alcoholism (most common cause in the United States)

- Protein-calorie malnutrition or starvation

- Endocrine disorders including diabetic ketoacidosis

- Drugs such as loop or thiazide diuretics, aminoglycoside antibiotics, amphotericin B, cyclosporine

- Rapid administration of citrated blood (banked blood)

- Kidney disease

Hypermagnesemia

- Renal failure

- Administration of parenteral or oral magnesium-containing drugs (e.g., magnesium-containing antacids or laxatives)

- Use of over-the-counter laxatives and preparations containing magnesium

Manifestations

Hypomagnesemia

- Neuromuscular: tremors, hyperreactive reflexes, positive Chvostek's and Trousseau's signs, tetany, paresthesias, and seizures

- CNS: confusion, mood changes (apathy, depression, agitation), hallucinations, and possible psychoses

- Cardiovascular: tachycardia, ventricular dysrhythmias; cardiac arrest and sudden death

- GI: nausea, vomiting, anorexia, diarrhea, abdominal distention

Hypermagnesemia

Mild elevation:

- Nausea and vomiting
- Hypotension
- Facial flushing, sweating, and a feeling of warmth

Moderate elevation:

- CNS depression with weakness, lethargy, drowsiness
- Weak or absent deep tendon reflexes

Marked elevation:

- Respiratory depression
- Coma
- Electrocardiogram (ECG) changes, bradycardia, heart block, cardiac arrest

Diagnostic Tests

- Serum magnesium levels are outside the normal range.
- ECG changes:
    1. Hypermagnesemia—prolonged Q-T interval, heart block
    2. Hypomagnesemia—prolonged Q-T interval, wide QRS complex, low or inverted T wave, and depressed ST segment

Interdisciplinary Management

Hypomagnesemia

- If possible, a mild deficiency is corrected by increasing intake of magnesium-rich foods (e.g., green leafy vegetables, seafood, citrus fruits, bananas, and chocolate).
- Oral magnesium supplements may be ordered, but their use is limited by risk for diarrhea.
- Parenteral magnesium sulfate can be given intravenously (IV) or by deep intramuscular injection. The IV route is used for severe magnesium deficiency or if neurologic changes or cardiac dysrhythmias are present.

Hypermagnesemia

- Identification and treatment of the underlying cause is vital.

- All medications or compounds containing magnesium (e.g., antacids, IV solutions, or enemas) are withheld.

- If renal failure is present, dialysis is instituted to remove the excess magnesium.

- Calcium gluconate is given IV to reverse the neuromuscular and cardiac effects of hypermagnesemia. Mechanical ventilation and a pacemaker may be required to support respiratory function and cardiac output.

Selected Nursing Diagnoses with Interventions

Hypomagnesemia
Risk for Injury

- Monitor serum electrolytes, including magnesium, potassium, and calcium.

- Monitor GI function, including bowel sounds and abdominal distention.

- Initiate cardiac monitoring, reporting and treating (as indicated) ECG changes and dysrhythmias. In patients receiving digitalis, monitor for digitalis toxicity.

- Assess deep tendon reflexes frequently during intravenous magnesium infusions and before each intramuscular dose.

- Maintain a quiet, darkened environment. Institute seizure precautions.

Hypermagnesemia
Decreased Cardiac Output, Risk for Ineffective Breathing Pattern

- Monitor serum magnesium levels every 6 hours.

- Monitor vital signs, level of consciousness, and deep tendon reflexes hourly.

- Administer loop diuretics as prescribed.

- Monitor cardiovascular and respiratory status, promptly reporting changes.

M

Risk for Injury

- Avoid use of magnesium-containing medications (e.g., Maalox, Mylanta, milk of magnesia).

- Encourage fluid intake.

- Administer IV calcium gluconate as prescribed.

- Observe for flushing of skin and diaphoresis.

Community-Based Care

- Instruct the patient with hypomagnesemia to increase dietary intake of foods high in magnesium, and provide information about magnesium supplements.

- Teach the patient with hypermagnesemia to avoid magnesium-containing medications, including antacids, mineral supplements, cathartics, and enemas. Provide a list of foods rich in magnesium, which should be restricted.

- If alcohol abuse has precipitated a magnesium deficit, discuss alcohol treatment options, including inpatient treatment and support groups such as Alcoholics Anonymous, Al-Anon, and/or Alateen.

For more information about magnesium imbalances, see Chapter 10 in *Medical-Surgical Nursing,* Fifth Edition, by LeMone, Burke, and Bauldoff.

MELANOMA

Overview

- Melanoma is a malignant neoplasm of melanocytes, the pigment-producing cells.

- It usually affects the skin, but can also occur in the eye.

- It is generally a highly malignant lesion, although different growth patterns exist.

  - The *superficial spreading type* consists of radial and shallow growth. It is a flat lesion; areas of growth are restricted to the epidermis and papillary dermis.

- The *nodular type* usually begins superficially; it has a vertical growth pattern, and involves the dermis and deeper tissues.

- *Lentigo maligna* melanomas are slow growing and flat. They occur most often on sun-exposed skin of older adults.

- Metastasis is via regional lymph nodes; hematologic spread to all organs is possible.

- The usual sites involved are areas of sun exposure, but melanoma can occur on the palms, soles of feet, groin, subungual areas, or in the eye.

Causes

The cause is unknown; however, risk factors are as follows:

- European American race, fair skin
- Excess sun exposure in childhood
- Positive family history
- Nevi (congenital giant, dysplastic, changing)
- Age: adolescents to older adults, with the greatest rates in those over the age of 80

Manifestations

- Change in the appearance of a preexisting skin lesion or mole
- Rapid growth of a new pigmented skin lesion with irregular borders
- Appearance of new pigmented lesion on palm, sole, or under fingernail
- Itchiness, tenderness, redness
- Ulceration, crusting, or bleeding

Diagnostic Tests

- Biopsy will determine the type and stage of invasion.
- Liver function tests and computed tomography scan of the liver may be done to determine whether the tumor has metastasized to the liver.
- A chest x-ray, bone scan, and computed tomography scan or magnetic resonance imaging of the brain may be conducted to assess for metastasis to these organs.

- Biopsy of tissue from lymph nodes or other skin lesions is done to identify metastases.

Interdisciplinary Management

- Surgical excision is the preferred treatment for malignant melanoma.

- Chemotherapy is used to treat metastatic melanoma or as an adjunct to other therapies.

- Immunotherapeutic agents, such as interferons, interleukins, and monoclonal antibodies, are used.

- Radiation frequently is used for palliation of symptoms resulting from metastasis.

Selected Nursing Diagnoses with Interventions

Impaired Skin Integrity (Following Surgery)

- Monitor for manifestations of infection: fever, tachycardia, malaise, and incisional erythema; swelling, pain, or drainage that increases or becomes purulent.

- Keep the incision line clean and dry by changing dressings as necessary.

- Follow principles of medical and surgical asepsis when caring for the incision. Teach the importance of careful hand hygiene. Maintain universal precautions if drainage is present.

- Encourage and maintain adequate kilocalorie and protein intake in the diet. Suggest a consultation with the dietitian if the patient does not want to eat.

Hopelessness

- Provide an environment that encourages expression of feelings, concerns, and goals.

- Explore perceptions and modify or clarify them if necessary by providing information and correcting misconceptions.

- Encourage the patient to identify and use support systems and sources of strength and coping in the past.

- Encourage activity in self-care and in mutual decision making and goal setting.

- Encourage focus not only on the present but also on the future. Review past occasions for hope, discuss the patient's personal meaning of hope, establish and evaluate short-term goals with the patient and significant others, and encourage them to express hope for the future.

Anxiety

- Provide reassurance and comfort by setting aside time to sit quietly with the patient, speaking slowly and calmly, conveying empathic understanding, and avoiding making demands or expecting the patient to make decisions.

- Decrease sensory stimuli by using short, simple sentences, focusing on the here and now, and providing concise information.

- Provide interventions that decrease anxiety levels and increase coping:
  - Provide accurate information about the illness, treatment, and prognosis.
  - Encourage discussion of expected physical changes and coping strategies.
  - Include significant others in teaching sessions.
  - Provide the patient with strategies for participating in the recovery process.

Community-Based Care

- Review techniques for avoiding sun exposure such as wearing sunscreen of at least 15 SPF, wearing protective clothing and sunglasses, and avoiding tanning booths.

- Show how to conduct monthly skin self-examinations, and suggest that significant others check hard-to-see areas such as the back of the neck.

- Encourage wound care and the importance of contacting the physician immediately if the patient notices signs of infection.

- Teach patient who has had a lymph node dissection about protecting the extremity from bleeding, trauma, and infection. Describe the manifestations and side effects of chemotherapy and radiation and provide information on how to decrease nausea, vomiting, anorexia, and fatigue, and how to care for irradiated skin areas.

- Provide the patient with a brochure explaining the various types of skin cancer, treatment, and prevention, and showing photographs of cancerous lesions.

- Encourage patients to continue regular medical check-ups every 3 months for 2 years following the initial diagnosis and treatment.

- A referral to a local cancer support group or psychologist may be helpful.

For more information about melanoma, see Chapter 16 in *Medical-Surgical Nursing,* Fifth Edition, by LeMone, Burke, and Bauldoff.

MÉNIÈRE'S DISEASE

Overview

- Ménière's disease is a recurrent disorder of the vestibular apparatus in the ear, producing severe vertigo, tinnitus, and sensorineural hearing loss.

- An accumulation of endolymph within the vestibular apparatus, due to an increased rate of production or a decreased rate of reabsorption, destroys vestibular and cochlear hair cells.

- Attacks occur in a paroxysmal pattern. Repeated attacks may result in permanent sensorineural deafness and tinnitus.

- It usually affects people aged 35 to 60 but can strike any age.

Causes

- Viral injury to the fluid transport system of the inner ear. Risk factors include trauma and bacterial infections such as syphilis, autoimmune processes, and vascular disorders. There is a possible genetic link.

Manifestations

- Vertigo, severe and usually disabling
- Sensorineural hearing loss
- Tinnitus
- Nystagmus

- Ataxia/falling: toward the affected side
- Nausea/vomiting

Diagnostic Tests

- Audiometric studies show sensorineural hearing loss involving the low tones.
- Caloric testing (electronystagmography) demonstrates blunting or absence of the normal nystagmus response.
- X-rays and computed tomography scans of the petrous bones may show vestibular aqueducts that are shorter and straighter than normal.
- Glycerol test produces an acute temporary hearing improvement in Ménière's disease.

Interdisciplinary Management

- Antivertigo/antiemetic medications are prescribed to reduce the whirling sensation and nausea. An oral diuretic may help maintain lower labyrinthine pressure between attacks. Central nervous system depressant drugs such as diazepam (Valium) or lorazepam (Ativan) may halt an attack of vertigo. Parenteral droperidol (Inapsine) is useful for acute attacks.
- A very low-sodium diet (1 Gm.), and in severe cases a salt-free neutral ash diet, may be prescribed. Alcohol, caffeine, and smoking are also prohibited.
- Surgical endolymphatic decompression and shunting relieves excess pressure in the labyrinth and relieves vertigo in about 70% of patients. Destruction of a portion of the acoustic nerve is an alternative to shunting procedures. A labyrinthectomy is used only when hearing loss is nearly complete and vertigo is persistent.

Selected Nursing Diagnoses with Interventions

Risk for Trauma

- Assess for manifestations of vertigo, nystagmus, nausea and vomiting, and hearing loss.
- Place the patient experiencing an acute attack of vertigo on bed rest with the side rails elevated and the call light readily accessible. Instruct the patient not to get up without assistance.

M

- Teach the patient to avoid sudden head movements or position changes.

- Administer prescribed medications, including antiemetics, diuretics, and sedatives.

- Instruct the patient who senses an impending attack to respond by taking the prescribed medication and lying down in a quiet, darkened room.

- If an attack occurs while driving, advise the patient to pull to the side of the road and wait for the symptoms to subside.

- Discuss the importance of wearing a MedicAlert bracelet or necklace.

- Discuss the effect of unilateral hearing loss on the ability to identify the direction from which sounds come.

Disturbed Sleep Pattern

- Discuss options for masking tinnitus to promote concentration and sleep:

  a. Ambient noise from a radio or sound system

  b. Masking device or white-noise machine

  c. Hearing aid that produces a tone to mask the tinnitus

  d. Hearing aid that amplifies ambient sound

Community-Based Care

- Review the disease process, causes, treatment options, medication regimen, methods to reduce the frequency of attacks, and prognosis.

- Explain safety measures, such as slowly turning the body rather than just the head to change position. Sit or lie down immediately with the onset of vertigo. Do not walk alone unless in a safe environment.

- Surgical intervention may result in permanent hearing loss in the affected ear. Teach alternative communication strategies for use postoperatively.

- Provide a referral to a dietitian as indicated to assist the patient with implementing a low-salt or salt-free ash diet.

- Support groups for the hearing impaired may provide information and emotional support.

For more information on Ménière's disease, see Chapter 46 in *Medical-Surgical Nursing,* Fifth Edition, by LeMone, Burke, and Bauldoff.

MENINGITIS (BACTERIAL, VIRAL, FUNGAL)

Overview

- Meningitis is an inflammation of the meninges of the central nervous system.

- Bacterial meningitis is the most common type, but meningitis can also be due to viruses, fungi, or chemical irritation.

- It usually involves all three meningeal layers (pia, arachnoid, and dura).

- The most common pathway for meningeal infection is via sepsis secondary to infections such as pneumonia, sinusitis, mastoiditis, otitis, pharyngitis, or osteomyelitis. Primary infections may occur with head trauma such as compound, especially basilar, skull fracture, or following surgery or lumbar puncture.

- Organisms multiply rapidly, especially within arachnoid space, and are spread readily via the cerebrospinal fluid (CSF) to all areas of the brain and spinal cord. Bacteria and their exudate accumulate and may result in increased intracranial pressure (ICP).

Causes

Bacterial (Acute Pyogenic)

- *Haemophilus influenzae:* usually in infants and children, vaccination has greatly reduced incidence

- *Streptococcus pneumoniae:* usually in very young or very old

- *Neisseria meningitidis:* second most common organism; usually in children, adolescents, and young adults; causes meningococcal (epidemic) meningitis

- *Escherichia coli:* usually in infants

Viral (Aseptic)

- Childhood disease viruses: mumps, measles, chickenpox

- Echo virus
- Arbovirus (epidemic): usually with encephalitis
- Coxsackievirus
- Epstein-Barr virus
- Herpes simplex virus, type I or II
- Cytomegalovirus
- Varicella zoster virus
- Polio virus
- Rabies virus: 100% fatal if untreated
- Human immunodeficiency virus
- West Nile virus

Fungal

- Usually seen only in immunocompromised patients
- Cryptococcus
- *Candida albicans*
- Aspergillus

Manifestations

- Fever, chills, malaise
- Irritability; photophobia; seizures; petechiae, purpura, ecchymosis (meningococcus); rash; deafness and joint pain (*H. influenzae*); increased deep tendon reflexes
- Stiff neck/back (nuchal rigidity), positive Brudzinski sign, positive Kernig's sign
- Increased ICP/herniation:
  - Severe headache
  - Decreased level of consciousness; decreasing Glasgow coma scale, coma
  - Projectile vomiting
  - Pupils: decreased response, inequality, dilation
  - Vital sign changes: increased systolic blood pressure, increased pulse pressure, decreased heart rate, irregular respiratory pattern

Diagnostic Tests

- Lumbar puncture for CSF culture and sensitivity (C&S):

    1. Bacterial: increased pressure; cloudy fluid; white cell count up to 90,000 polymorphonuclear leukocytes/μL; elevated protein; decreased glucose; C&S positive for specific organism

    2. Viral: clear fluid; normal glucose; increased pressure; increased lymphocytes; negative bacterial C&S; positive or negative viral culture

- Cultures of blood, nose and throat mucous membranes, or urine to locate primary infection site

- X-rays of the chest, for pneumonia; of the head, for sinusitis; or cranial osteomyelitis

- Computed tomography scan or magnetic resonance imaging to rule out abscess, hematoma, hemorrhage, or tumor

Interdisciplinary Management

- A broad-spectrum antibiotic (usually penicillin or cephalosporin) is prescribed until the results of the culture and Gram stain are available, at which time a specific antibiotic is prescribed as appropriate. Vancomycin may be used for resistant strains of bacteria.

- Anticonvulsant medications may be prescribed to prevent seizure activity, and antipyretics and nonopiate analgesics may be given for symptom relief.

- An Ommaya reservoir may be surgically implanted into a lateral ventricle of the brain to enhance CSF absorption of antibiotics.

Selected Nursing Diagnoses with Interventions

Ineffective Protection

- Assess neurologic status and vital signs, including temperature, on a regular basis.

- Assess for and report decreasing levels of consciousness. Assess orientation, memory, attention span, and response to overall stimuli.

- Assess for and report manifestations of seizures and institute seizure precautions.

- Assess for and report manifestations of cranial nerve damage; monitor extraocular movements, facial movement, dizziness, ability to hear, double vision, drooping upper eyelids, and pupillary changes.

- Assess for and report manifestations of increased ICP: decreased pulse, increased systolic blood pressure, widening pulse pressure, respiratory changes, and vomiting.

- Administer prescribed medications and fluids.

Risk for Deficient Fluid Volume

- Measure intake and output every 2 to 4 hours; weigh daily.

- Assess condition and turgor of skin and mucous membranes.

- Monitor urine specific gravity, blood urea nitrogen, and serum creatinine.

- When administering fluids, either orally or parenterally, consider other illnesses that are occurring concurrently.

Community-Based Care

Include patient, significant others, and caregivers as appropriate:

- Review the disease process, treatment, and ways to prevent future occurrences and spread of the disease to others.

- Teach the names, dosages, and purposes of all prescribed medications, and stress the importance of taking all medication until completely gone.

- Instruct to report any manifestations of ear infection, sore throat, or upper respiratory tract infection.

For more information about meningitis, see Chapter 43 in *Medical-Surgical Nursing,* Fifth Edition, by LeMone, Burke, and Bauldoff.

METHICILLIN-RESISTANT *Staphylococcus Aureus* (MRSA) INFECTION

Overview

- Methicillin-resistant *staphylococcus aureus* (MRSA) infections are resistant to broad-spectrum antibiotics and spread by direct contact with the bacteria or with contaminated equipment.

- This potentially fatal disease is divided into two types:

  1. Healthcare-associated infections (HA-MRSA), which are acquired in hospitals and other healthcare settings. They may lead to infections of wounds, skin around invasive tubes or catheters, the blood, the lungs, or the urinay system. An estimated 1.2 million hospitalized patients acquire HA-MRSA.

  2. Community associated infections (CA-MRSA), which are acquired in the community in otherwise healthy people. They are often manifested as skin infections and a potentially life-threatening pneumonia.

- The rates of both types are highest in healthcare workers, in males, in those over age 65, in Blacks, and in those with HIV and AIDS. The risk for CA-MRSA is increased in those who participate in contact sports, and in people sharing personal items and/or living in crowded or unsanitary conditions.

Cause

- Infection with *S. aureus*.

Manifestations

- Begins as a small, raised, red nodule on the skin resembling a pimple or spider bite.

- Nodule increases in size, becomes dark red, is painful; contains pus, and may become a deep abscess.

- Cellulitis involving the area containing the initial infection (such as an extremity) is common.

Diagnostic Tests

- Positive blood culture for *S. aureus* from draining lesions.

- Culture from external nares of healthcare workers or people with repeated bacterial skin infections can determine whether they are carriers of MRSA.

Interdisciplinary Management

MRSA infections may be treated with antimicrobial therapy, including trimethoprim-sulfamethoxazole (Bactrim), minocycline (Minocin), doxycycline (Vibramycin), or clindamycin (Cleocin).

Selected Nursing Diagnoses with Interventions

Risk for Infection

- Practice good hand hygiene and teach its importance.

- Teach how to identify an increase in infection (fever, tachycardia, chills, malaise, increase in erythema, lesion size, and drainage).

- Cover draining lesions with a sterile dressing, and handle soiled dressings or linens according to standard precautions. When changing dressings, always wear disposable rubber gloves and masks.

Community-Based Care

- Follow CDC guidelines and state laws for reporting and treating CA-MRSA.

- Focus patient teaching on facilitating tissue healing and eliminating the infection. Address the following topics:

  - The importance of maintaining good nutrition

  - The importance of maintaining cleanliness through careful hand hygiene and proper handling and disposal of dressings

  - Preventing the spread of infection by not sharing linens and towels, and washing clothing and linens in hot water

  - The importance of not squeezing or trying to open a pimple or boil

  - The importance of taking the full course of prescribed antibiotics

For more information on methicillin-resistant *staphylococcus aureus* infections, see Chapters 12 and 16 in *Medical-Surgical Nursing,* Fifth Edition, by LeMone, Burke, and Bauldoff.

MONONUCLEOSIS

Overview

- Infectious mononucleosis is characterized by invasion of B cells in the oropharyngeal lymphoid tissues by the Epstein-Barr virus (EBV).

- EBV is thought to spread via saliva, as with kissing.
- Infection spreads from oral mucosa to pharynx and lymphatic vessels, nodes, and spleen to enter B lymphocytes. The lymph nodes and spleen enlarge.
- It occurs primarily in young adults (15 to 30).
- Symptoms last an average of 2 weeks but fatigue may linger for months.
- EBV is associated with Burkitt's lymphoma and nasopharyngeal carcinoma.

Cause
- Infection with EBV.

Manifestations
- Fever, diaphoresis, chills, malaise
- Sore throat
- Lymphadenopathy
- Left upper quadrant abdominal tenderness
- Fatigue, often profound; anorexia
- Headache, generalized myalgia
- Rash, red papular

Diagnostic Tests
- White blood cell count shows elevated lymphocytes; atypical lymphocytes.
- Monospot is positive.
- Liver enzymes show an abnormal profile.

Interdisciplinary Management
- Treatment includes rest and analgesics. Corticosteroids may be used to treat severe cases of pharyngotonsillitis.

Selected Nursing Diagnoses with Interventions

Fatigue

- Assess physical limitations and toleration of activities of daily living. Assess sleep pattern and number of sleep hours per 24-hour period. Assess dietary intake to ensure adequate nutrition for healing.

- Encourage frequent rest and activity restrictions to diminish fatigue. Discuss strategies for increasing rest time, prioritizing daily tasks, and relinquishing tasks when fatigued.

Risk for Ineffective Role Performance

- Assess need for assistance in caring for self or family. Assist the patient to identify coping mechanisms and personal strengths and to acknowledge limitations.

Acute Pain

- Encourage to take analgesics as prescribed, and corticosteroids if prescribed for pharyngotonsillitis.

Community-Based Care

- Explain the disease process, treatment, and strategies to avoid relapse. Symptoms normally last 2 to 3 weeks, but some degree of lethargy and debility may remain for several months.

- A referral to social or community services may be appropriate to assist the patient with self-care and care of family in the initial stages of the disease.

For more information on mononucleosis, see Chapter 33 in *Medical-Surgical Nursing,* Fifth Edition, by LeMone, Burke, and Bauldoff.

MULTIPLE MYELOMA

Overview

- Multiple myeloma is a malignancy in which plasma cells (mature B cells that produce antibodies) multiply uncontrollably and infiltrate the bone marrow, lymph nodes, spleen, and other tissues.

- Multiple myeloma affects more Blacks than Whites, and more men than women. Its incidence increases with age.

- Malignant plasma cells produce large amounts of an abnormal immunoglobin called the *M protein*.

- M protein impairs normal antibody production and the humoral immune response. It increases blood viscosity and may damage kidney tubules.

- Myeloma cells proliferate, replacing bone marrow and infiltrating bone. Cortical bone is progressively destroyed by the tumor and enzymes it produces.

- Affected bones (vertebrae, ribs, skull, pelvis, femur, clavicle, and scapula) are weakened and may break without trauma (*pathologic fracture*).

- Course of disease is usually chronic, progressing more rapidly after remissions.

Causes

- The cause of multiple myeloma is unknown.

- Possible contributing factors include genetic alterations, radiation exposure, oncogenic virus, inflammatory stimuli, and chronic antigenic stimulation.

Manifestations

- Bone pain (usual presenting symptom)
- Hypercalcemia with lethargy, confusion, and weakness
- Recurrent infections
- Bence Jones proteins in the urine
- Possible renal failure and azotemia
- Anemia

Diagnostic Tests

- X-rays and other radiologic bone studies may reveal multiple punched-out lesions.
- Bone marrow examination shows an abnormal number of immature plasma cells.

- Complete blood cell count shows moderate to severe anemia.
- Urinalysis shows Bence Jones protein.
- Biopsy of myeloma lesions confirms the presence of malignant cells.

Interdisciplinary Management

- There is no cure for multiple myeloma.
- Standard treatment includes induction chemotherapy followed by stem cell transplant and maintenance chemotherapy to control disease progression, and to reduce bone pain, hypercalcemia, anemia, and the number of infections.
- Localized radiation therapy may be used to treat painful bone lesions.
- Supportive care includes hydration; bisphosphonate therapy to reduce bone loss; and calcium, vitamin D, and fluoride supplements to support bone structure. Plasmapheresis is used as needed to remove circulating M proteins in acute renal failure. Infections are treated promptly.

Selected Nursing Diagnoses with Interventions

Chronic Pain

- Assess pain using a standard pain scale; include onset, duration, precipitating factors, and effective relief measures.
- Determine position of comfort, and assist as needed into this position. Support position with pillows.
- Provide uninterrupted rest periods.
- Teach adjunctive pain relief strategies such as relaxation or guided imagery.
- Teach effective analgesic use, including the family in instruction.
- Report unrelieved pain to the physician.

Impaired Physical Mobility

- Gently support extremities during repositioning.
- Assist to change position at least every 2 hours.
- Provide a trapeze to assist in repositioning.

Risk for Injury

- Place needed items close at hand.

- Provide safety measures to prevent falls from bed: place the bed in a low position, use side rails as indicated, and place the call bell within reach.

- Provide shoes with nonskid soles, a clear pathway, adequate lighting, and a level surface free of scatter rugs or other hazards when ambulating. Provide a walker as needed for support and security.

Risk for Infection

- Ensure meticulous hand hygiene of all persons coming in contact with the patient.

- Restrict visitors with colds, flu, or other infections.

- Provide a high-protein, high-vitamin diet.

- Provide oral hygiene after every meal.

- Use strict aseptic technique for invasive procedures.

- Assess vital signs including temperature every 4 hours. Report changes to the physician.

- Monitor white blood cell count and differential to detect increasing risk of infection.

- Institute protective isolation if the neutrophil count is less than 500/µL.

- Restrict fresh flowers and plants from the patient's room, as insects may harbor microorganisms that could cause infection.

Community-Based Care

- Teach about the disease process, treatment options, pain control, and prognosis.

- Teach manifestations of complications to report to the physician (e.g., symptoms of vertebral and extremity fractures).

- Discuss manifestations of infection to report: fever and chills; increased malaise, fatigue, or weakness; cough with or without sputum; sore throat; dysuria, nocturia, frequency, urgency, or malodorous urine.

- Discuss strategies for home maintenance management with the patient and family.

- Provide referrals for home health and home maintenance services, physical or occupational therapy, social services, and hospice care as appropriate.

For more information on multiple myeloma, see Chapter 33 in *Medical-Surgical Nursing,* Fifth Edition, by LeMone, Burke, and Bauldoff.

Multiple Sclerosis

Overview

- Multiple sclerosis (MS) is characterized by inflammatory demyelination and gliosis (scarring) of the central nervous system.

- Myelin is a fatty substance that insulates axons and speeds conduction of action potentials. In MS, myelin is lost in scattered patches of the central nervous system; rapid transmission of impulses is impaired, producing progressive motor, sensory, and visual neurologic deficits.

- MS follows a progressive, relapsing-remissing course. During remission, remyelination can occur and symptoms improve. The disease usually progresses slowly with long periods of remission, but may progress rapidly in some people.

- Permanently lost myelin is replaced by sclerotic plaques (scar tissue); conduction is permanently impaired, eventually leading to severe neurologic disability.

- Classifications of MS: relapsing-remitting, primary progressive, secondary progressive, and progressive-relapsing. Most people present with relapsing-remitting MS.

- The disease is usually diagnosed in young adults between the ages of 20 and 50.

Causes

- MS is believed to result from an autoimmune response to a prior viral infection in a genetically susceptible person. The target antigen has not been identified, but is suggested to be an immune response to a protein in the central nervous system. Episodes may be triggered by fever, pregnancy, extreme physical exertion, and exhaustion.

- Risk factors are family history, age 20 to 40, and residence in a temperate climate (e.g., the northern United States) before age 15.

Manifestations

Motor

- Paresis, fatigue
- Paralysis, spastic type (upper motor neuron lesion)
- Intention tremor, ataxia
- Eyes: diplopia (eye muscles); nystagmus (cerebrum/brainstem)
- Head: slurred speech; dysphagia
- Incontinence: urinary and/or fecal
- Positive Babinski's reflex

Sensory

- Reduced general senses: touch, vibration, temperature, pain
- Special senses: eyes—diplopia, clouding, blurring, scotoma, loss of acuity, with eye pain due to optic neuritis; vestibular—loss of proprioception, vertigo, tinnitus
- Paresthesias: numbness, tingling, "pins and needles" sensation
- Hypesthesia
- Trigeminal neuralgia

Emotional

- Euphoria
- Irritability/hyperexcitability
- Apathy/depression
- Emotional lability: uncontrollable laughter or crying

Cognitive

- Memory loss

- Poor judgment
- Inappropriate responses

Diagnostic Tests

- Magnetic resonance imaging can demonstrate sclerotic lesions and is the most definitive test available.

- Cerebrospinal fluid analysis reveals an increased number of T lymphocytes and often elevated levels of immunoglobulin G.

- Computed tomography scan of the brain shows atrophy and white matter lesions; the ventricles may be enlarged.

- Positron emission tomography scan reveals areas with altered glucose metabolism.

- Evoked response testing of visual, auditory, or somatosensory impulses may show delayed conduction.

Interdisciplinary Management

- A combination of adrenocorticotrophic hormone and glucocorticoids is used to decrease inflammation and suppress the immune system. Immunosuppressive agents, including azathioprine (Imuran) and cyclophosphamide (Cytoxan), are also used.

- Interferon (interferon alpha, beta, and gamma) and glatiramer acetate are used to reduce exacerbations with relapsing-remitting MS.

- Natalizumab (Tysabri) is given to patients with relapsing forms of MS to delay physical disability and reduce the frequency of exacerbations.

- Physical and rehabilitative therapies are individualized to the patient's level of functioning.

Selected Nursing Diagnoses with Interventions

Fatigue

- Assess degree of fatigue and identify contributing factors.
- Arrange daily activities to include rest periods.
- Help the patient set priorities.

M

- Encourage doing tasks in the morning hours when energy levels are higher.

- Advise to avoid temperature extremes, such as hot showers or exposure to cold.

- Refer to professional services such as stress management groups, physical therapists.

Self-Care Deficit

- Fully assess the extent of self-care abilities and deficits.

- Help maintain as much independence in activities as possible.

- Provide adaptive devices as needed.

- Assist with meal preparation and eating as needed.

- Teach routine inspection of skin.

- Teach interventions related to altered bowel and bladder function.

Community-Based Care

In addition to the teaching previously discussed, do the following:

- Teach the disease process and how to reduce the risk of exacerbations. Stress the importance of avoiding respiratory and urinary tract infections. If appropriate, tell the patient that pregnancy may exacerbate the condition.

- Review treatment options and their side effects.

- Explain how to make the home environment safe, such as removing scatter rugs and using handrails in the shower.

- Emphasize the importance of long-term follow-up care.

- Tell the patient how to obtain assistive devices.

- If unable to prepare meals, refer to Meals on Wheels.

- Refer to the local chapter of the Multiple Sclerosis Society.

For more information on multiple sclerosis, see Chapter 44 in *Medical-Surgical Nursing,* Fifth Edition, by LeMone, Burke, and Bauldoff.

MUSCULAR DYSTROPHY

Overview

- Muscular dystrophy (MD) is a group of genetic muscle diseases with a variety of genetic inheritance patterns that result in progressive symmetrical skeletal muscle wasting.

- Duchenne's muscular dystrophy (DMD), the most common form, results from mutation of the gene that codes for dystrophin, a protein necessary for stability of the sarcolemma.

- The disease occurs in about 1 in 3,500 live births.

- Skeletal and cardiac muscles show patchy necrosis; muscle is replaced by fibrous or fatty tissue.

- Symptoms are evident by early childhood (3 to 4 years).

Cause

- The disease is hereditary in two-thirds of cases; the defective gene is present in both parents, while in one-third of cases, MD is thought to be due to spontaneous mutation in the maternal gamete.

M

Manifestations

Weakness is evident by age 3 and is symmetric. Early on, it involves pelvic and shoulder girdles; later in the course of the disease, it involves all muscles.

Additional manifestations are as follows:

- Delayed walking, waddling gait, frequent falls.

- Muscle pain.

- Muscle wasting/pseudohypertrophy.

- Cardiac signs and symptoms: tachycardia; dysrhythmias.

- Progressive muscle weakness ultimately leads to death from respiratory and cardiac muscle involvement by the late teens or early adulthood.

Diagnostic Tests

- Muscle biopsy shows increased muscle fat and fibrosis.
- Electromyography shows deficiency of electric activity.
- Serum enzymes show increased creatine kinase (CK-MM).

Interdisciplinary Management

- Therapy is usually supportive and rehabilitative, involving physical and occupational therapy.

Selected Nursing Diagnoses with Interventions

Self-Care Deficit

- Assess for complications of immobility. Provide active and passive range-of-motion exercises, foot support, and adequate nutrition and hydration.
- Teach how to turn, cough, deep breathe, and use the incentive spirometer. Encourage independence as much as possible.

Risk for Impaired Skin Integrity

- Assess skin frequently. Provide pressure relief for both bed and wheelchair, and keep skin clean and dry. Change position every 2 hours.

Ineffective Coping

- Encourage the patient and caregivers to verbalize their feelings about this progressive, often fatal, disease. Refer them to psychological, spiritual, or religious counseling as appropriate.
- Assess the patient and caregivers' coping strategies for long-term needs.

Community-Based Care

- Explain the disease process, supportive therapies, and prognosis. Listen actively to questions and concerns and provide accurate information.
- Teach basic care skills. Involve the patient in decision making as much as possible. Provide positive reinforcement for independent activities such as self-care, eating, and asking questions.
- Refer to the local chapter of the Muscular Dystrophy Association for resources and support.

For more information on muscular dystrophy, see Chapter 40 in *Medical-Surgical Nursing,* Fifth Edition, by LeMone, Burke, and Bauldoff.

MYASTHENIA GRAVIS

Overview

- Myasthenia gravis (MG) is a chronic neuromuscular disease that causes progressive weakness and easy fatigability of skeletal muscles.

- Motor neurons transmit impulses to skeletal muscle by releasing acetylcholine (ACh) from the axon endplate into the synaptic cleft. The ACh crosses the synaptic cleft, attaches to receptors on the muscle fibers, and stimulates the muscle. In MG, antibodies destroy or block receptor sites, decreasing the number of ACh receptors. ACh uptake also is reduced. The net result is a decrease in the muscle's ability to contract despite sufficient ACh.

- Muscles supplied by cranial nerves are particularly susceptible, but MG may affect any skeletal muscle.

- Manifestations usually begin after age 50, with men affected more often than women.

- The course is unpredictable, with remissions and exacerbations.

Causes

- Autoimmune: destruction of ACh receptors on skeletal muscle cell membrane of myoneural junction; most common form.

- Rare genetic types.

- Other autoimmune disorders, thymomas, and small (oat) cell carcinoma of lung may coexist with MG.

Manifestations

- Skeletal muscle weakness

- Easy fatigability of skeletal muscles, especially following repetitive movements

- Eyes: ptosis, diplopia, incomplete closure

M

- Cranial muscles: reduced facial expression, difficult vocalization, difficulty chewing and swallowing
- Respiratory muscles: respiratory distress or failure, which can be life threatening

Diagnostic Tests

- Electromyographic studies show fatigue following repeated muscle stimulation.
- Tensilon test: intravenous injection of edrophonium chloride (Tensilon), a short-acting anticholinesterase, brings dramatic improvement of muscle function within 30 to 60 seconds and lasts about 5 minutes.
- Increased serum level of circulating ACh receptor antibodies is strongly diagnostic of MG.

Interdisciplinary Management

- Anticholinesterases (e.g., neostigmine, ambenonium, pyridostigmine) are used to promote ACh concentration at receptor sites.
- Immunosuppression with glucocorticoids (e.g., prednisone) improves muscle strength.
- Drugs such as beta-adrenergic blockers, aminoglycoside antibiotics, and narcotic analgesics are used with caution as they may exacerbate muscle weakness or depress respiratory function.
- Plasmapheresis may be used in conjunction with other therapies to remove ACh receptor antibodies
- Thymectomy is often recommended for patients younger than 60 to prevent the release of an autoantigen that is believed to trigger an autoimmune response in MG.

Selected Nursing Diagnoses with Interventions

Ineffective Airway Clearance

- Assist with turning, deep breathing, and coughing at least every 2 hours. Teach proper coughing techniques. Use an incentive spirometer every 2 hours while awake.
- Place in semi-Fowler's position.
- Maintain hydration status and monitor for dehydration. Use a humidifier as needed.

- Assess lung sounds, rate and character of respirations, and pulse oximetry readings at least every 4 hours.

Impaired Swallowing

- Assess ability to manage safely various consistencies of foods.
- Instruct to eat slowly, using small bites of food. Schedule mealtimes during periods when the patient is adequately rested.
- If necessary, give cues while eating; for example, "Chew your food thoroughly; now swallow."
- Teach caregivers the Heimlich maneuver and how to suction.

Community-Based Care

- Review the disease process, treatment options, and prognosis.
- Explain medication side effects and scheduling, and instruct to avoid nonprescription drugs without first consulting the physician.
- Encourage strategies to avoid fatigue and undue stress. Teach strategies for avoiding upper respiratory tract infections. Stress the importance of avoiding extreme heat or cold.
- Discuss family planning as appropriate, since pregnancy can exacerbate symptoms, and medications used to control MG can cross the placenta.
- Refer to a physical or occupational therapist and/or social services as appropriate.
- Provide information on local MG support groups.
- Refer significant others to local cardiopulmonary resuscitation certification classes.

For more information on myasthenia gravis, see Chapter 44 in *Medical-Surgical Nursing,* Fifth Edition, by LeMone, Burke, and Bauldoff.

MYOCARDIAL INFARCTION

Overview

- Myocardial infarction (MI) is necrosis (death) of myocardial cells.
- Heart disease is the leading cause of death in the United States. MI and other forms of ischemic heart disease cause

the majority of these deaths, usually within the first hour of the onset of symptoms.

- MI occurs when blood flow to a portion of cardiac muscle is blocked, causing prolonged tissue ischemia and irreversible cell damage. Coronary occlusion is usually caused by ulceration or rupture of a complicated atherosclerotic lesion.

- Prolonged tissue ischemia causes irreversible hypoxemic damage, with cell death and tissue necrosis. Cellular acidosis develops, and intracellular enzymes are released through damaged cell membranes into interstitial spaces.

- Acute cell injury and infarction affect impulse conduction and myocardial contractility, increasing the risk of dysrhythmias and reducing stroke volume, cardiac output, blood pressure, and tissue perfusion.

- The subendocardium suffers the initial damage, progressing to the epicardium within 1 to 6 hours (*transmural infarction*).

- Infarcted tissue is surrounded by potentially viable tissue. This tissue may be stunned, with impaired contractility. Rapid restoration of blood flow limits these changes.

- The size of the occluded vessel and available collateral circulation determine the extent of myocardial damage. The area of damage is determined by the affected coronary artery.

- Cocaine intoxication can lead to acute myocardial infarction (AMI) by increasing sympathetic nervous system activity and the workload of the heart.

- Common complications of MI include dysrhythmias, pump failure, infarct extension, structural defects, and pericarditis.

Causes

No specific cause has been identified. Risk factors include the following:

- Preexisting coronary heart disease
- Age, gender, heredity, race
- Smoking
- Obesity, hyperlipidemia, diet

- Hypertension, diabetes
- Sedentary lifestyle

Manifestations

- Sudden onset of chest pain, usually not associated with activity; crushing and severe; a pressure, heavy, or squeezing sensation; or chest tightness or burning; often substernal, radiating to shoulders, neck, jaw, or arms; duration of more than 15 to 20 minutes, not relieved by rest or nitroglycerin

- Women and older adults usually present with atypical chest pain: possible indigestion, heartburn, nausea, and vomiting

- Anxiety

- Tachycardia, tachypnea; possible bradycardia

- Cool, clammy, mottled skin

- Sense of impending doom and death

- Hypertension or hypotension

- Signs of heart failure

- Nausea and vomiting, hiccupping

Diagnostic Tests

- Levels of serum cardiac markers such as creatine kinase (CK) and its isoenzyme CK-MB (most sensitive indicator of MI), and cardiac-specific troponins (cT_nT and cT_nI) rise in AMI.

- Myoglobin is a cardiac marker released shortly after symptom onset.

- Complete blood cell count shows elevated white blood cells and sedimentation rate due to inflammation of the injured myocardium.

- The electrocardiogram (ECG) reflects characteristic changes, including T-wave inversion, ST-segment elevation, and possible Q-wave development.

- Echocardiography shows decreased contractility and ventricular wall motion in the infarcted area.

- Radionuclide imaging may show ischemic areas of the myocardium.

- Hemodynamic monitoring may be initiated when AMI significantly affects cardiac output and hemodynamic status.

Interdisciplinary Management

- Fibrinolytic drugs to dissolve or break up blood clots are first-line drugs used to treat AMI. These drugs limit infarct size, reduce heart damage, and improve outcomes.

- Sublingual or intravenous nitroglycerin is given to relieve pain and reduce cardiac work. Intravenous morphine sulfate is given in small doses until pain is relieved. Antianxiety agents may be given to promote rest. Antidysrhythmics may be used as needed to prevent and treat dysrhythmias. Beta blockers and angiotensin-converting enzyme inhibitors reduce mortality associated with AMI.

- Aspirin, a platelet inhibitor, is recommended at the onset of symptoms or given by emergency personnel. Anticoagulants and other antiplatelet medications often are prescribed as well.

- Immediate or early percutaneous coronary revascularization may follow thrombolytic therapy or be used in place of thrombolytic therapy. Coronary artery bypass grafting may be done.

- With pump failure accompanying MI, invasive devices such as the intra-aortic balloon pump or a ventricular assist device may be used to temporarily support myocardial function.

- Cardiac rehabilitation begins with admission and continues through transition to independent exercise and exercise maintenance.

Selected Nursing Diagnoses with Interventions

Acute Pain

- Assess for verbal and nonverbal signs of pain. Document characteristics and the intensity of the pain, using a standard pain scale. Verify nonverbal indicators of pain with the patient.

- Administer oxygen at 2 to 5 L/min per nasal cannula.

- Promote physical and psychologic rest. Provide information and emotional support.

- Titrate intravenous nitroglycerin as ordered to relieve chest pain, maintaining a systolic blood pressure greater than 100 mmHg.

- Administer 2 to 4 mg morphine by intravenous push for chest pain as needed.

- Reassess for relief of chest pain.

Ineffective Tissue Perfusion

- Assess and document vital signs. Report increases in heart rate and changes in rhythm, blood pressure, and respiratory rate.

- Assess for changes in level of consciousness; decreased urine output; moist, cool, pale, mottled or cyanotic skin; dusky or cyanotic mucous membranes and nail beds; diminished to absent peripheral pulses; delayed capillary refill.

- Auscultate heart and breath sounds. Note abnormal heart sounds (S_3 or S_4 gallop or murmur) or adventitious lung sounds.

- Monitor ECG rhythm continuously.

- Obtain a 12-lead ECG to assess complaints of chest pain. Report marked changes to the physician.

- Monitor oxygen saturation levels. Administer oxygen as ordered. Obtain and assess arterial blood gases as indicated.

- Administer antidysrhythmic medications as needed.

- Obtain serial CK, isoenzyme, and troponin levels as ordered.

- Plan for invasive hemodynamic monitoring.

- Continuously evaluate the response to interventions such as thrombolytic therapy, drugs to improve cardiac output and tissue perfusion, and drugs to reduce cardiac work.

Ineffective Coping

- Establish an environment of caring and trust. Encourage the patient to express feelings.

- Accept denial as a coping mechanism, but do not reinforce it.

- Note aggressive behaviors, hostility, or anger. Document any failure to comply with treatments.

- Help identify and reinforce use of positive coping skills (e.g., problem-solving skills, verbalization of feelings, asking for help, prayer).

- Provide opportunities for the patient to make decisions about the plan of care, as possible.

- Provide privacy for the patient and significant other to share their questions and concerns.

Fear

- Identify the patient's level of fear, noting verbal and nonverbal signs.

- Acknowledge the patient's perception of the situation.

- Encourage questions and provide consistent, factual answers. Repeat information as needed.

- Encourage self-care. Allow the patient to make decisions regarding the plan of care.

- Administer antianxiety medications as ordered.

- Teach nonpharmacologic methods of stress reduction (e.g., relaxation techniques, mental imagery, music therapy, breathing exercises, meditation, massage).

Community-Based Care

- Teach about the disease process; treatments, including medications, dosage, effects, and side effects; and prescribed risk factor modifications.

- For the patient who has had percutaneous transluminal coronary angioplasty, advise a return to moderate activities in 1 to 2 weeks, per the physician's recommendation. Instruct to avoid heavy lifting, and to apply manual pressure if bleeding occurs at the insertion site. Instruct to call the physician if bleeding is extensive or lasts for more than 15 minutes.

- Emphasize the importance of continuing the medical regimen and keeping follow-up appointments. Provide telephone numbers and addresses of resource personnel who are available to respond to questions and concerns after discharge.

- Discuss and provide referral to a community cardiac rehabilitation program.

- Provide information about community resources, such as the local chapter of the American Heart Association.

- Encourage significant others to learn cardiopulmonary resuscitation in the event of an emergency, and provide information on community agencies that offer cardiopulmonary resuscitation classes.

For more information on myocardial infarction, see Chapter 30 in *Medical-Surgical Nursing,* Fifth Edition, by LeMone, Burke, and Bauldoff.

MYOCARDITIS

Overview

- Myocarditis is inflammation of the heart muscle.

- It usually is self-limited but may progress to become chronic, leading to dilated cardiomyopathy.

- The inflammatory process in myocarditis causes local or diffuse swelling and damage. Abscesses may form. Myocardial cells may be further damaged by immune responses.

Causes

- Usually viral (coxsackievirus B)

- May be bacterial or parasitic

- Immunologic response (e.g., associated with rheumatic fever)

- Effects of radiation, toxins, or drugs

- Risk factors include malnutrition, alcohol use, immunosuppressive drugs, exposure to radiation, stress, and advanced age

Manifestations

- May be asymptomatic

- Fever, fatigue, general malaise

- Dyspnea, palpitations

- Arthralgias

- Muffled S_1, S_3, murmur, and pericardial friction rub

- Manifestations of heart failure or myocardial infarction

Diagnostic Tests

- Electrocardiography may show transient ST segment and T wave changes, dysrhythmias, and possible heart block.

- Cardiac markers, such as creatine kinase, troponin T, and troponin I, may be elevated.

- Endomyocardial biopsy shows patchy cell necrosis and inflammation.

Interdisciplinary Management

- If appropriate, antimicrobial or antiviral therapy is initiated. Immunosuppressive therapy may be used to minimize the inflammatory response. Heart failure is treated as needed, using angiotensin-converting enzyme inhibitors and drugs.

- Bed rest and activity restrictions are ordered during the acute period; activities may be limited for 6 to 12 months.

Selected Nursing Diagnoses with Interventions

Decreased Cardiac Output

- Monitor ECG and hemodynamic parameters closely.

- Administer antidysrhythmic agents, antiplatelets, or ACE inhibitors as ordered. Use digitalis with caution.

- Administer antimicrobial, antiviral, corticosteroid or immunosuppressive medications if prescribed.

- Assess level of pain. Administer pain medications as prescribed.

Activity Intolerance

- Encourage bed rest and activity restriction until fever and cardiac symptoms subside.

- Discuss with the patient and significant others the change in the patient's role performance, their questions, and concerns. Assess the need for home care, social services, or other community assistance to provide for patient's and significant others' immediate needs.

Community-Based Care

- Teach about the disease process; treatment, including medications; strategies for preventing recurrences; and prognosis.

- Stress the importance of reporting manifestations of streptococcal pharyngitis to the physician immediately for antibiotic therapy.

- Explain that prophylactic antibiotic therapy may be necessary to prevent streptococcal infection or bacterial endocarditis for the remainder of the patient's life.

- Provide referral to social or community services as appropriate for the patient experiencing altered role performance due to activity restrictions.

For more information on myocarditis, see Chapter 31 in *Medical-Surgical Nursing,* Fifth Edition, by LeMone, Burke, and Bauldoff.

M

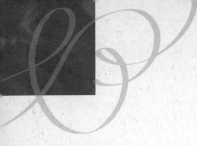

NEAR-DROWNING

Overview

- About 5,500 people die of drowning every year in the United States.
- Asphyxiation and aspiration are the primary problems associated with drowning and near-drowning.
- Hypoxia causes loss of consciousness within 3 to 5 minutes, and brain death within 5 to 10 minutes.
- Delayed death from near-drowning may be attributed to the effects of water aspiration on blood cells, fluid and electrolyte balance, and respiratory tissues.
- Aspiration of freshwater leads to hypervolemia, hemodilution, and hemolysis.
- Aspiration of saltwater draws fluid into the alveoli, leading to hypovolemia and hemoconcentration.
- Pneumonia and acute respiratory distress syndrome may develop due to aspirated microorganisms and debris.

Causes

- Prolonged immersion in a body of water
- Alcohol ingestion is a significant risk factor, implicated in 25% of adult drowning deaths.

Manifestations

- Altered level of consciousness, restlessness, apprehension
- Headache, chest pain
- Vomiting
- Cyanosis
- Apnea or tachypnea, wheezing
- Pink froth in the mouth and nose

- Tachycardia, dysrhythmias
- Hypotension, shock, cardiac arrest
- Hypothermia

Diagnostic Tests

- Arterial blood gases evaluate gas exchange and effects on acid–base balance.
- Serum electrolytes and serum osmolality show hemodilution in freshwater drowning and possible hemoconcentration in salt-water drowning.
- Chest x-ray may not show significant changes for several hours.

Interdisciplinary Management

- Hypothermia or barbiturate-induced coma, corticosteroids, and osmotic diuretics may be used to help prevent neurologic damage.
- Oxygen is administered; intubation and mechanical ventilation may be used to support respiratory function.
- Intravenous fluids are administered to restore fluid and electrolyte balance; packed red blood cells may be given if significant hemolysis has occurred.

Selected Nursing Diagnoses with Interventions

N

Ineffective Airway Clearance

- Frequently assess respiratory status, including rate, depth, effort, and breath sounds; amount, color, and consistency of sputum.
- Assist to cough frequently; suction the intubated patient as needed.
- Elevate the head of the bed unless otherwise ordered.
- Stabilize endotracheal tube with tape and ties.
- Report pink, frothy, or purulent sputum.
- Administer bronchodilators as ordered.
- Perform percussion and postural drainage as ordered.

Impaired Gas Exchange

- Administer supplemental oxygen as ordered.
- Frequently assess oxygen saturation, skin color, and mental status.
- Monitor exhaled carbon dioxide, arterial blood gases, and pulmonary artery pressures. Report changes.

- Provide frequent mouth care.
- Work with respiratory therapy to maintain effective oxygen delivery with mechanical ventilation.

Ineffective Tissue Perfusion: Cerebral

- Monitor vital signs, intracranial pressure, and neurologic status frequently. Report changes promptly to the physician.
- Maintain seizure precaution.
- Elevate the head of the bed; keep the head in neutral position.
- Maintain effective ventilation and oxygenation.
- Administer sedation, osmotic diuretics, or corticosteroids as ordered to reduce cerebral edema.
- Maintain fluid restriction.
- Space activities and promote rest to reduce metabolic demands.

Community-Based Care

- Teach patients never to swim alone when fatigued or immediately following a meal.
- Instruct to always wear flotation devices while boating, water-skiing, surfing, or windsurfing. Wet suits help prevent hypothermia during activities in very cold water.
- If hospitalization is not required, teach about symptoms of possible complications to report: increasing dyspnea, cough productive of purulent or pink frothy mucus, confusion, or other changes.
- Advise covering or fencing swimming pools, hot tubs, and ponds to prevent inadvertent entry and drowning.
- Encourage all people to be trained and regularly update cardiopulmonary resuscitation skills.
- If permanent neurologic deficits result from near-drowning, work with the family to develop communication techniques and identify remaining strengths. Assist to identify future care needs.
- Refer for services such as home health, personal care aides, social services, and support groups as indicated.

For more information about near-drowning, see Chapter 36 in *Medical-Surgical Nursing,* Fifth Edition, by LeMone, Burke, and Bauldoff.

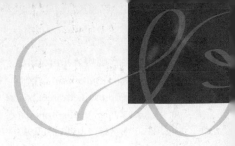

Occupational Lung Disease

Pneumoconiosis

Hypersensitivity pneumonitis

Overview

- Pneumoconiosis is chronic fibrotic lung disease caused by exposure to inorganic dusts and particulate matter. The most common types include asbestosis, silicosis, and coal worker's pneumoconiosis (black lung disease).

- Hypersensitivity pneumonitis is an allergic pulmonary disease caused by exposure to inhaled organic dusts and gases. Some common types include byssinosis, bagassosis, and farmer's lung.

- Dusts are deposited within alveoli and ingested by pulmonary macrophages. The resulting inflammatory process damages lung tissue, resulting in replacement of normal elastin fibers by fibrotic tissue.

- Fibrotic lung tissues are stiff and noncompliant, reducing lung volumes, increasing the work of breathing, and impairing alveolar-capillary diffusion.

Causes

Pneumoconiosis

- Asbestosis is caused by exposure to asbestos; people involved in asbestos mining, milling, manufacturing, application, and removal are at risk.

- Coal worker's pneumoconiosis is caused by exposure to coal dust.

- Silicosis is caused by exposure to silica; mining, stonecutting, sandblasting, and quarrying increase the risk.

- Other inorganic dusts implicated include talc, beryllium, and graphite.

Hypersensitivity Pneumonitis

- Byssinosis results from exposure to cotton dust.
- Bagassosis results from exposure to moldy sugar cane.
- Farmer's lung results from exposure to molds or fungi on grain, hay, or straw, or from exposure to bird droppings.

Manifestations

- Exertional dyspnea, exercise intolerance
- Tachypnea
- Progressive dyspnea
- Inspiratory crackles
- Chronic productive cough
- Possible acute response to organic dusts: malaise, chills, fever, dyspnea, cough, nausea

Diagnostic Tests

- Chest x-ray can show characteristic changes of the disorder.
- Pulmonary function testing shows restrictive impairment of lung ventilation with reduced vital capacity and total lung capacity.
- Bronchoscopy may be done to visually identify lung tissue changes and obtain a tissue sample for biopsy.

Interdisciplinary Management

- There is no specific treatment for occupational lung diseases.
- Eliminating further exposure to the offending agent is vital.
- Anti-inflammatory drugs (e.g., corticosteroids) may slow the progress of the disease. Pneumococcal and influenza vaccines are recommended to reduce the risk for lower respiratory infections.

Selected Nursing Diagnoses with Interventions

Ineffective Breathing Pattern

- Teach controlled cough techniques (e.g., huff cough, controlled cough).
- Teach effective breathing techniques (e.g., pursed-lip and diaphragmatic breathing).

Activity Intolerance

- Discuss energy conservation measures.
- Encourage rest periods between activities and treatments.

Ineffective Family Coping

- Encourage verbalization of fears and concerns. Listen and answer questions in a nonjudgmental manner.

- Provide support and reassurance—focus on positive ways of handling stress.

- Provide realistic hope by focusing on short-term goals.

Community-Based Care

- Provide information about occupational lung diseases and risk-reduction measures to workers, including measures to reduce dust in work areas and use of personal protective devices such as masks.

- Instruct to avoid exposure to cigarette smoke, environmental pollutants, and other respiratory irritants. Advise to avoid further exposure to the offending agent.

- Recommend immunizations for influenza and pneumococcal pneumonia.

- Recommend yearly tuberculin testing for patients with silicosis.

- Teach pulmonary hygiene measures such as maintaining good fluid intake, coughing, and deep-breathing exercises.

- If home oxygen therapy is ordered, discuss its use and care of equipment.

- Teach about any prescribed or recommended over-the-counter medications.

- Referral to a smoking cessation program may be appropriate.

- Refer to the local chapter of the American Lung Association for information and support.

For more information about occupational lung diseases, see Chapter 37 in *Medical-Surgical Nursing,* Fifth Edition, by LeMone, Burke, and Bauldoff.

OSTEOARTHRITIS

Overview

- Osteoarthritis (OA) is a degenerative disorder characterized by loss of articular cartilage in joints and hypertrophy of the bones at joint margins.

- OA is the most common form of arthritis. It may be either primary or secondary in nature.

- In OA, collagen fibers and proteoglycans in joint cartilage are destroyed by enzymes, reducing its tensile strength. The cartilage ulcerates, and as the disease progresses, large areas are lost, exposing underlying bone. Exposed bone thickens and is deformed by cysts and cartilage-coated outgrowths called osteophytes (spurs). Small pieces of osteophytes may break off, leading to mild synovitis.

- Localized OA affects only one or two joints. Generalized OA affects three or more joints.

- OA usually involves the major weight-bearing joints (vertebrae, hips, knees); it is also seen in the distal and proximal interphalangeal joints of the hands.

- The incidence of OA increases with age.

Causes

- Primary: idiopathic; genetic and/or metabolic factors may contribute

- Risk factors include obesity and inactivity

- Secondary: trauma, mechanical stress, inflammation of joint structures, joint instability, neurologic disorders, endocrine disorders, and selected medications

Manifestations

- Insidious onset

- Joint stiffness/chronic pain: deep, aching, worse in morning and with exercise, and from weather changes

- Crepitus: grating type, with motion

- Decreased range of motion (ROM)

- Joint spurs/deformity: Heberden's and Bouchard's nodes in finger; enlargement of large joints

Diagnostic Test

- X-ray or MRI of joint shows joint-space narrowing, bone cysts, osteophytes, subchondral sclerosis, and absence of the gross inflammation typical of rheumatoid arthritis.

- Synovial fluid examination helps determine the type of arthritis.

Interdisciplinary Management

- Mild analgesics such as acetaminophen and nonsteroidal anti-inflammatory drugs typically are used to manage the pain of OA. Topical medications such as counterirritants, salicylates and capsaicin are available over-the-counter to improve comfort.

- Corticosteroids may be injected into the joint space to relieve severe pain. However, frequent injections can hasten the rate of cartilage breakdown. Hyaluronidase may be injected into the joint each week for 3 to 5 weeks to increase joint lubrication.

- Surgery may be indicated for chronic pain and loss of joint function. Arthroscopy may be used to débride the joint. Osteotomy may be done to realign an affected joint. Arthroplasty reconstructs or replaces a joint.

Selected Nursing Diagnoses with Interventions

Chronic Pain

- Assess level of pain, including intensity, location, quality, and aggravating and relieving factors.

- Encourage use of prescribed analgesic or anti-inflammatory medication as needed.

- Encourage rest of painful joints.

- Apply heat to painful joints using the shower, a tub or sitz bath, warm packs, hot wax baths, heated gloves, or diathermy.

- Emphasize the importance of maintaining a moderate level of physical activity.

- Encourage the overweight patient to reduce weight.

- Teach the patient to use splints or other devices on affected joints as needed.

- Encourage use of nonpharmacologic pain relief measures such as progressive relaxation, meditation, visualization, and distraction.

Impaired Physical Mobility

- Assess the ROM of affected joints.

- Assess functional mobility, evaluating gait and ability to sit and rise from a chair, step into or out of a tub or shower, and negotiate stairs.

- Teach active and passive ROM exercises, as well as isometric, progressive resistance, and low-impact aerobic exercises.

- Provide analgesics or other pain relief measures prior to exercise or ambulation.

Community-Based Care

- Explain the disease process and its chronic degenerative nature, treatments including medication regimen, and ways to slow joint destruction, as discussed.

- Assess the home environment for hazards to safe mobility, such as scatter rugs. Encourage use of devices such as hand rails and grab bars.

- Teach how to use ambulatory aids such as a cane or a walker as prescribed.

- Following arthroplasty, teach proper use and weight bearing of the affected limb. Teach the proper use of splints, braces, and assistive devices such as walkers or canes.

- Discuss possible complications, including signs of infection or dislocation, and instruct the patient to notify the physician promptly if these occur.

- Provide referrals to physical or occupational therapy, or other community agencies as indicated.

- The obese patient may benefit from a referral to a weight-reduction program.

For more information on osteoarthritis, see Chapter 40 in *Medical-Surgical Nursing,* Fifth Edition, by LeMone, Burke, and Bauldoff.

OSTEOMALACIA (RICKETS)

Overview

- Osteomalacia (adult rickets) is a metabolic bone disorder characterized by inadequate mineralization.

- In osteomalacia, the bone matrix is not mineralized due to insufficient calcium or phosphate. Bones become spongy, weak, and soft, leading to skeletal deformity and pathologic fractures.

- It usually affects weight-bearing bones: pelvis, spine, legs.

- It is more common later in life, and affects women more than men.

Causes

- Lack of vitamin D activity from inadequate ingestion, inadequate sunlight exposure, or altered metabolism, as in renal disease, or hereditary disorders.

- Hypophosphatemia due to insufficient intake, excessive losses through the urine or stool, or a shift into the cells. Alcohol abuse is the most common cause of hypophosphatemia.

Manifestations

- Bone pain and tenderness

- Skeletal deformity: scoliosis, kyphosis, bowed legs; waddling gait

- Muscle weakness may be an early sign of vitamin D deficiency

- Pathologic fracture, usually of the distal radius or proximal femur

Diagnostic Tests

- Serum calcium may be within normal limits or low, depending on the cause.

- Alkaline phosphatase usually is elevated; parathyroid hormone levels also may be elevated.

- X-rays demonstrate the effects of generalized bone demineralization.

Interdisciplinary Management

- Therapy typically includes vitamin D supplementation. Calcium and phosphorus supplements also may be prescribed.

Selected Nursing Diagnoses with Interventions

Imbalanced Nutrition: Less than Body Requirements

- Teach about dietary sources of calcium, phosphorus, and vitamin D. Encourage patients to maintain adequate milk intake as a good dietary source of vitamin D.

- Refer to appropriate specialists, especially the dietitian and gastroenterologist.

Risk for Injury

- Evaluate the home environment for hazards that could lead to falls.

- Teach safety measures and ways to acquire safety aids for the home.

- Consult with a physical therapist regarding the use of ambulatory or gait devices.

Community-Based Care

- Explain the disease process, treatments, and expected outcomes. Discuss foods high in vitamin D and calcium, including dairy products. Encourage appropriate, regular exercise.

- Instruct patients taking vitamin D supplements to report to their primary care provider symptoms such as anorexia, nausea and vomiting, frequent urination, muscle weakness, and constipation.

- Teach safety measures to prevent falls, such as eliminating scatter rugs and clutter from living areas to prevent tripping, placing a night light in hallways and the bathroom, and installing grab bars in the shower and tub and next to the toilet.

- Teach appropriate use of splints, braces, and ambulatory aids as indicated.

- Encourage daily brief exposure to the sun, even in winter.

- Stress the importance of follow-up visits with the physician.

- A referral to a home health nurse may be appropriate.

For more information on osteomalacia (rickets), see Chapter 40 in *Medical-Surgical Nursing,* Fifth Edition, by LeMone, Burke, and Bauldoff.

OSTEOMYELITIS

Overview

- Osteomyelitis is an acute, subacute, or chronic infection of bone.

- Pathogens can infect the bone directly from compound fractures, penetrating injuries, or surgery; or secondarily from hematogenous spread of bacteria or extension of local soft-tissue infection.

- The infection usually remains localized, but may spread within marrow to the cortex and periosteum.

- Acute osteomyelitis is the more common form; the chronic form is rare.

- Early diagnosis and treatment of osteomyelitis is important to prevent bone necrosis.

Causes

- *Staphylococcus aureus* is the most common organism. Others include *Escherichia coli, Pseudomonas, Klebsiella, Proteus,* or

Salmonella. Although less common, fungi, parasites, and viruses can also cause bone infection.

- Risk factors include a penetrating wound or open trauma, aging, immunosuppression, compromised circulation (e.g., peripheral vascular disease), chronic diseases such as diabetes or chronic obstructive pulmonary disease, and pressure ulcers.

Manifestations

Local

- Pain, swelling, erythema, and warmth at infection site
- Drainage and ulceration of the involved site
- Local tenderness, reduced weight-bearing on affected extremity

Systemic

- Fever, chills, malaise, usually sudden onset
- Anorexia, nausea, and vomiting
- Tachycardia
- Lymphadenopathy of involved extremity

Diagnostic Tests

- White blood cell count and erythrocyte sedimentation rate are elevated.
- Bone scan, ultrasound, computed tomography scan and magnetic resonance imaging are used to identify subperiosteal fluid collections, abscesses, sinus tracts, and bone changes associated with osteomyelitis.
- Needle aspiration or percutaneous needle biopsy may be performed to obtain a specimen for culture in acute cases.
- Blood cultures frequently are positive.

Interdisciplinary Management

- Parenteral antibiotic therapy is begun as soon as cultures are obtained. Antibiotics (intravenous or oral) are continued for at least 4 to 6 weeks.
- Surgical debridement is the primary treatment for the patient with chronic osteomyelitis.

Selected Nursing Diagnoses with Interventions

Risk for Infection

- Maintain strict hand hygiene practices and standard precautions to prevent the spread of infection.
- Administer antimicrobial therapy as ordered.
- Maintain optimal dietary kilocalorie and protein intake.

Hyperthermia

- Monitor temperature every 4 hours and if chills are present.
- Maintain a cool environment and provide light clothing and bedding during temperature elevation.
- Ensure a daily fluid intake of 2,000 to 3,000 mL.

Impaired Physical Mobility

- Maintain a functional position of the affected limb when immobilized.
- Maintain rest and avoid subjecting the affected extremity to weight-bearing activities.
- Ensure active or passive range-of-motion exercises every 4 hours.

Community-Based Care

- Discuss the disease process, treatment, and prognosis, and general principles of infection control.
- Stress the importance of follow-up care with the physician.
- When the patient is on bed rest, teach the importance of shifting position frequently to relieve pressure on skin areas. Instruct to maintain the joint in a position of function as well as comfort.
- Provide information to prevent yeast infections and diarrhea often associated with prolonged antibiotic therapy by eating 8 oz of live-culture yogurt each day.
- Provide information on community agencies and social services that can provide financial assistance during the prolonged recuperative period.
- A referral to a home healthcare provider may be appropriate.

For more information on osteomyelitis, see Chapter 40 in *Medical-Surgical Nursing*, Fifth Edition, by LeMone, Burke, and Bauldoff.

OSTEOPOROSIS

Overview

- Osteoporosis is a metabolic bone disorder characterized by loss of bone mass, increased bone fragility, and an increased risk of fractures.

- Osteoporosis involves an imbalance of the activity of osteoblasts that form new bone and osteoclasts that resorb bone. As a result, the outer supporting cortex of the bone thins and becomes more porous.

- A major health problem in the United States, an estimated 10 million adults have osteoporosis and another 34 million have low bone mass.

- A woman's lifetime risk of having an osteoporosis-related fracture is 1 in 2 after age 50; a man's risk is 1 in 4 after age 50.

Causes

- Risk factors:
  - Nonmodifiable: female gender; advanced age; European American or Asian American race; genetic factors
  - Modifiable: sedentary lifestyle; vitamin D or calcium deficiency; low estrogen (amenorrhea or postmenopausal females) or testosterone (aging males); high alcohol intake; smoking; medications such as glucocorticosteroids; some anticonvulsants; prolonged use of antacids (phosphate binders), proton pump inhibitors, and heparin
  - Malabsorption disorders: celiac disease, pancreatic disorders, inflammatory bowel disease
  - Endocrine disorders: hyperthyroidism, hyperparathyroidism, Cushing's syndrome, diabetes mellitus

Manifestations

- May be asymptomatic until fracture occurs
- Loss of height, progressive curvature (dorsal kyphosis, cervical lordosis) of the spine
- Fractures (may be pathologic) of the forearm, spine, or hip
- Pain, often low back; may be acute or chronic; may radiate around the flank into the abdomen

O

Diagnostic Tests

- Bone mineral density (BMD) to estimate skeletal mass or density for at-risk patients.
- Dual-energy x-ray absorptiometry (DEXA) measures bone density in the lumbar spine or hip.
- Ultrasound of the heel of the foot to measure bone density is used to screen for osteoporosis.
- X-ray will show fracture if present.
- Serum alkaline phosphatase may be elevated following a fracture.

Interdisciplinary Management

- Hormone replacement therapy in postmenopausal women may be used to preserve existing bone mass. Raloxifene, a selective estrogen receptor modulator, appears to prevent bone loss by mimicking estrogen's beneficial effects on bone density.
- Biphosphonates such as alendronate (Fosamax), risedronate (Actonel), and ibandronate (Boniva), are current drugs of choice used to prevent and treat osteoporosis.
- Teriparatide, a synthetic parathyroid hormone, may be used to decrease the risk of bone fracture in postmenopausal women and in men with primary or secondary hypogonadism.
- Other pharmacologic agents include calcium supplements and calcitonin to increase bone formation and decrease resorption.

Selected Nursing Diagnoses with Interventions

Readiness for Enhanced Self- Health Management

- Assess health habits, including diet, exercise, smoking, and alcohol use.
- Teach women and men of all ages the importance of maintaining an adequate calcium intake. Provide a list of calcium-rich foods, and discuss the use of calcium supplements with patients who do not consume adequate dietary calcium.
- Discuss the importance of maintaining a regular schedule of weight-bearing exercise, either through an exercise program or regular physical activity.
- Refer patients to smoking-cessation programs and alcohol treatment programs as appropriate.

- Refer patients with significant risk factors for osteoporosis to primary care providers or clinics for bone-density evaluation as indicated.

Risk for Injury

- Implement safety precautions as necessary: maintain the bed in low position; use side rails if indicated; provide nighttime lighting to toilet facilities.
- Avoid using restraints (if hospitalized or a resident in a long-term care facility) if at all possible.
- Encourage older adults to use assistive devices to maintain independence in activities of daily living.
- Teach older patients about safety and fall precautions.

Imbalanced Nutrition: Less than Body Requirements

- Teach adolescents, pregnant or lactating women, and adults through age 35 to eat foods high in calcium and to maintain a daily calcium intake of 1,200 to 1,500 mg.
- Encourage postmenopausal women to maintain a calcium intake of 1,000 to 1,500 mg daily, either through diet or a calcium supplement.
- Teach patients taking calcium supplements the importance of taking the medication at the proper time and the side effects that may occur.

Community-Based Care

O

- Explain the disease process, and how to limit its progression through diet, activity, supplements, and medications as appropriate.
- Teach about prescribed medications, their appropriate use, precautions, and intended and potential adverse effects.
- Review the effects of smoking; encourage the patient not to smoke.
- Advise to maintain a regular schedule of weight-bearing activity.
- Encourage moderate exposure to sunlight.
- Assess home environment for fall risk and discuss safety measures to prevent falls.
- Suggest anti-inflammatory pain medications for acute or chronic pain. Instruct about appropriate dose and frequency, advising the patient to take the medication regularly, not just as needed for pain.
- Suggest the application of heat to relieve pain.
- A dietary consult may be appropriate.
- Provide the name and address of a local osteoporosis support group.

For more information on osteoporosis, see Chapter 40 in *Medical-Surgical Nursing,* Fifth Edition, by LeMone, Burke, and Bauldoff.

Otitis, Otitis Externa (Swimmer's Ear), Otitis Media

Overview

- Otitis is inflammation of the ear, usually due to infection.

Otitis Externa

- Otitis externa is inflammation of the ear canal.
- *Pseudomonas aeruginosa* or other bacterial infection is the usual cause; may also be due to fungal infection, mechanical trauma, or a local hypersensitivity reaction.

Otitis Media

- Otitis media is an inflammation of the middle ear. There are two primary forms: serous and acute or suppurative. Both are associated with upper respiratory infection and eustachian tube dysfunction.
- Acute (suppurative) otitis media occurs when edema of the auditory tube impairs drainage of the middle ear, causing mucus and serous fluid to accumulate. This fluid is an excellent environment for the growth of bacteria, which may enter from the oronasopharynx via the eustachian tube. Bacterial growth and the immune response cause pus formation, increasing pressure, potentially rupturing the tympanic membrane.
- Serous otitis media occurs when the eustachian tube is obstructed for a prolonged period, preventing air from entering the middle ear. The resulting negative pressure causes sterile serous fluid to move from the capillaries into the space, forming a sterile effusion of the middle ear.

Causes

Otitis Externa

- Bacteria: *Pseudomonas aeruginosa, Proteus vulgaris, Streptococcus, Staphylococcus aureus*
- Fungi: *Aspergillus niger, Candida albicans*
- Skin diseases: psoriasis, seborrhea, hypersensitivity reaction
- Risk factors: competitive swimming, diving, surfing; using ear plugs or a hearing aid; inserting object into ear

Otitis Media

- Suppurative: associated with upper respiratory tract infection; bacteria (usually *Streptococcus pneumoniae, Haemophilus influenzae,* or *Streptococcus pyogenes*) ascend the eustachian tube
- Serous: inadequately treated acute otitis media, viral infection, allergy, barotrauma

Manifestations

Otitis Externa

- Sensation of fullness in the ear
- Pain, possibly severe, aggravated by manipulation of the auricle
- Odorless watery or purulent drainage
- Inflammation and edema of the ear canal

Otitis Media

- Acute suppurative:
  - Mild to severe pain in the affected ear
  - Diminished hearing, dizziness, vertigo, and tinnitus
  - Red and inflamed or dull and bulging tympanic membrane on otoscopic exam; decreased tympanic membrane movement
  - Fever
  - Mastoid tenderness
- Acute serous:
  - Decreased hearing in the affected ear
  - Complaints of "snapping" or "popping" in the ear
  - Otoscopic exam reveals decreased tympanic membrane mobility; may appear retracted or bulging; clear fluid or air bubbles may be visible behind the membrane

Diagnostic Tests

Otitis Externa

- No diagnostic tests usually are required. Culture and sensitivity can identify specific organism.

Otitis Media

- Impedance audiometry(tympanometry) shows reduced compliance of the tympanic membrane and middle ear.

- Complete blood cell count may show an elevated white blood cell count and increased numbers of immature cells indicative of acute bacterial infection.
- If the tympanic membrane has ruptured or a tympanocentesis or myringotomy is performed, drainage is cultured to determine the infecting organism.

Interdisciplinary Management

- Otitis externa is usually treated with a topical antibiotic, often in combination with a topical corticosteroid to promote comfort.
- Systemic antibiotics and analgesics are prescribed for acute otitis media. A short course of oral corticosteroid therapy may be ordered for serous otitis media that does not spontaneously resolve within several days.
- Surgical myringotomy or tympanocentesis may be performed to prevent spontaneous rupture of the tympanic membrane. Antibiotic eardrops may be prescribed postoperatively.

Selected Nursing Diagnoses with Interventions

Acute Pain

- Assess severity, quality, and location of pain.
- Instruct the patient to use mild analgesics such as aspirin or acetaminophen every 4 hours as needed to relieve pain and fever.
- Advise applying heat to the affected side unless contraindicated.
- Instruct to avoid air travel, rapid changes in elevation, or diving until the condition is completely resolved.
- Instruct to report promptly an abrupt relief of pain.

Impaired Tissue Integrity

- Stress the importance of completing the full prescribed course of antibiotics.
- Discuss the desired and potential adverse effects of the prescribed antibiotic. Tell the patient to report any adverse effects to the physician.
- Instruct the patient who has ventilation tubes inserted or a ruptured tympanic membrane to avoid swimming, diving, or submerging the head while bathing.
- Instruct to avoid air travel, rapid changes in elevation, or diving, all of which can cause bruising, hematoma, or hemorrhage.

- Encourage to rest, drink ample amounts of fluid, and consume a nutritious diet.

Community-Based Care

Do the following in addition to the above mentioned teaching:

- Review the disease process, causes and prevention, treatments, and expected recovery time.

- As indicated, teach the patient with eustachian tube dysfunction to autoinflate the middle ear by performing the Valsalva maneuver or by forcefully exhaling against closed nostrils.

- If surgery is necessary, teach about the procedure and postoperative care. Provide instruction about any special postoperative precautions, such as avoiding water in the ear canals.

- Teach to avoid inserting foreign objects into the ear canal.

- Contact the healthcare provider if symptoms recur or persist despite therapies.

For more information on otitis, see Chapter 46 in *Medical-Surgical Nursing,* Fifth Edition, by LeMone, Burke, and Bauldoff.

OVARIAN CANCER

Overview

- Ovarian cancer is a malignant tumor of the ovary.

- Most ovarian tumors arise from surface epithelium; germ cell or stromal types account for most other cases.

- Ovarian cancer usually spreads by shedding cancer cells into the peritoneal cavity and by direct invasion of the bowel and bladder. Tumor cells also spread through the lymph and blood to such organs as the liver, and across the diaphragm to involve the lungs. Pelvic and para-aortic lymph nodes may be involved.

- Ovarian cancer is the fourth most common gynecologic cancer, but the most lethal.

- The incidence increases with age, peaking between ages 40 and 80.

- It is usually found in advanced stages because it is asymptomatic in early stages.

Causes

- Risk factors: family history of ovarian cancer, breast-ovarian cancer syndrome, genetic mutations such as those in BRCAI

and BRCAII (breast and ovarian cancer) and Lynch syndrome (colorectal cancer).
- Other risk factors include increasing age, having no children or giving birth after age 35, early menarche and late menopause, infertility drugs, obesity, eating a high fat diet, and a personal history of breast cancer. Polycystic ovarian disease and hormone replacement therapy after menopause may also place a woman at risk.
- More common in White women than in other races.

Manifestations
- Usually asymptomatic in early stages; fatigue, back pain
- Feeling full quickly, urinary urgency and/or frequency, abdominal bloating, constipation
- Pain during intercourse, and menstrual changes in women prior to menopause
- Possible abnormal vaginal bleeding, pelvic or abdominal pain
- Enlarged abdomen with ascites in later-stage disease

Diagnostic Tests
- Transvaginal or abdominal ultrasound may reveal location and size of the tumor.
- Computed tomography scan of the pelvis or abdomen may show the tumor and possible metastasis.
- CA-125 is a tumor marker that is highly specific to epithelial ovarian cancer.

Interdisciplinary Management
- Combination chemotherapy may be used to achieve remission of the disease; it is not, however, curative for ovarian cancer.
- Surgery is the treatment of choice, usually involving total hysterectomy with bilateral salpingo-oophorectomy and removal of the omentum.
- Radiation therapy may be performed for palliative purposes only.

Selected Nursing Diagnoses with Interventions
Acute/Chronic Pain
- Assess level of pain, characteristics, and duration. Provide pain medications as prescribed and monitor for effects.
- Teach nonpharmacologic measures to reduce pain, including meditation, guided imagery, and distraction.

Disturbed Body Image

- Encourage the patient to express feelings of anxiety. Discuss coping strategies that have worked in the past. Make her a part of the decision-making process when feasible. Provide diversion through television, radio, games, and occupational therapies when possible.

- Assess interaction between patient and significant others. Teach significant others as well as the patient about the disease process, treatment options, and prognosis. Also teach skills required for patient care.

- Provide referral to home health services, financial assistance, psychologic counseling, clergy, and social services as appropriate.

Anticipatory Grieving

- Assess past experience of the patient and her significant others with loss, existing support systems, and current grief work. Discuss the phases of the grieving process with the patient and significant others. Refer them to appropriate resources, including religious or spiritual counselors, legal assistance, or financial assistance.

- Encourage active participation in cancer support groups. Arrange for visits from cancer survivors. Provide positive reinforcement for behaviors that demonstrate initiative, including self-disclosure, self-care, and increased appetite.

Community-Based Care (For Surgery)

- Explain pre- and postoperative procedures.

- Relate side effects of chemotherapy and/or radiation therapy, and their management.

- Explain the importance of planned rest periods.

- Explain the importance of involving family members or significant others in dealing with the body image changes.

- Stress the importance of follow up with outpatient care for further treatment of cancer as necessary.

- Refer to home care, cancer support groups, social services, legal services, psychologic counselors, hospice care, and/or spiritual counselors as appropriate.

For more information on ovarian cancer, see Chapter 49 in *Medical-Surgical Nursing*, Fifth Edition, by LeMone, Burke, and Bauldoff.

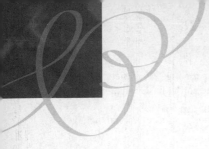

PANCREATIC CANCER

Overview

- Pancreatic cancer is primary malignant tumor of the pancreas, usually in the head of the gland.
- Most pancreatic cancers occur in the exocrine pancreas, are adenocarcinomas, and are fatal within 1 to 3 years after diagnosis.
- Pancreatic cancer accounts for only about 3% of all cancers, but the 5-year survival rate is only about 5%. It causes over 35,000 deaths annually in the United States.

Causes

- Unknown; risk factors include the following:
  - Smoking, exposure to industrial chemicals or environmental toxins, obesity, high-fat diet, possibly red meat consumption, pancreatitis, diabetes mellitus, and cirrhosis.
  - Age (after 50), genetic predisposition, and race (higher in Blacks than in Whites)

Manifestations

- Insidious onset
- Early manifestations: Anorexia, nausea, weight loss, flatulence
- Dull epigastric pain, gradually increasing in severity; may increase with eating or lying down
- Jaundice, clay-colored stools, dark urine, and pruritus may occur with tumors of head of pancreas
- Late manifestations: palpable abdominal mass, ascites

Diagnostic Tests

- Biopsy is diagnostic for malignant cells.

P

- Carcinoembryonic antigen may be elevated.
- CA 19-9 tumor marker may be positive.

Interdisciplinary Management

- Early tumors of the head of the pancreas may be resectable; a pancreatoduodenectomy (Whipple's procedure) is performed.
- Advanced pancreatic cancer is usually treated with palliative chemotherapy and radiation for pain and symptom relief.

Selected Nursing Diagnoses with Interventions

Pain

- Maintain bed rest in position of comfort.
- Assess pain using a standard pain scale and noting characteristics of the pain.
- Administer analgesics as prescribed. Use a regular schedule and prn doses to maintain comfort and treat breakthrough pain.
- Administer chemotherapy as prescribed.
- Teach and assist with alternative pain management techniques, such as progressive relaxation, therapeutic touch, guided imagery, and music.
- Encourage to change position every 2 hours, to cough, and to deep breathe.

Imbalanced Nutrition: Less than Body Requirements

- Administer total parenteral nutrition via a central or Hickman catheter as prescribed.
- Monitor intake and output.
- Administer medications as prescribed: antiemetics, antacids, pancreatic enzymes, bile salts, and insulin.

Anticipatory Grieving

- Ask about past experience of the patient and family with loss. Assess support systems and current grief work. Discuss phases of the grieving process with the patient and significant others. Assist them to verbalize their fears and concerns, and provide referrals to appropriate resources.

Impaired Skin Integrity

- Keep fingernails short to avoid injury from scratching. Apply hand mitts if necessary.

- Avoid the use of soap. Use bath oils, creams, and lotions to keep skin soft and to reduce itching.

- Use protective barriers around drainage tubes to prevent excoriation.

Community-Based Care

- Teach about the disease process, treatment options, and prognosis.

- Discuss skin care and measures to manage adverse effects of chemotherapy and radiation therapy if prescribed.

- Teach effective use of analgesics and nonpharmacologic comfort measures such as guided imagery, distraction, and meditation.

- If surgery has been performed, teach wound care and activity restrictions to reduce the risk for infection or injury to the incision site.

- Refer the patient and significant others to support groups such as the American Cancer Society, social services, psychologic counselors, and religious/spiritual caregivers as appropriate.

- Referral to hospice services may be appropriate.

For more information about pancreatic cancer, see Chapter 25 in *Medical-Surgical Nursing,* Fifth Edition, by LeMone, Burke, and Bauldoff.

PANCREATITIS

Acute

Chronic

Overview

- Pancreatitis is inflammation of the pancreas characterized by release of pancreatic enzymes into the tissue of the pancreas itself, with resulting hemorrhage and necrosis.

Acute Pancreatitis

- Acute pancreatitis involves self-destruction of the pancreas by its own enzymes through autodigestion. It often is self-limiting and may be relatively mild (*interstitial edematous pancreatitis*), with inflammation and edema of pancreatic tissue; or more severe (*necrotizing pancreatitis*), characterized by inflammation, hemorrhage, and necrosis of pancreatic tissue.

Chronic Pancreatitis

- Chronic pancreatitis is an irreversible process characterized by gradual destruction of functional pancreatic tissue with eventual pancreatic insufficiency.

Causes

Acute Pancreatitis

Specific cause is unknown. Risk factors include the following:

- Alcoholism (more common in men)
- Cholelithiasis (more common in women)
- Tissue ischemia or anoxia
- Trauma, surgery, or invasive procedures (e.g., endoscopic retrograde cholangiopancreatography)
- Pancreatic tumors
- Third-trimester pregnancy
- Infectious agents (viral, bacterial, or parasitic)
- Hypercalcemia, hyperlipidemia
- Drugs, including thiazide diuretics, estrogen, steroids, salicylates, and nonsteroidal anti-inflammatory drugs

Chronic Pancreatitis

- Alcoholism is the primary risk factor in the United States.
- Malnutrition is a major worldwide risk factor.
- About 10% to 20% of cases are idiopathic, with no identified cause, although they may have a genetic link.
- Cystic fibrosis is a risk factor.

P

Manifestations

Acute Pancreatitis

- Abrupt onset of continuous severe epigastric and abdominal pain, often initiated by a fatty meal or excessive alcohol intake.
- Pain commonly radiates to the back, and may be relieved by sitting up and leaning forward.
- Nausea, vomiting.
- Abdominal distention and rigidity; decreased bowel sounds.
- Tachycardia; hypotension; cold, clammy skin.
- Fever.
- Mild jaundice.
- Possible retroperitoneal bleeding with bruising in the flanks (Turner's sign) or around the umbilicus (Cullen's sign).

Chronic Pancreatitis

- Recurrent episodes of epigastric and left upper quadrant abdominal pain that radiates to the back
- Anorexia, nausea, vomiting
- Weight loss
- Flatulence, constipation, steatorrhea (fatty, frothy, foul-smelling stools)

Diagnostic Tests

- Serum amylase and serum lipase levels are elevated in acute pancreatitis.
- Urine amylase levels also are high in acute pancreatitis.
- Serum calcium may be low.
- White blood cell count is elevated in acute pancreatitis.
- Abdominal ultrasound may show gallstones or a pancreatic pseudocyst; endoscopic ultrasound can identify changes indicative of chronic pancreatitis in the pancreatic duct and parenchyma.
- Computed tomography scan can show pancreatic enlargement, fluid collections, and areas of necrosis.
- Endoscopic retrograde cholangiopancreatography is used to diagnose chronic pancreatitis.

- Magnetic resonance cholangiopancreatography (MRCP) is a noninvasive test that allows visualization of the bile and pancreatic ducts.

Interdisciplinary Management

- A narcotic analgesic is prescribed to relax smooth muscle and decrease pain. Antibiotics may be given to prevent or treat infection. Antacids and H_2 antagonists or proton pump inhibitors are given to neutralize or decrease gastric secretions. In chronic pancreatitis, pancreatic enzyme supplements are given to reduce steatorrhea, and octreotide (Sandostatin) may be given to suppress pancreatic enzyme secretion and relieve pain.

- Oral intake is withheld in acute pancreatitis; a nasogastric tube is inserted and connected to suction. Total parenteral nutrition is initiated.

- Surgical resection of all or part of the pancreas may be done to treat chronic pancreatitis. A cholecystectomy may be performed to remove gallstones.

Selected Nursing Diagnoses with Interventions

Acute Pain

- Administer prescribed analgesics on a regular schedule. Assess the location, radiation, duration, character, and intensity of the pain using a standard pain scale. Assess nonverbal indicators of pain.

- Maintain NPO status and nasogastric tube drainage as prescribed.

- Maintain bed rest in a calm, quiet environment.

- Encourage position of comfort, such as side-lying with knees flexed and head elevated to 45 degrees.

- Encourage relaxation and use guided imagery or other nonpharmacologic methods to reduce pain.

- Provide careful explanations of all procedures and care. Listen to concerns and evaluation of pain relief.

Risk for Imbalanced Nutrition: Less than Body Requirements

- Monitor nutritional parameters, including serum albumin, serum transferrin, total lymphocyte count, blood urea nitrogen, hematocrit, and hemoglobin.

P

- Weigh daily using consistent timing and technique.
- Maintain stool chart; include frequency, color, odor, and consistency of stools.
- Assess the presence and character of bowel sounds.
- Administer prescribed intravenous fluids and/or total parenteral nutrition.
- Provide oral hygiene before and after meals. Offer small, frequent feedings.

Community-Based Care

- Explain the disease process, treatments, medications, effects, side effects, prognosis, and strategies for preventing further attacks of pancreatitis.
- Discuss foods to meet nutritional needs and to maintain a high-carbohydrate, low-protein, low-fat diet. Include foods to avoid, such as alcohol, caffeine, spicy foods, and gas-producing foods. Emphasize the need to avoid large meals and to restrict dietary fats.
- Advise that smoking and stress stimulate the pancreas and should be avoided.
- Since an abscess may form months after the initial attack, stress the importance of reporting symptoms of infection, including fever, pain, rapid pulse, and malaise.
- Emphasize the importance of follow-up with the physician.
- Provide referrals to a smoking cessation program or to Alcoholics Anonymous as appropriate.
- A referral for home care may be appropriate.

For more information about pancreatitis, see Chapter 25 in *Medical-Surgical Nursing,* Fifth Edition, by LeMone, Burke, and Bauldoff.

PARKINSON'S DISEASE

Overview

- Parkinson's disease (PD) is a progressive, degenerative neurologic disorder characterized by resting tremor, muscle rigidity, and bradykinesia.

- In PD, degenerative changes in the substantial nigra and other portions of the brain lead to decreased production of dopamine (a neurotransmitter that helps regulate motor function). The usual balance of activity between dopamine and acetylcholine in the brain is disrupted; acetylcholine is no longer inhibited by dopamine. This imbalance leads to manifestations of the disorder.

- PD is relatively common; it usually develops after age 50 (late-onset PD), but can occur in younger adults (early-onset PD).

Causes

- The cause is unknown, although there is a genetic link, about 15% of PD having a family history of the disease.

- Secondary parkinsonism may result from trauma, encephalitis, tumors, toxins, carbon monoxide or cyanide poisoning, and drugs (e.g., neuroleptics, antiemetics, antihypertensives, and illegal designer drugs containing MPTP, a toxic chemical). Drug-induced parkinsonism often is reversible.

Manifestations

- Akinesia: loss of spontaneous movement (arm swinging, eye blinking)
- Bradykinesia: slowing of voluntary movement
- Rigidity: cogwheel type; of limb muscles
- Rhythmic "pill-rolling" movements of fingers seen mostly during rest
- Tremor of the hands, feet, head, neck, face, lips, tongue
- Stooped posture
- Shuffling gait with difficult starting and stopping movement
- Loss of facial expression, staring
- Monotonous vocalization
- Dementia in about 20% of cases (occurs in latter stages of the disease)

Diagnostic Tests

- There is no test that clearly differentiates PD from other neurological disorders.

P

Interdisciplinary Management

- At present there is no cure for PD, but medications bring dramatic improvement in manifestations. Throughout the disease process, drugs and combinations of drugs such as anticholinergics, monoamine oxidase B inhibitors (MOA-B), dopamine precursors, and dopamine agonists may be used for symptom control.

- Implantation of an electrical deep brain stimulator to block selected neural impulses or surgical destruction of tissue may improve symptoms in patients who do not respond to drug therapy.

- Stem cell transplantation is a surgical procedure still under investigation by the FDA.

- Patients frequently benefit from rehabilitation therapy.

Selected Nursing Diagnoses with Interventions

Impaired Physical Mobility

- Perform range-of-motion exercises at least twice a day, emphasizing the trunk, neck, arms, hips, and legs.

- Consult with a physical therapist to develop an individualized exercise program.

- Ambulate at least four times a day.

- Incorporate assistive devices such as canes, splints, or braces as indicated.

Impaired Verbal Communication

- Assess current communication abilities: speech, hearing, and writing.

- Develop methods of communication appropriate to the patient, such as a write-on, wipe-off slate; flash cards with common phrases; pointing to objects, and so on.

- Refer to a speech pathologist for oral exercises and interventions to facilitate speaking.

- Remind the patient to speak more loudly, if possible.

Imbalanced Nutrition: Less than Body Requirements

- Assess nutritional status and self-feeding abilities.

- Provide foods of proper consistency as determined by the patient's swallowing function.

- Weigh weekly and notify the physician of significant weight loss.

- Teach eating methods to decrease tremors, such as holding a piece of bread in the hand that is not holding an eating utensil.

- Encourage fluid intake and a diet high in fiber and low in saturated fat.

Community-Based Care

In addition to the previous teaching provide the following:

- The disease process, treatment options including medication regimen, and prognosis.

- Measures to prevent falls, malnutrition, constipation, skin breakdown, and joint contracture.

- Coordinate referrals for speech therapy, physical therapy, occupational therapy, psychotherapy, and social services as appropriate.

- Referral to a home health nurse for home care and a home safety check may be appropriate.

- A referral to respite care for caregiver relief may be required. Alternatively, a referral to a long-term care facility may be necessary if significant others are absent or unable to provide the appropriate level of care.

- Provide the name and address of local support groups.

For more information on Parkinson's disease, see Chapter 44 in *Medical-Surgical Nursing,* Fifth Edition, by LeMone, Burke, and Bauldoff.

PELVIC INFLAMMATORY DISEASE

Overview

- Pelvic inflammatory disease (PID) is infection of the pelvic organs, including the fallopian tubes (*salpingitis*), ovaries (*oophoritis*), cervix (*cervicitis*), endometrium (*endometritis*), pelvic peritoneum, and the pelvic vascular system.

- PID is usually caused by organisms entering the vagina and endocervical canal during sexual activity. From there, organisms ascend to the fallopian tubes and ovaries.

- Organisms can also be acquired during childbirth, abortion, or surgery of the reproductive tract.

- Complications of PID include pelvic abscess, infertility, ectopic pregnancy, pelvic adhesions, dyspareunia, and chronic pelvic pain.

Causes

- Infection due to *Neisseria gonorrhoeae* and *Chlamydia trachomatis* accounts for most cases.

- Other causative organisms include *Staphylococcus, Haemophilus influenzae,* and enteric Gram-negative rods.

- Risk factors include current sexual activity, a history of sexually transmitted infection (especially gonorrhea and chlamydia), bacterial vaginitis, multiple sexual partners, douching, and previous PID.

Manifestations

Acute Infection
- Fever
- Purulent vaginal discharge
- Abnormal bleeding
- Severe lower abdominal or back pain
- Dyspareunia
- Painful cervical movement

Subacute Infection
- Generally asymptomatic
- Infertility a presenting complaint

Diagnostic Tests

- Complete blood cell count with differential reveals a markedly elevated white blood cell count.

- The sedimentation rate is elevated.
- Gram stain and culture and sensitivity of secretions identify the causative organisms.
- Ultrasound is used to rule out ectopic pregnancy.
- Laparoscopy may reveal inflammation of the fallopian tubes and, possibly, generalized pelvic involvement, abscesses, and scarring.

Interdisciplinary Management

- Combination antibiotic therapy with broad-spectrum antibiotics is the typical treatment for PID.
- Surgical procedures may be performed to drain an abscess or treat a life-threatening complication such as rupture of a fallopian tube or abscess.

Selected Nursing Diagnoses with Interventions

Risk for Injury

- Encourage completion of antibiotic therapy as prescribed; monitor closely for adverse effects.
- Teach to recognize and report side effects of medications, as well as manifestations of ectopic pregnancy.

Readiness for Enhanced Knowledge

- Caution the patient about using tampons. Instruct the patient to change tampons or pads at least every 4 hours.
- Provide information about safer sex practices and family planning. Instruct patient to remove diaphragm within 6 hours after use. Intrauterine devices are contraindicated. Latex condoms offer the most protection against infection.
- Teach to report any unusual vaginal discharge or odor to the healthcare provider.
- Explain the treatment options, emphasizing those that could preserve fertility, if this is desired.
- Suggest a support group or counselor as needed.

Acute Pain

- Assess the level, characteristics, and duration of pain. Note verbal and nonverbal indicators of pain. Encourage analgesic use as prescribed.

- Encourage use of sitz baths and apply heat to lower back or abdomen. Teach other nonpharmacologic pain relief measures, including guided imagery, meditation, and distraction.

- Maintain bed rest in semi-Fowler's position.

Community-Based Care

- Review the disease process, causes, prevention, treatment options, medication regimen, and prognosis.

- Discuss how to prevent recurrences, the importance of completing the full course of antibiotics, and the need for meticulous personal hygiene.

- Explain the importance of treating sexual partners.

- Encourage the use of latex condoms during sexual intercourse.

- Stress the importance of regular medical examinations, including Pap smears to detect neoplastic changes.

- Provide referrals to fertility counselors, psychologic counselors, and/or spiritual counselors as appropriate.

- Referral to support groups, such as RESOLVE for infertile couples, may be helpful.

For more information on pelvic inflammatory disease, see Chapter 50 in *Medical-Surgical Nursing,* Fifth Edition, by LeMone, Burke, and Bauldoff.

PEPTIC ULCER DISEASE

Overview

- Peptic ulcer disease (PUD) is characterized by a break in the mucous lining of the gastrointestinal tract where it comes in contact with gastric juice.

- The mucosal barrier, a thin coating of mucous gel and bicarbonate, protects gastric mucosa. An ulcer develops when the mucosal barrier is unable to protect the mucosa from damage by hydrochloric acid and pepsin, the gastric digestive juices.

- *H. pylori* bacteria produce enzymes that impair the mucosal barrier; the inflammatory response to *H. pylori* infection contributes to gastric epithelial cell damage.

- Nonsteroidal anti-inflammatory drugs (NSAIDs) contribute to PUD by interrupting prostaglandin synthesis (prostaglandins help support the gastric mucosal barrier) and by directly damaging gastric epithelial cells.

- The ulcers of PUD may be superficial or deep, affecting the mucosa, submucosa, muscular layers of the stomach, or duodenum.

- Duodenal ulcers, the most common, usually develop in the proximal portion of the duodenum, close to the pylorus. They are more common in younger adults and men.

- Gastric ulcers often develop on the lesser curvature near to the pylorus.

Causes
- Chronic *H. pylori* infection
- Use of aspirin, NSAIDS, or corticosteroid drugs
- Probable genetic factors
- Cigarette smoking
- Zollinger-Ellison syndrome (a type of PUD) caused by a gastrinoma or gastrin-secreting tumor of the pancreas, stomach, or intestines
- Unrelated to alcohol and dietary intake; stress may contribute

Manifestations
- Pain: gnawing, burning, aching, or hungerlike; epigastric, may radiate to the back; occurs 2 to 3 hours after meals and at night; relieved by eating
- Heartburn or regurgitation
- Possible vomiting

- Vague and poorly localized discomfort in the older adult; dysphagia, weight loss, or anemia
- Possible black, tarry stools
- Manifestations of hemorrhage and shock: pallor, tachycardia, hypotension, cool and clammy skin
- Manifestations of perforation: sudden, sharp pain; rigid abdomen; shallow breathing; absent bowel sounds; shock

Diagnostic Tests

- Upper gastrointestinal series detects 80% to 90% of peptic ulcers, but may miss small or very superficial ones.
- Endoscopy allows visualization of the ulcers.
- Biopsy specimens obtained during endoscopy can be tested for *H. pylori* infection using a biopsy urease test (90% accurate in diagnosing the infection).
- Fecal *H. pylori* antigen and urea breath tests are noninvasive measures to detect *H. pylori* infection and evaluate effectiveness of treatment.
- Gastric analysis shows very high gastric acid levels in Zollinger-Ellison syndrome.

Interdisciplinary Management

- Drugs used to treat PUD include antacids, which neutralize hydrochloric acid and reduce pepsin activity; H_2 receptor antagonists and proton pump inhibitors, which reduce gastric acid secretion.
- Sucralfate and bismuth subsalicylate may be used to provide a protective coating and promote wound healing; antibiotics are used to eradicate *H. pylori*.
- Surgery may be required to treat complications of PUD such as perforation or obstruction of the gastric outlet.

Selected Nursing Diagnoses with Interventions

Pain

- Assess pain, including location, type, severity, frequency and duration, and its relationship to food intake or other contributing factors.

- Administer antacids, H_2 receptor antagonists, or mucosal protective agents as prescribed. Monitor for effectiveness and side effects.
- Provide and teach adjunctive relief measures such as distraction, relaxation, and breathing exercises.

Imbalanced Nutrition: Less than Body Requirements

- Assess current diet, including pattern of food intake, eating schedule, and foods that precipitate pain or are being avoided in anticipation of pain.
- Arrange consultation with a dietitian to identify a meal plan that minimizes PUD symptoms yet meets the nutritional needs of the patient.
- Monitor for complaints of anorexia, fullness, nausea, and vomiting or symptoms of dumping syndrome. Adjust dietary intake or medication schedule as indicated.
- Assess and monitor laboratory values for indications of anemia or other specific nutritional deficits. Monitor for therapeutic and side effects of measures such as oral iron replacement. If oral iron supplements are ordered, separate administration of iron and antacids by at least 1 to 2 hours.

Risk for Bleeding

- Monitor vital signs every 15 to 30 minutes until stable if hemorrhage occurs. Monitor hemodynamic parameters as indicated. Insert a Foley catheter and monitor urinary output hourly.
- Monitor stools and gastric drainage for obvious and occult blood.
- Maintain intravenous fluid volume and electrolyte replacement solutions; administer whole blood or packed cells as prescribed.
- Insert a nasogastric tube and maintain its position and patency; irrigate with sterile normal saline as needed or prescribed. Initially, measure gastric output hourly, then every 4 to 8 hours.
- Monitor hemoglobin and hematocrit, serum electrolytes, blood urea nitrogen, and creatinine. Report abnormal findings.
- Assess abdomen, including bowel sounds, distention, girth, and tenderness, every 4 hours and record findings.
- Maintain bed rest with the head of the bed elevated.

Community-Based Care

- Teach about the disease process as well as preventive and therapeutic strategies.

- Provide written and verbal instruction about prescribed medications, including dosage, effects, and side effects. Stress the importance of continuing medications even when symptoms are relieved, and of avoiding aspirin and other NSAIDs.

- Provide information about the relationship between PUD and smoking.

- Teach the symptoms that may indicate complications, such as increased abdominal pain or distention, vomiting, black or tarry stools, lightheadedness, or fainting.

- Refer to a smoking cessation or alcohol treatment program as appropriate.

- Referral for counseling, classes, or support groups for stress reduction may be appropriate.

For more information on peptic ulcer disease, see Chapter 23 in *Medical-Surgical Nursing,* Fifth Edition, by LeMone, Burke, and Bauldoff.

PERICARDITIS

Overview

- Pericarditis is inflammation of the visceral and parietal pericardium.

- Pericarditis may be primary or develop secondarily to another cardiac or systemic disorder.

- Acute pericarditis is usually viral and affects men (usually under the age of 50) more frequently than women.

- Pericardial tissue damage triggers an inflammatory response and exudate formation. The exudate may be fibrinous or serofibrinous, and may contain red blood cells or purulent material.

- The inflammatory process may resolve without long-term effects, or lead to scar tissue and adhesion formation between the pericardial layers.

- Fibrosis and scarring of the pericardium may restrict diastolic filling and impair cardiac function.

- Pericardial effusions may develop as exudate collects in the pericardial sac. Significant pericardial effusion can interfere with cardiac filling and output (cardiac tamponade).

Causes

- Frequently idiopathic.
- Viral or bacterial infection; fungi; parasites.
- Immune mediated (hypersensitivity or autoimmune): rheumatic fever, rheumatoid arthritis, scleroderma, systemic lupus erythematosus.
- Chest trauma, surgery, or radiation.
- Post myocardial infarction.
- Drugs: procainamide, hydralazine.
- Uremia; myxedema.
- Constrictive pericarditis may follow viral infection, radiation therapy, or heart surgery.

Manifestations

Acute

- Chest pain: abrupt onset; usually sharp, steady or intermittent, may radiate to the back or neck; aggravated by respiratory movements, position changes, or swallowing; relieved by sitting upright, leaning forward
- Pericardial friction rub (a leathery, grating sound) heard most clearly at the left lower sternal border
- Low-grade fever
- Dyspnea, tachycardia
- Manifestations of pericardial effusion: distant or muffled heart sounds; dyspnea; enlarged cardiac silhouette on x-ray
- Manifestations of cardiac tamponade: narrowed pulse pressure, hypotension, increased central venous pressure; paradoxical pulse; muffled or inaudible heart sounds

Chronic Constrictive

- Weakness, fatigue
- Anorexia, weight loss, cachexia

P

- Dyspnea on exertion, orthopnea
- Jugular vein distention
- Positive Kussmaul's sign (failure of central venous pressure to fall during inspiration)
- Manifestations of right heart failure

Diagnostic Tests

- Complete blood cell count shows elevated white blood cells and an erythrocyte sedimentation rate greater than 20 mm/h in acute pericarditis.
- Cardiac enzymes may be slightly elevated but are typically much lower levels than in myocardial infarction.
- Electrocardiography shows diffuse ST segment elevation and possible decreased QRS amplitude with pericardial effusion.
- Echocardiography shows pericardial effusion (if present), and the extent of restriction.
- Hemodynamic monitoring demonstrates elevated pulmonary artery pressures and venous pressures with pericardial effusion or constrictive pericarditis.
- Chest x-ray shows cardiac enlargement if pericardial effusion is present.
- Computed tomography scan or magnetic resonance imaging can identify pericardial effusion or constrictive pericarditis.

Interdisciplinary Management

- Aspirin, acetaminophen, and other nonsteroidal anti-inflammatory drugs (NSAIDs) are used to relieve pain and reduce inflammation. In severe cases, corticosteroids may be used.
- Pericardiocentesis, removal of fluid from the pericardial sac, may be necessary with large pericardial effusions.
- A partial or total pericardiectomy, removal of part or all of the pericardium, may be required in chronic constrictive pericarditis.

Selected Nursing Diagnoses with Interventions

Acute Pain

- Assess complaints of chest pain using a standard pain scale and noting the quality and radiation of the pain. Ask about factors that aggravate or relieve pain. Note nonverbal cues of pain and validate them with the patient.

- Administer NSAIDs on a regular basis as ordered with food.
- Provide supportive measures: Maintain a calm, quiet environment; provide position changes, back rubs, heat/cold therapy, diversional activity, and emotional support.

Ineffective Breathing Pattern

- Assess respiratory rate, depth, and effort, and breath sounds every 2 to 4 hours. Note and report the presence of adventitious or diminished breath sounds.
- Encourage to breathe deeply and use the incentive spirometer. Provide pain medication at least 30 minutes before respiratory therapy treatments, as needed.
- Administer oxygen as needed.
- Elevate the head of the bed to Fowler's or high Fowler's position. Assist to assume position of comfort.

Risk for Decreased Cardiac Output

- Document vital signs hourly during an acute inflammatory process.
- Assess heart sounds and peripheral pulses, and observe for neck vein distention and pulsus paradoxus, hourly. Promptly report distant, muffled heart sounds, new murmurs or extra heart sounds, decreasing quality of peripheral pulses, and distended neck veins.
- Monitor trends of hemodynamic parameters and cardiac rhythm. Notify physician of changes.
- Promptly report other signs of decreased cardiac output: changes in level of consciousness; decreased urine output; cold, clammy, mottled skin; delayed capillary refill; and weak peripheral pulses.
- Ensure that at least one intravenous access line is established, and maintain its patency.
- If emergency pericardiocentesis and/or surgery is needed to evacuate pericardial fluid, prepare the patient for the procedure, providing appropriate explanations and reassurance. Observe the patient during the procedure for adverse effects.

Community-Based Care

- Teach about the disease process; treatments, including any procedures such as pericardiocentesis; medications, activity restrictions, and so on.

- If surgery is scheduled, provide preoperative and postoperative teaching as appropriate.

- Stress the importance of continuing anti-inflammatory medications as prescribed. Instruct to take the medications with food to minimize gastric distress, and to monitor weight at least weekly, as these drugs may cause fluid retention. Advise to avoid aspirin and over-the-counter preparations containing aspirin while taking other NSAIDs. Encourage a fluid intake of at least 2500 mL per day.

- Teach about specific activity restrictions if prescribed.

- Teach manifestations of recurrence that should be promptly reported to the physician.

For more information on pericarditis, see Chapter 31 in *Medical-Surgical Nursing*, Fifth Edition, by LeMone, Burke, and Bauldoff.

PERIPHERAL VASCULAR DISEASE

Overview

- Peripheral vascular disease is a general term for disease of arteries to the extremities that impairs the blood supply to peripheral tissues.

- Atherosclerosis, characterized by thickening, loss of elasticity, calcification of arterial walls, and plaque formation, is the usual cause of peripheral vascular disease.

- Atherosclerotic lesions typically develop in large and midsize arteries, particularly the abdominal aorta and iliac arteries, the femoral and popliteal arteries, and more distal arteries.

- Plaque tends to form at arterial bifurcations, gradually obstructing the vessel and impairing blood flow to the lower extremities; tissue hypoxia or anoxia results.

- Although collateral circulation often develops, it is usually not adequate to supply tissue needs.

Causes

- Atherosclerosis; risk factors: older age, diabetes mellitus, hypercholesterolemia, hypertension, cigarette smoking, and high homocystine levels; possibly male gender
- Vasculitis
- Trauma to legs
- Buerger's disease
- Raynaud's phenomenon

Manifestations

- *Intermittent claudication,* cramping or aching pain that occurs with activity and is relieved by rest; often accompanied by weakness
- *Rest pain,* a burning sensation in the lower legs during periods of inactivity; increases with leg elevation, decreases with dependent positioning; cold or numb feeling
- Diminished sensation
- Muscle atrophy
- Weak or absent peripheral pulses
- Bruit over large arteries (e.g., femoral artery, abdominal aorta)
- Pallor with leg elevation; dependent rubor when dependent
- Thin, shiny, hairless skin with discolored areas; thickened toenails
- Areas of skin breakdown and ulceration
- Possible edema

Diagnostic Tests

- Segmental pressure measurements may show a lower blood pressure in legs and in the distal extremities.
- Stress testing often shows a further decline in blood pressure at the ankle with exercise.
- Doppler ultrasound evaluates blood flow within affected blood vessels. Duplex Doppler ultrasound and color-flow Doppler ultrasound provide images of the vessel and blood flow.

- Transcutaneous oximetry evaluates oxygenation of tissues.
- Angiography or magnetic resonance angiography locates and evaluates the extent of arterial obstruction.

Interdisciplinary Management

- Medications to inhibit platelet aggregation (e.g., aspirin, clopidogrel [Plavix]) are given to reduce the risk of arterial thrombosis; cilostazol (Pletal) and pentoxifylline (Trental) improve blood flow and claudication. Parenteral vasodilator prostaglandins may be given to decrease pain and facilitate healing when limb ischemia is severe.
- Smoking cessation is vital. Other conservative measures include progressive daily walking, weight reduction, and meticulous foot care.
- Surgical (e.g., endarterectomy) or nonsurgical (e.g., angioplasty with stent placement) revascularization may be done if symptoms are progressive, severe, or disabling, or for pregangrenous or gangrenous lesions.

Selected Nursing Diagnoses with Interventions

Ineffective Tissue Perfusion: Peripheral

- Assess peripheral pulses, pain, color, temperature, and capillary refill of extremities with each home visit; every 4 hours or more often when hospitalized. Use a Doppler device to locate and assess pulses that cannot be palpated; mark location with an indelible marker.
- Teach the importance of avoiding extremity elevation.
- Keep extremities warm using lightweight blankets, socks, and slippers. Do not use electric heating pads or hot water bottles to warm extremities.
- Encourage frequent position changes; instruct to avoid leg crossing.
- Provide meticulous leg and foot care daily, using mild soaps and moisturizing lotions.

Impaired Skin Integrity

- Assess skin of the extremities with each home visit and at least once each shift; more often if needed. Document findings and changes with each assessment.

- Provide meticulous daily skin care, being sure to keep skin clean, dry, and supple.

- Apply a bed cradle.

Community-Based Care

- Provide information about the disease process and conservative management strategies. Stress the importance of smoking cessation, progressive exercise, maintaining a healthy weight, and taking medications as prescribed.

- Teach care of the legs and feet: Keep legs and feet clean, dry, and well lubricated. Inspect the feet and legs daily, using a mirror as needed. Wear well-fitting shoes. Keep toenails trimmed straight across. Avoid exposure to extremes of temperature. Avoid constricting leg garments.

- Referral to a smoking cessation program, cardiac rehabilitation, and/or weight reduction program may be appropriate.

- Provide a list of support groups, public health services, and other community agencies.

For more information on peripheral vascular disease, see Chapter 32 in *Medical-Surgical Nursing,* Fifth Edition, by LeMone, Burke, and Bauldoff.

PERITONITIS

P

Overview

- Peritonitis is inflammation of the peritoneum, a serious complication of many acute abdominal disorders.

- Peritonitis usually results from enteric bacteria entering the peritoneal cavity through a perforated ulcer, ruptured appendix, or perforated diverticulum.

- Chemical peritonitis (from gastric secretions or bile) often precedes bacterial peritonitis.

- Fibrinogen-rich plasma exudate forms fibrin clots to segregate the bacteria, limiting and localizing the infection.

- Continued contamination leads to generalized inflammation of the peritoneal cavity. This causes third spacing of fluid, depletion of blood volume, and hypovolemia.
- Septicemia, systemic disease caused by pathogens or their toxins in the blood, may follow.

Causes

- Contamination with *Escherichia coli, Klebsiella, Proteus,* or *Pseudomonas* bacteria
- Perforated ulcer or diverticulum, ruptured appendix or gallbladder
- Necrotic bowel
- Abdominal surgery or trauma
- Pelvic inflammatory disease

Manifestations

- Abrupt onset of diffuse, severe abdominal pain increased by movement
- Abdominal tenderness with guarding or rigidity of abdominal muscles
- Possible rebound tenderness
- Markedly diminished or absent bowel sounds
- Progressive abdominal distention
- Nausea and vomiting
- Fever, malaise
- Tachycardia, tachypnea
- Restlessness, possible disorientation
- Possible oliguria and shock

Diagnostic Tests

- White blood cell count is elevated, often to > 20,000/μL, with increased numbers of immature cells.
- Paracentesis is performed to extract fluid for analysis or culture and sensitivity.

- Abdominal x-ray may show air-fluid levels indicative of bowel obstruction, and free air under the diaphragm indicative of gastrointestinal perforation.

Interdisciplinary Management

- A beta-lactam antibiotic such as imipenem (Primaxin) or meropenem (Merrem), which have a very broad spectrum of action, may be used until the infecting organism has been identified. Antibiotic therapy is modified for specific organisms to treat the infection; narcotic analgesics are given to promote comfort and rest.
- Surgery may be required to repair the source of contamination. Peritoneal lavage may be done during surgery.
- Intestinal decompression may be initiated to relieve abdominal distention, facilitate closure, and minimize postoperative respiratory problems.

Selected Nursing Diagnoses with Interventions

Acute Pain

- Assess pain, noting its location, severity, and type.
- Place in Fowler's or semi-Fowler's position with the knees and feet elevated.
- Once the diagnosis has been established, administer analgesics as prescribed.
- Teach and assist the patient to use alternative pain management techniques along with pharmacologic interventions.
- Frequently evaluate response to analgesics.

Deficient Fluid Volume

- Record intake and output carefully. Measure urine output every 1 to 2 hours; report output of less than 30 mL per hour to the physician. Measure gastrointestinal output at least every 4 hours.
- Monitor vital signs and hemodynamic parameters hourly or as indicated.
- Weigh daily using standard technique.
- Assess skin turgor, color, temperature, and mucous membranes at least every 8 hours.

P

- Measure or estimate fluid losses through abdominal drains and on dressings.
- Monitor laboratory values, including hemoglobin and hematocrit, urine specific gravity, serum osmolality, serum electrolytes, and blood gases. Report changes to the physician.
- Provide intravenous fluid and electrolyte replacement as prescribed.
- Provide good skin care and frequent oral hygiene.

Delayed Surgical Recovery

- Monitor for manifestations of infection, including increased temperature, increased pulse, redness and increased swelling around incisions and drain sites, increased or purulent drainage, and changes in the character of urine output.
- Obtain cultures of purulent drainage from any site.
- Monitor white blood cell count and differential, serum protein, and albumin.
- Practice meticulous hand hygiene on entering and leaving the patient's room.
- Use strict aseptic technique when performing dressing changes and wound or peritoneal irrigations.
- Maintain fluid balance and adequate nutrition through enteral or parenteral feedings, as indicated.

P

Anxiety

- Assess anxiety level of the patient and significant others and their present coping skills.
- Present a calm, reassuring manner. Encourage the patient and significant others to express their concerns. Listen carefully, and acknowledge their validity.
- Minimize changes in caregiver assignments.
- Explain all treatments, procedures, tests, and examinations.
- Reinforce and clarify information provided by physicians.
- Teach and assist to use relaxation techniques such as meditation, visualization, and progressive relaxation.

Community-Based Care

- Explain the disease process, manifestations, treatment including medication regimen, and prognosis.

- Teach wound care procedures, including dressing changes or irrigations that will be required.

- Describe manifestations of further infection and other potential complications. Stress the importance of reporting these immediately to the physician.

- Discuss the need to consume a diet with adequate kilocalories and protein to meet the needs of the body for healing and optimal immune function.

- Instruct to avoid heavy lifting, strenuous labor, and driving a car until wound healing has occurred.

- Provide information on where to obtain necessary supplies.

- A referral to home health care for assessment, wound care, and further teaching may be appropriate.

For more information on peritonitis, see Chapter 24 in *Medical-Surgical Nursing,* Fifth Edition, by LeMone, Burke, and Bauldoff.

PERTUSSIS (WHOOPING COUGH)

Overview

- Pertussis (whooping cough) is a highly contagious, acute upper respiratory infection caused by *Bordetella pertussis*.

- Although thought of as a childhood disease, up to 45% of people affected by pertussis are adolescents and adults.

- *B. pertussis* produces bacterial toxins that damage respiratory mucosa and paralyze the cilia, impairing clearance of respiratory secretions and increasing the risk for pneumonia; the toxins also cause an inflammatory response and inhibit immune defenses.

- The disease tends to be milder in adolescents, adults, and people who have been immunized.

Cause

- *B. pertussis* infection
- Reservoir is humans; spread by respiratory droplets

Manifestations

- Manifestations of upper respiratory infection (coryza, sneezing, low-grade fever, and mild cough)
- Persistent cough (longer than 7 days)
- Possible paroxysms of coughing ending with an audible whoop (less common in adolescents and adults)
- Vomiting following coughing episodes
- Cough often worse at night

Diagnostic Tests

- Culture of nasopharyngeal secretions is positive for *B. pertussis*.
- Serologic testing for antibodies to the organism confirms the diagnosis.
- Lymphocytosis (elevated lymphocyte count) may be present.

Interdisciplinary Management

- Active immunization with pertussis vaccine is the primary preventive strategy for pertussis.
- Erythromycin is prescribed to eradicate *B. pertussis* infection; trimethoprim-sulfamethoxazole is an alternate antibiotic. Prophylactic antibiotics are prescribed for all household and close contacts of the patient.
- If hospitalized, respiratory isolation is maintained for 5 days after antibiotic therapy is started.

Selected Nursing Diagnoses with Interventions

Risk for Infection

- Promote effective immunization of all infants and young children against pertussis.
- Discuss potential long-term adverse consequences of the vaccine.
- Recommend that parents request acellular vaccine due to its lower risk of adverse effects.
- Recommend nasopharyngeal culture for patients complaining of persistent cough, especially when the cough is accompanied by vomiting or significantly worse at night, or if other members of the household or close contacts have a similar illness.

- Report all probable and confirmed cases of pertussis to the local health department and Centers for Disease Control and Surveillance.

Community-Based Care

- Teach respiratory isolation measures to be used until the disease is no longer communicable to others.
- Discuss ways to control respiratory secretions, and the importance of disposing of tissues and secretions personally to prevent exposure of others.
- Stress the importance of prophylactic treatment for all household and close contacts.
- Discuss measures to maintain fluid and nutrient intake, and use of a cough suppressant at night to promote rest.
- Encourage increased fluid intake to promote expectoration of respiratory secretions.
- Teach about the prescribed antibiotic, including its potential adverse effects and measures to reduce them, such as taking erythromycin with meals to prevent gastric upset.
- Contact the local county health department for follow-up of contacts and compliance with prescribed treatment.

For more information about pertussis, see Chapter 35 in *Medical-Surgical Nursing*, Fifth Edition, by LeMone, Burke, and Bauldoff.

P

PHEOCHROMOCYTOMA

Overview

- Pheochromocytomas are tumors of chromaffin tissues in the adrenal medulla.
- Pheochromocytomas produce catecholamines (epinephrine, norepinephrine); manifestations are due to this excess secretion.
- These small tumors are usually benign and unilateral.

Causes

- Sporadic, unknown
- Genetics: 5% due to an autosomal-dominant trait

Manifestations

- Manifestations occur in paroxysms, varying in duration and frequency.
- Hypertension: often severe or malignant; unresponsive to conventional treatment; can be episodic or constantly elevated.
- Tachycardia, dysrhythmia, or angina.
- Headache.
- Profuse diaphoresis.
- Extreme anxiety.
- Nausea or vomiting.
- Pallor or flushing.
- Hypotension/shock: may occur during anesthetic induction, due to down regulation (decrease) in catecholamine receptors.

Diagnostic Tests

- Magnetic resonance imaging or computed tomography scan may localize the tumor.
- Serum and/or urine chemistries may reveal an elevation of vanillylmandelic acid and free catecholamines.

Interdisciplinary Management

- Surgical removal of the tumor(s) by adrenalectomy is the treatment of choice.
- Inoperable tumors may be managed with alpha- and beta-adrenergic blocking agents.

Selected Nursing Diagnoses with Interventions

Risk for Ineffective Tissue Perfusion

- Remain with the patient during episodes of hypertension.
- Monitor blood pressure every 10 to 15 minutes.
- Observe for any neurologic or respiratory changes.
- Provide a calm, restful environment.

Risk for Imbalanced Nutrition: Less than Body Requirements

- Assess nutritional status and food preferences.
- Assist in selecting daily menu (help incorporate basic food groups).
- Ask family or significant others to bring favorite foods from home, within the limits of the prescribed diet.
- Consult with a dietitian to reduce tyramine-containing foods in the diet.
- Monitor daily kilocalorie intake and patient's weight.

Anxiety

- Explain the basic concepts of the disease and potential risk factors.
- Encourage the patient and significant others to ask questions and express their fears and concerns.
- Encourage the patient to avoid dietary stimulants (e.g., caffeine, chocolate).

Community-Based Care

- *See* Nursing Interventions.
- Emphasize the importance of ongoing outpatient care.
- Provide information on obtaining a MedicAlert bracelet and card if necessary.
- Explain the need to avoid over-the-counter medications without first consulting a physician.

For more information on pheochromocytoma, see Chapter 19 in *Medical-Surgical Nursing,* Fifth Edition, by LeMone, Burke, and Bauldoff.

Phosphate Imbalance

Hypophosphatemia

Hyperphosphatemia

Overview

- Phosphate is the primary intracellular anion, essential for adenosine triphosphate production.

- Most phosphate (85%) is found in bones, about 14% is in intracellular fluid, and the remainder (1%) is in extracellular fluid.
- The normal serum phosphate (or phosphorus) level in adults is 2.5 to 4.5 mg/dL.
- Phosphate helps maintain red blood cell function and oxygen delivery, neuromuscular function, nutrient metabolism, and acid–base balance.
- Phosphorus is ingested in the diet, absorbed in the jejunum, and primarily excreted by the kidneys.
- An inverse relationship exists between phosphate and calcium levels; mechanisms for regulating calcium levels (parathyroid hormone, calcitonin, and vitamin D) also influence phosphate levels.
- *Hypophosphatemia* is a serum phosphorus < 2.5 mg/dL.
- Hypophosphatemia causes adenosine triphosphate depletion and impaired oxygen delivery to the cells. Severe hypophosphatemia affects virtually every major organ system.
- *Hyperphosphatemia* is a serum phosphate > 4.5 mg/dL.
- Hyperphosphatemia can cause calcification and impaired function of soft tissues in the kidneys and other organs.
- Hypocalcemia develops secondary to hyperphosphatemia as the phosphate combines with ionized calcium, lowering the ionized serum calcium level.

P

Causes

Hypophosphatemia

- Shift of phosphate from extracellular to intracellular space: refeeding syndrome, hyperventilation and respiratory alkalosis
- Medications: intravenous glucose solutions, antacids (aluminum- or magnesium-based antacids), anabolic steroids, and diuretics
- Alcoholism
- Other causes: diabetic ketoacidosis; stress responses; extensive burns

Hyperphosphatemia

- Acute or chronic renal failure (impaired phosphate excretion)
- Rapid administration of phosphate-containing solutions
- Shift of phosphate from the intracellular to extracellular space: chemotherapy, sepsis, hypothermia, extensive trauma, heat stroke
- Disruption of calcium-regulating mechanisms: hypoparathyroidism, hyperthyroidism, or vitamin D intoxication

Manifestations

Hypophosphatemia

- Neurologic: irritability, apprehension, weakness, paresthesias, lack of coordination, confusion, seizures, and coma
- Hematologic: cellular hypoxia, possible hemolytic anemia
- Musculoskeletal: muscle weakness; release of creatinine phosphokinase; possible acute rhabdomyolysis (muscle cell breakdown)
- Respiratory: chest muscle weakness, impaired ventilation; possible respiratory failure
- Cardiovascular: decreased cardiac output; chest pain and dysrhythmias
- Gastrointestinal: anorexia; dysphagia (difficulty swallowing); nausea and vomiting; decreased bowel sounds and possible ileus

Hyperphosphatemia

- Primarily the result of secondary hypocalcemia
- Muscle cramps and pain
- Paresthesias, tingling around the mouth
- Muscle spasms, tetany
- Soft-tissue calcification and impaired organ function

Diagnostic Tests

- Serum phosphate will be outside the normal range of 2.5 to 4.5 mg/dL (1.7 to 2.6 mEq/L).

- Parathyroid hormone levels may be abnormal if this is the cause of phosphate imbalance.

- Blood urea nitrogen and serum creatinine are measured to evaluate renal function as a cause of phosphate imbalance.

- X-rays may show bone changes indicative of hypophosphatemia, or osteodystrophy.

Interdisciplinary Management

- Hypophosphatemia treatment focuses on treating the underlying cause and replacing phosphate. Mild to moderate deficiencies are treated with diet and oral phosphate supplements; intravenous phosphate is given when serum phosphate levels are < 1 mg/dL.

- Treating the underlying disorder often corrects hyperphosphatemia. Phosphate-containing drugs are eliminated and phosphate-rich foods are restricted. Calcium-containing antacids may be prescribed to bind phosphate. Intravenous normal saline may be given to promote renal excretion; dialysis may be required in renal failure.

Selected Nursing Diagnoses with Interventions

Hypophosphatemia
Risk for Injury

- Encourage the patient to ask for assistance when ambulating.

- Monitor respiratory rate and oxygen saturation.

Decreased Cardiac Output

- Monitor electrocardiogram for any changes or abnormalities.

Imbalanced Nutrition: Less than Body Requirements

- Offer nutritional snacks, such as Ensure.

- Provide phosphorus-rich foods, such as dairy products and organ meats.

- Monitor serum phosphate levels frequently.

Hyperphosphatemia
Imbalanced Nutrition: More than Body Requirements

- Instruct to reduce intake of dairy products and organ meats.

- Provide adequate hydration to enhance renal excretion of phosphorus.
- Administer phosphate-binding agents as prescribed.

Community-Based Care

- Teach about the disorder, including causes, treatment, and prevention of recurrences.
- For the patient with hypophosphatemia, discuss the importance of avoiding phosphorus-binding antacids. Provide a list of foods high in phosphorus (e.g., organ meats, milk, and milk products).
- For the patient with hyperphosphatemia, discuss the importance of avoiding phosphate enemas and over-the-counter medications containing phosphorus. Encourage the patient to eliminate foods high in phosphorus from the diet, and provide a list of these foods.
- Referral to a dietitian may be appropriate.

For more information about phosphate imbalances, see Chapter 10 in *Medical-Surgical Nursing,* Fifth Edition, by LeMone, Burke, and Bauldoff.

PLEURAL EFFUSION

Overview

- Pleural effusion is collection of excess fluid in the pleural space (between the visceral and parietal pleural membranes).
- The collected fluid may be transudate, exudate, or other substances such as pus from an empyema, blood (hemothorax), or a mixture of blood and pleural fluid (hemorrhagic pleural effusion).
- Transudate contains few cells and has a low specific gravity, whereas exudate, associated with inflammation or malignancy, is rich in proteins.
- A large pleural effusion compresses adjacent lung tissue, impairing ventilation and gas exchange.

Causes

Systemic Disorders

- Heart failure

- Cirrhosis, liver failure
- Nephrotic syndrome, renal failure
- Connective tissue disorders: rheumatoid arthritis, systemic lupus erythematosus, Sjögren's syndrome

Local Conditions

- Pneumonia
- Atelectasis
- Tuberculosis
- Lung cancer
- Chest trauma

Manifestations

- Progressive dyspnea
- Cough
- Pleuritic chest pain
- Decreased breath sounds, decreased tactile fremitus, dull percussion tone

Diagnostic Tests

- Chest x-ray shows the presence of an effusion.
- Computed tomography scan or ultrasonography assists in localizing and differentiating the type of effusion.
- Thoracentesis obtains aspirated fluid for analysis to determine the type of fluid and cause.

Interdisciplinary Management

- Thoracentesis to remove the fluid is the treatment of choice for significant pleural effusion.
- Recurrent pleural effusions, often due to cancer, may be prevented by instilling an irritant such as doxycycline, bleomycin, or talc into the pleural space to cause adhesion of the parietal and visceral pleura.

Selected Nursing Diagnoses with Interventions

Impaired Gas Exchange

- Prepare for thoracentesis by ensuring that informed consent for the procedure has been given, providing patient teaching, obtaining a thoracentesis tray and supplies, and placing the patient in an upright position, leaning forward, with the arms and head supported on an anchored over-bed table.

- Following thoracentesis:

  1. Frequently monitor vital signs, color, and respiratory status including oxygen saturation and breath sounds.

  2. Assess the puncture site for bleeding or presence of crepitus.

  3. Apply a dressing over the puncture site and position patient on the unaffected side for 1 hour.

  4. Label the obtained specimen with the name, date, source, and diagnosis. Send the specimen to the laboratory for analysis.

  5. Obtain a chest x-ray.

  6. If chest tube is inserted, monitor function of the drainage system and maintain gravity flow. Document the color and amount of drainage.

Community-Based Care

- Teach abdominal breathing technique and encourage its use.

- Teach about the disease process, its relationship to the underlying disorder, and treatments, including thoracentesis and prescribed medications.

- Instruct the patient to report to the physician increasing dyspnea or shortness of breath, cough, hemoptysis, and pleuritic pain.

- A referral to a smoking cessation program may be appropriate.

- The patient may obtain information from the American Lung Association and the American Cancer Society.

For more information on pleural effusion, see Chapter 36 in *Medical-Surgical Nursing,* Fifth Edition, by LeMone, Burke, and Bauldoff.

PNEUMONIA

Overview

- Pneumonia is inflammation of the respiratory bronchioles and alveoli (called the lung parenchyma).
- Pneumonia may be either infectious or noninfectious; bacterial pneumonia is the most common type; aspiration of gastric contents is an important noninfectious cause.
- Pathogens usually enter the lungs by aspiration of oropharyngeal secretions containing the organism. Colonization of the alveoli initiates inflammatory and immune responses, which can further damage bronchial and alveolar mucous membranes.
- Infectious debris and exudate can fill alveoli (*consolidation*), interfering with ventilation and gas exchange.
- Lobar consolidation is typical of pneumococcal pneumonia.
- Bronchopneumonia is patchy consolidation of several lobules, and is characteristic of other bacterial pneumonias.
- Viral pneumonia is characterized by inflammation of the alveolar septum and interstitial spaces.

Causes

Bacterial

- Community-acquired: *Streptococcus pneumoniae, Haemophilus influenzae, Staphylococcus aureus, Mycoplasma pneumoniae, Chlamydia pneumonia*
- Nosocomial: *Klebsiella pneumoniae, Pseudomonas aeruginosa, Escherichia coli*

Viral

- Influenza virus, adenovirus, respiratory syncytial virus
- Childhood disease viruses: measles, varicella

Opportunistic

- *Pneumocystis carinii*
- Cytomegalovirus

Noninfectious

- Aspiration of gastric contents
- Inhalation of toxic smoke or gases

Manifestations

- Chills and fever
- Pleuritic chest pain
- Cough; productive of rust-colored or purulent sputum in bacterial pneumonia
- Possible dyspnea and cyanosis
- Diminished breath sounds, fine crackles or rales, pleural friction rub
- Malaise, fatigue, headache, muscle aching
- Atypical manifestations seen in older adults or debilitated patients include little cough, scant sputum, and minimal evidence of respiratory distress. Fever, tachypnea, and altered mentation or agitation may be primary presenting symptoms.

Diagnostic Tests

- Chest x-ray determines the extent and pattern of lung involvement.
- Sputum gram stain and culture and sensitivity are used to detect the causative organism and direct therapy.
- In acute bacterial pneumonia, the white blood cell count is generally elevated to 15,000 to 21,000/μL.
- Arterial blood gases may be ordered to evaluate gas exchange.
- Fiberoptic bronchoscopy may be done to obtain a sputum specimen or remove secretions.

Interdisciplinary Management

- Medications include antibiotics to eradicate the causative organism and bronchodilators to reduce bronchospasm and facilitate ventilation. An agent to break up mucus or reduce its viscosity may be prescribed.
- Oxygen therapy may be prescribed if the patient is tachypneic or hypoxemic.

- Chest physiotherapy, postural drainage, incentive spirometry, and endotracheal suctioning may be ordered.

Selected Nursing Diagnoses with Interventions

Ineffective Airway Clearance

- Assess respiratory status, including vital signs, breath sounds, and skin color, as well as cough and sputum, at least every 4 hours.
- Monitor arterial blood gases and oxygen saturation levels.
- Place in Fowler's position. Encourage frequent turning, sitting, and ambulation.
- Assist to cough, deep breathe, and use assistive devices. Provide endotracheal suctioning using aseptic technique as prescribed.
- Provide a fluid intake of at least 2,500 to 3,000 mL per day.
- Work with the physician and respiratory therapist to provide pulmonary hygiene measures.
- Administer prescribed medications and monitor for their effects.
- Administer oxygen therapy as prescribed.

Ineffective Breathing Pattern

- Assess and document pleuritic discomfort. Administer analgesics as prescribed.
- Remain present and provide reassurance during periods of respiratory distress.
- Enlist the help of significant others to minimize the patient's level of anxiety.
- Instruct to use slow abdominal breathing.
- Teach relaxation techniques such as visualization and meditation.

Activity Intolerance

- Assess activity tolerance, noting any increase in pulse, respirations, dyspnea, diaphoresis, or cyanosis with activities.
- Assist with self-care as needed.
- Schedule activities, planning for rest periods.
- Provide assistive devices such as an overhead trapeze.

- Provide emotional support and reassurance that the patient's strength and activity level will return to normal.

Community-Based Care

- Encourage patients in high-risk groups to obtain immunizations against influenza and pneumococcal pneumonia.

- Stress the importance of following the prescribed medication regimen and completing the entire prescription.

- Instruct to limit activity and increase rest. Explain the importance of maintaining a high fluid intake.

- Tell the patient to report to the physician any increase in or recurrence of shortness of breath, dyspnea, temperature, fatigue, headache, sleepiness, or confusion. Stress the importance of keeping follow-up appointments.

- Referral to a smoking cessation program may be appropriate.

- Provide information on obtaining influenza and pneumococcal pneumonia vaccinations.

- Home health care may be appropriate for elderly patients or those with additional chronic conditions.

For more information about pneumonia, see Chapter 36 in *Medical-Surgical Nursing,* Fifth Edition, by LeMone, Burke, and Bauldoff.

PNEUMOTHORAX

Overview

- Pneumothorax is an accumulation of air in the pleural space that impairs lung expansion and causes some degree of lung collapse.

- It can be caused by an opening of the parietal pleura (chest wall) or through the visceral pleura (lung rupture).

- A *spontaneous pneumothorax* develops when an air-filled bleb, or blister, on the lung surface ruptures. Air accumulates in the pleural space until pressures are equalized or until collapse of the involved section seals the leak.

- *Primary pneumothorax* generally is a benign condition that affects previously healthy people, usually tall, slender young men.
- *Secondary pneumothorax* results from overdistention and rupture of an alveolus. It results from underlying lung disease, usually chronic obstructive pulmonary disease.
- *Traumatic pneumothorax* occurs when chest trauma disrupts the pleural membrane.
- *Tension pneumothorax* develops when air enters the pleural space with inspiration, but is unable to exit with expiration, and is trapped in the chest cavity. The lung on the affected side collapses and pressure on the mediastinum causes thoracic organs to shift to the unaffected side, placing pressure on the opposite lung as well. Ventilation is severely compromised and venous return to the heart is impaired. Tension pneumothorax is a medical emergency.

Causes
- Idiopathic
- Preexisting lung disease
- Blunt or penetrating chest trauma
- Iatrogenic: positive pressure ventilation, thoracentesis, liver biopsy

Manifestations
- Pleuritic chest pain, may be severe, sharp, and stabbing
- Dyspnea, shortness of breath
- Tachypnea, tachycardia
- Unequal chest excursion
- Diminished or absent breath sounds on affected side
- Hyperresonant percussion tone on affected side
- Open: air movement through wound
- Tension: hypotension, shock; distended neck veins; severe dyspnea; tachypnea, tachycardia; tracheal deviation to unaffected side

Diagnostic Tests
- Chest x-ray shows air in the pleural space, its location and amount, and mediastinal shift, if present.

- Oxygen saturation monitoring and arterial blood gases are evaluated for the effect on gas exchange.

Interdisciplinary Management

- In small pneumothorax no treatment other than close observation may be required as the air will gradually reabsorb.

- Significant pneumothorax requires placement of a closed-chest catheter to allow the lung to reexpand. The tube is sealed with a one-way valve (Heimlich valve) or water-seal system to prevent air from reentering the chest cavity.

- A chemical such as doxycycline may be instilled into the pleural space to create adhesions between the parietal and visceral pleura, or a thoracotomy may be done to excise blebs in patients with recurrent spontaneous pneumothorax.

Selected Nursing Diagnoses with Interventions

Impaired Gas Exchange

- Assess vital signs and respiratory status at least every 4 hours.
- Place in Fowler's or high Fowler's position.
- Administer oxygen as prescribed.
- Provide emotional support.
- Monitor drainage and function of chest tube.
- Assist with position changes and ambulation as needed.

Risk for Injury

- Assess chest tube and drainage system at least every 2 hours.
- Avoid occluding or placing tension on chest tubes during turning or care activities.
- Keep the drainage system lower than the chest. Suction usually can be discontinued during ambulation.
- Observe the insertion site for redness, swelling, pain, or drainage. Report signs of infection, including fever, to the physician.
- Should a connection come loose, reconnect it as soon as possible.
- For inadvertent chest tube removal or an open chest wound, seal the wound with a sterile occlusive dressing taped on three sides only.

Community-Based Care

- Discuss the risk for reoccurrence of spontaneous pneumothorax. Stress the importance of smoking cessation. Advise to avoid exposure to significant pressure differences (e.g., mountain climbing, scuba diving) and contact sports.

- Instruct to gradually increase exercise and activity to previous levels.

- Advise to report to the physician upper respiratory infection, fever, cough, or difficulty breathing; sudden, sharp chest pain; or redness, pain, swelling, tenderness, or drainage from the chest tube puncture wound.

- Provide referral to a smoking cessation program as appropriate.

- Referral to the local chapter of the American Lung Association may be helpful for information and support.

For more information on pneumothorax, see Chapter 36 in *Medical-Surgical Nursing*, Fifth Edition, by LeMone, Burke, and Bauldoff.

POLIOMYELITIS, POSTPOLIOMYELITIS SYNDROME

Overview

- Poliomyelitis is an infection of motor neurons with the poliovirus. It especially affects the anterior horn cells in the spinal cord.

- Infection is usually mild and self-limiting, producing transitory meningitis with no sequelae. Less commonly, paralytic poliomyelitis occurs.

- Poliovirus enters, often from contaminated water, and colonizes the nasopharynx and gastrointestinal mucosa. Resulting viremia spreads the organisms to the spinal cord.

- Acute infection is endemic in underdeveloped nations, and occurs more commonly in warm months (summer, autumn).

- Postpoliomyelitis syndrome, developing years after the initial infection, affects approximately 25% to 50% of patients who had the acute disease. Postpolio syndrome usually develops between the ages of 45 and 65. The incidence is slightly higher in women.

Causes

- Acute episode is caused by infection with poliovirus.
- Cause of postpoliomyelitis syndrome is unknown.

Manifestations

Acute Infection

- Fever, malaise.
- Nausea, vomiting.
- Generalized muscle pain.
- Spasms in unaffected muscle groups.
- Decreased deep tendon reflexes.
- Paralysis may precede or follow the above manifestations: asymmetric; flaccid; may affect muscles of respiration, cranial nerves, or somatic motor nerves.
- Sensory changes: hypersensitivity to touch, paresthesias.
- Meningeal irritation: headache, stiff neck, Brudzinski's sign, Kernig's sign.

Postpoliomyelitis Syndrome

- Fatigue
- Muscle and joint weakness
- Loss of muscle mass
- Respiratory distress
- Pain, headache
- Cold intolerance
- Dizziness
- Urinary incontinence
- Sleep disorders

Diagnostic Tests

- Viral cultures of the throat and stool will identify poliovirus.
- Cerebrospinal fluid analysis will reveal excess leukocytes; pressure and protein may be slightly elevated.

- Other diagnostic studies include nerve conduction, muscle strength, and pulmonary function.

Interdisciplinary Management

- Treatment is symptomatic.
- Analgesics may be prescribed to relieve pain.
- Respiratory status is carefully monitored and supported as indicated.
- Physical therapy also may be indicated.

Selected Nursing Diagnoses with Interventions

Risk for Infection (Patient Contacts)

- Collect fecal and nasopharyngeal specimens for laboratory analysis.
- Use enteric precautions.
- Participate in follow-up of patient contacts to ensure immunization.
- Make a report to the local health authority.

Ineffective Breathing Pattern

- Monitor patient for dyspnea.
- Initiate ventilatory assistance if needed.
- Monitor for inability to swallow.
- Feed the patient via a nasogastric tube if necessary.

Impaired Physical Mobility

- Position the patient in a dorsal position with the extremities extended (maintain body alignment).
- Turn the patient every 2 hours, or more often as needed.
- Perform range-of-motion exercises every 8 hours.

Self-Care Deficit

- Feed the patient, and increase diet from fluids to solids as tolerated.
- Assist with bowel and bladder elimination.
- Refer patient to home health care prior to discharge.

P

Community-Based Care

- Provide preventive teaching, including information about immunization.

- Explain the disease process, treatments, activity restrictions, medication regimen, use of braces and other assistive devices, and prognosis.

- Teach how to prevent fatigue, promote optimal respiratory function, meet self-care needs, modify activities of daily living, and maintain safety.

- Stress the importance of follow-up care with nurses, physicians, physical therapists, respiratory therapists, and psychologic counselors as indicated.

- Emphasize the importance of lifelong follow-up with the physician. Long-term physical therapy also may be necessary.

- Referral to a support group can make a positive difference in the patient's ability to cope with the disorder. March of Dimes and Polio Network News provide information and support for patients and families.

For more information on postpoliomyelitis syndrome, see Chapter 43 in *Medical-Surgical Nursing,* Fifth Edition, by LeMone, Burke, and Bauldoff.

POLYCYSTIC KIDNEY DISEASE

P

Overview

- Polycystic kidney disease is a hereditary disease characterized by formation of fluid-filled cysts and massive kidney enlargement.

- Autosomal dominant polycystic kidney disease (ADPKD) affects adults; it is relatively common, affecting 1 in every 400 to 1,000 people.

- The autosomal recessive form is present at birth and is rare; renal failure generally develops during childhood.

- Renal cysts (fluid-filled sacs) develop in tubular epithelium of the nephron, affecting the renal cortex and medulla of both kidneys. The cysts may be microscopic to several centimeters in diameter, compressing and obstructing renal blood vessels and nephrons and destroying functional tissue.

- Cysts often develop elsewhere, including the liver, spleen, pancreas, lungs, and reproductive organs; subarachnoid hemorrhage is a risk, as is cardiac valve incompetence.

Cause

- Genetic mutations: ADPKD type 1 (chromosome 16) accounts for approximately 85% of cases. ADPKD type 2 (chromosome 4) is responsible for most remaining cases. Infantile type is autosomal recessive.

Manifestations

- Flank pain
- Microscopic or gross hematuria
- Proteinuria
- Polyuria, nocturia
- Manifestations of urinary tract infection (UTI) or renal calculi
- Palpable, enlarged, and knobby kidneys
- Manifestations of renal insufficiency and chronic renal failure

Diagnostic Tests

- Renal ultrasonography shows enlarged kidneys and the presence of cysts.
- Computed tomography scan provides detailed picture of renal cysts and masses.
- Genetic testing for ADPKD type 1 and type 2 is available, and is particularly important when a family member is being considered as a potential kidney donor.
- Serum creatinine and blood urea nitrogen are used to evaluate and monitor renal function.

Interdisciplinary Management

- Management is largely supportive, including avoidance of nephrotoxins, prevention of UTI, and treatment of hypertension using a multidrug regimen that includes an angiotensin-converting enzyme (ACE) inhibitor or angiotensin receptor blocker (ARB). A fluid intake of 2,000 to 2,500 mL per day is encouraged.

- Ultimately, dialysis or renal transplantation is required.

Selected Nursing Diagnoses with Interventions

Excess Fluid Volume

- Administer medications as prescribed. Avoid nephrotoxic drugs and aspirin products, which could cause bleeding.

- Monitor intake and output, daily weight, and abdominal girth. Notify the physician of any abnormalities.

- If salt intake is restricted, provide dietary instruction about a low-sodium diet and foods to avoid.

- Stress the importance of maintaining fluid intake of at least 2,500 mL per day.

- Increase intake of fluid and fiber to prevent constipation, unless contraindicated.

Readiness for Enhanced Knowledge

- Teach the importance of blood pressure management and instruct how to measure blood pressure.

- Teach measures to prevent UTI.

- Discuss genetic counseling and screening of family members for evidence of the disease.

Community-Based Care

- Explain the importance of continuing care.

- Instruct to notify the physician if the urine becomes foul-smelling, contains blood, or if other symptoms of UTI develop, and if a persistent or severe headache or visual disturbances occur.

- Explain the importance of checking with the physician before taking any new drug, including over-the-counter medications, as some may be toxic to the kidneys.

- Refer the patient to the Polycystic Kidney Research Foundation, the National Kidney Foundation, and the American Association of Kidney Patients for further information and support.

For more information on polycystic kidney disease, see Chapter 28 in *Medical-Surgical Nursing,* Fifth Edition, by LeMone, Burke, and Bauldoff.

POLYCYTHEMIA

Overview

- Polycythemia (erythrocytosis) is an excess of red blood cells (RBCs) characterized by a hematocrit higher than 55%.

- *Primary polycythemia* (polycythemia vera, or PV) is an uncommon stem cell disorder that usually affects men of European Jewish ancestry between the ages of 40 and 70.

- In PV, colonies of endogenous erythroid stem cells that produce RBCs in the absence of erythropoietin develop, leading to excess RBC production.

- *Secondary polycythemia,* the most common form of polycythemia, occurs in response to elevated erythropoietin levels, usually as a compensatory response to chronic hypoxia.

- *Relative polycythemia* is due to fluid deficit; the total RBC count is normal but the hematocrit is elevated.

Causes

- The cause of PV is unknown; genetic risk factors contribute.

- Secondary polycythemia: chronic hypoxia due to living at high altitudes, chronic heart or lung disease, or smoking; kidney disease, erythropoietin-secreting tumors (e.g., renal cell carcinoma), or abnormal hemoglobin.

- Relative polycythemia: dehydration or third spacing.

Manifestations

- Often asymptomatic

- Hypertension; headaches, dizziness, vision and hearing disruptions

- *Plethora* (ruddy, red color) of the face, hands, feet, and mucous membranes

- Severe, painful itching of the fingers and toes

- Engorged retinal and cerebral vessels
- Hypermetabolism with weight loss and night sweats
- Altered mental status
- Possible thrombosis with ischemic attacks, angina, or manifestations of peripheral vascular disease

Diagnostic Tests

- The RBC count is elevated; the white blood cell and platelet counts also may be elevated.
- The hemoglobin and hematocrit are elevated.
- Serum erythropoietin levels are low in PV and elevated in secondary polycythemia.
- Bone marrow studies show hyperplasia of all hematopoietic elements in PV and only red stem cell hyperplasia in secondary polycythemia.

Interdisciplinary Management

- Periodic phlebotomy, removing 300 to 500 mL of blood, may be performed to keep blood volume and viscosity within normal levels.
- For PV, chemotherapy may be used to suppress marrow function. Pruritus may be treated with antihistamines, interferon alpha, or other therapies; aspirin may be ordered to control thrombosis.
- Treatment for secondary polycythemia focuses on the underlying cause. Smokers are urged to quit; measures to raise oxygen saturations and reduce tissue hypoxia may relieve the polycythemia.

Selected Nursing Diagnoses with Interventions

Risk for Ineffective Tissue Perfusion

- Report early signs of bleeding or thrombosis to the physician.
- Prepare for phlebotomy as indicated.
- Instruct to avoid tight or constrictive clothing, especially garters or girdles.
- Discuss measures to prevent venous stasis: elevate feet when sitting, wear support hose while awake and ambulating, and exercise daily.

Acute/Chronic Pain

- Assess pain using a standard pain scale, including location and duration.
- Monitor effectiveness of prescribed analgesics and other medications.
- Teach nonpharmacologic pain relief measures, such as meditation, imagery, and progressive relaxation.
- Maintain a quiet environment.

Decisional Conflict: Smoking Cessation

- Teach about the disease process, its treatment, and prognosis.
- Emphasize the importance of smoking cessation to patients who smoke.
- Referral for a smoking cessation program may be appropriate.

Community-Based Care

- Encourage a generous fluid intake of at least 3,000 mL per day.
- Teach how to assess skin and peripheral pulses.
- Discuss symptoms of recurrence and complications to report to the physician.
- Explain the importance of regular follow-up care.

For more information on polycythemia, see Chapter 33 in *Medical-Surgical Nursing,* Fifth Edition, by LeMone, Burke, and Bauldoff.

POTASSIUM IMBALANCE

Hyperkalemia

Hypokalemia

Overview

- Potassium, the primary intercellular cation, plays a vital role in cell metabolism, cardiac, and neuromuscular function.
- The normal serum (extracellular fluid) potassium level is 3.5 to 5.0 mEq/L.
- Most potassium is within the cells (intracellular fluid); the significant difference in intracellular fluid and extracellular fluid

potassium concentrations (maintained by the sodium-potassium pump) helps maintain the resting membrane potential of nerve and muscle cells; either a deficit or an excess of potassium can adversely affect neuromuscular and cardiac function.

- Potassium is obtained through the diet and primarily eliminated by the kidneys; aldosterone helps regulate renal potassium excretion. A consistent potassium intake is necessary because it is poorly conserved by the kidneys.

- Potassium constantly shifts into and out of the cells in response to changes in serum levels, pH, and other factors such as glucocorticoid and insulin levels.

Hypokalemia (Serum Potassium < 3.5 mEq/L)

- Hypokalemia affects nerve impulse transmission, interfering with smooth, skeletal, and cardiac muscle contractility, and cardiac impulse regulation and transmission.

- Hypokalemia also can affect kidney function, particularly the ability to concentrate urine.

Hyperkalemia (Serum Potassium > 5.0 mEq/L)

- Hyperkalemia alters the cell membrane potential, affecting the heart, skeletal muscle function, and gastrointestinal tract.

- Its most harmful effect is on cardiac function; the conduction system is affected, leading to characteristic electrocardiogram (ECG) changes; severe hyperkalemia decreases the strength of myocardial contractions.

- Hyperkalemia increases smooth muscle activity; very high levels lead to skeletal muscle weakness and paralysis.

Causes

Hypokalemia

Increased Renal Excretion

- Drugs such as potassium-wasting diuretics, corticosteroids, amphotericin B, and some antibiotics
- Hyperaldosteronism
- Diabetes mellitus

Gastrointestinal Losses
- Severe vomiting or gastric suction
- Diarrhea or ileostomy drainage

Inadequate Intake
- Starvation, malnutrition; alcoholism
- Extended parenteral fluid therapy

Shift into Cells
- Alkalosis
- Rapid tissue repair
- Excess insulin
- Acute stress
- Hypothermia

Hyperkalemia

Impaired Renal Excretion
- Renal failure
- Adrenal insufficiency
- Drugs such as potassium-sparing diuretics, trimethoprim, and some nonsteroidal anti-inflammatory drugs

Excess Intake
- Rapid intravenous administration of potassium
- Transfusion of aged blood

Shift From Intracellular to Extracellular
- Acidosis, particularly metabolic acidosis
- Severe tissue trauma
- Chemotherapy
- Starvation

Manifestations

Hypokalemia
- Reduced nerve and muscle cell excitability
- Gastrointestinal: anorexia, reduced bowel sounds, abdominal distension, paralytic ileus

- Neurologic: paresthesias
- Musculoskeletal: muscle weakness, paralysis, poor tone
- Cardiac: dysrhythmias; ECG changes (ST depression, flat T wave, U wave); possible cardiac arrest
- Respiratory: shallow respirations, shortness of breath

Hyperkalemia

- Gastrointestinal: diarrhea, colic (abdominal cramping)
- Neurologic: anxiety, paresthesias, irritability
- Musculoskeletal: muscle tremors and twitching, progressing to muscle weakness and flaccid paralysis; lower extremities are affected first, progressing to the trunk and upper extremities
- Cardiac: bradycardia, possible heart blocks; peaked T waves, prolonged PR interval, and widened QRS complex on ECG; ventricular dysrhythmias, possible cardiac arrest

Diagnostic Tests

- Serum potassium level is outside normal range.
- Arterial blood gases may reveal acidosis, pH < 7.35; or alkalosis, pH > 7.45.
- ECG shows changes in the T-wave and conduction patterns.

Interdisciplinary Management

Hypokalemia

- Oral and/or parenteral potassium supplements are given to prevent and treat hypokalemia.
- A diet high in potassium-rich foods is prescribed.

Hyperkalemia

- For moderate to severe hyperkalemia, intravenous calcium gluconate is given to stabilize the cardiac conduction system; regular insulin and 50 g of glucose are administered to rapidly lower serum potassium levels; a β_2-agonist (e.g., albuterol) may be given by nebulizer to temporarily push potassium into the cells; sodium bicarbonate may be given to treat acidosis.

- Sodium polystyrene sulfonate (Kayexalate) may be administered orally or rectally; diuretics such as furosemide are given to promote potassium excretion.
- Hemodialysis or peritoneal dialysis may be necessary to lower potassium levels in renal failure.

Selected Nursing Diagnoses with Interventions

Activity Intolerance

- Monitor skeletal muscle strength and tone.
- Monitor respiratory rate, depth, and effort; heart rate and rhythm; and blood pressure at rest and following activity.
- Assist with self-care activities as needed.

Decreased Cardiac Output

- Monitor serum potassium levels, particularly in patients at risk for hypokalemia or hyperkalemia. Report abnormal levels to the physician.
- Monitor vital signs, including orthostatic vitals and peripheral pulses.
- Place patients with potassium imbalance on a cardiac monitor. Closely monitor cardiac rhythm and observe for characteristic ECG changes. Report rhythm changes and treat as indicated.
- Monitor patients taking digitalis for digitalis toxicity. Monitor response to antidysrhythmic drugs.
- Dilute intravenous potassium, and administer using an electronic infusion device no faster than 10 to 20 mEq/hour.

Risk for Imbalanced Fluid Volume

- Maintain accurate intake and output records and daily weight. Report urine output less than 30 mL/hour or a weight gain of more than 3 lb in 24 hours.
- Monitor bowel sounds and abdominal distention.
- Monitor patients receiving sodium bicarbonate or Kayexalate for fluid volume excess.

- Closely monitor serum potassium, blood urea nitrogen, and serum creatinine. Notify the physician if serum potassium level is greater than 5 mEq/L, or if serum creatinine and blood urea nitrogen levels are increasing.

Acute Pain

- When possible, administer intravenous KCl through a central line.
- Spread the total daily dose of KCl over 24 hours to minimize the concentration of intravenous solutions.
- Discuss with the physician using a small amount of lidocaine prior to or with the infusion.

Community-Based Care

- Teach about the imbalance, its causes, treatment, and strategies for preventing recurrence.
- Provide a list of potassium-rich foods, salt substitutes, and medications that contain potassium, with individualized instructions.
- Instruct to have blood potassium levels monitored as recommended by the physician.
- Stress the importance of taking medications as prescribed, and not changing the dose or frequency of diuretics or potassium supplements without notifying the physician.
- Provide a referral to a dietitian if appropriate.

For more information about potassium imbalances, see Chapter 10 in *Medical-Surgical Nursing,* Fifth Edition, by LeMone, Burke, and Bauldoff.

PROSTATE CANCER

Overview

- Prostate cancer is a primary malignant neoplasm of the prostate gland. It is the most common malignancy in men.
- Most prostate tumors are adenocarcinomas that arise at the periphery of the gland.

- Without treatment, the tumor invades local tissues, including the seminal vesicles. Tumors may grow slowly, however, posing little risk.
- Prostate cancer spreads by direct extension or via the lymph or blood.
- The disease rarely strikes men younger than 50; incidence rises with age.

Causes
- Risk factors:
  - Increasing age
  - Race: Blacks, followed by Whites, followed by Asian Americans and Hispanic/Latino men
  - Possible genetic and hereditary factors; vasectomy; and diet high in animal fat and excess supplemental vitamin A

Manifestations
- Asymptomatic in early stages, then much the same as benign prostatic hyperplasia
- Dysuria, urinary retention, frequency, nocturia, incontinence
- Recurrent urinary tract infection
- Hematuria; painless, gross or occult
- Bone pain is a late symptom

Diagnostic Tests
- Digital rectal examination reveals an enlarged, hard, irregularly shaped gland.
- Prostatic specific antigen is a sensitive test for detection of early prostate cancer.
- Transrectal sonography will show densities in the peripheral portion of the gland.
- Magnetic resonance imaging or computed tomography scan can localize the tumor for biopsy and show spread.
- Biopsy is diagnostic for the specific type of cancer.

P

Interdisciplinary Management

- Hormone therapy and chemotherapy are used to treat metastatic prostate cancer.
- Newly approved injectable drugs for treating prostate cancer include Degarelix (firmagon) and Lupron Depot (leuprolide acetate) to rapidly lower testosterone levels and decrease rate of prostate tumor growth.
- Surgery for patients with prostate cancer includes several types of prostatectomies and transurethral resection of the prostate.
- Radiation therapy is used in treatment of prostate cancer and also for palliative care.

Selected Nursing Diagnoses with Interventions

Urinary Incontinence (Reflex, Stress, Total)

- Assess the degree of incontinence and its impact on lifestyle.
- Teach Kegel exercises to help restore continence.
- Teach methods to control dampness and odor from stress incontinence.
- Teach control of occasional episodes of incontinence with absorbent pads worn inside the underwear and changed as needed.
- Explore options with the patient who has total incontinence.
- Help the patient to verbalize his feelings about the impact of incontinence on his quality of life.

Sexual Dysfunction

- Assess pretreatment sexual function.
- Discuss potential effects of treatment on sexual function.
- Assist the patient in choosing therapeutic options for erectile dysfunction.

Acute Pain/Chronic Pain

- Assess the intensity, duration, location, and quality of the pain.
- Teach the patient and family methods of pain control.
- Instruct the patient and significant others about the use of analgesic drugs to control pain.

Community-Based Care

- Explain the disease process, types of treatment, their side effects, and the prognosis with or without treatment.

- Because prostate cancer frequently metastasizes to the spinal cord, discuss early manifestations of spinal cord compression, such as back pain and lower extremity weakness.

- Following surgery, instruct to avoid strenuous activity, including sexual intercourse, for 6 to 8 weeks. Encourage long walks, and advise to continue dorsiflexion exercises to prevent blood clots in the legs. Driving is allowed after 2 weeks. Tub baths should be avoided while the catheter is in place.

- Instruct or promptly report to the physician excessive bleeding, chills, fever, abdominal pain, swollen or tender scrotum, calf or chest pain, or difficulty breathing.

- Provide the names and addresses of local cancer support groups. Special prostate cancer support groups may be available in the patient's area.

- Emphasize the importance of keeping all regularly scheduled follow-up appointments to detect metastasis or local recurrence.

For more information on prostate cancer, see Chapter 48 in *Medical-Surgical Nursing,* Fifth Edition, by LeMone, Burke, and Bauldoff.

PSORIASIS

Overview

- Psoriasis is a chronic inflammatory skin condition characterized by red, scaling plaques, mostly over the dorsal surfaces and joints.

- Psoriasis represents an abnormally increased rate of epidermal proliferation with polymorphonuclear leukocyte infiltration.

- It often occurs in a paroxysmal pattern; exacerbations may be precipitated by skin trauma, infection, or stress.

- Psoriasis is common, affecting 1% to 2% of the population; it can occur at any age, but usually begins in young adults.

Causes

- The cause is unknown; it may be a T-lymphocyte-mediated reaction resulting in the production of chemical messengers that stimulate the growth of keratinocytes and dermal blood vessels.

- Exacerbating factors include sunlight, seasonal changes, hormone fluctuations, steroid withdrawal, and certain drugs (beta blockers, lithium, and chloroquine), which may act as triggers.

- Trauma to the skin from surgery, sunburn, or excoriation are also common precipitating factors.

Manifestations

- Skin lesions: well-demarcated, reddish plaques covered by silvery scales

- Lesion locations: over extensor skin surfaces of elbows, knees; on scalp or trunk

- Bleeding: punctate, if scales scraped off

- Nails: pitted, discolored, thickened

- Joint pain, if arthritis is a feature

Diagnostic Tests

- Skin biopsy will distinguish between clinically similar disorders.

- Ultrasonography may be performed to measure skin thickness.

Interdisciplinary Management

- Topical corticosteroids, tar preparations, anthralin, and calcipotriene (a vitamin D derivative) and tazarotene (a synthetic retinoid) are typically used.

- Ustekinumab, an injectable monoclonal antibody that decreases the immune response, is in advanced clinical trials for severe psoriasis.

- Photochemotherapy is the preferred treatment for severe psoriasis.

- Phototherapy using Ultraviolet-B (UVB) light or narrow band UVB is used to treat generalized psoriasis.

P

Selected Nursing Diagnoses with Interventions

Impaired Skin Integrity

- Teach methods to reduce injury to the skin:
  - Use warm, not hot, water.
  - Gently rub lesions with a soft washcloth, using a circular motion.
  - Blot the skin dry with a soft towel.
  - Keep the skin lubricated at all times.
- Demonstrate application of topical medications:
  - Apply in a thin layer.
  - Avoid getting medication in the eyes, on mucous membranes, or in skinfolds.
  - Cover the medicated areas as ordered, usually for no more than 12 hours, often during the evening and night. Choose plastic wrap that covers the area well.
- Teach manifestations of infection to report to the physician.
- Teach to assess for treatment complications: excoriation, increased erythema, increased peeling, blister formation.

Disturbed Body Image

- Establish a trusting relationship by expressing acceptance of the patient, both verbally and nonverbally.
- Encourage the patient to verbalize feelings about self-perception in view of the chronic nature of psoriasis, and to ask questions about the disease and its treatment.
- Promote social interaction through family involvement in care, referral to support groups, and referral to the National Psoriasis Foundation.

Community-Based Care

In addition to the previous teaching:

- Eat a healthy, well-balanced diet, use relaxation techniques to reduce stress, get adequate rest and exercise, and avoid exposure to contagious illnesses.
- Avoid extremely cold or hot temperatures.
- Expose the skin to sunlight, but avoid sunburn.
- Avoid skin trauma; use only an electric shaver.

- Instruct to discuss all medications, including nonprescription drugs, with the physician. Some medications may precipitate exacerbations of psoriasis.

- Provide with simply written self-care instructions.

- Refer to the National Psoriasis Foundation and local support groups for people with chronic skin conditions.

For more information on psoriasis, see Chapter 16 in *Medical-Surgical Nursing,* Fifth Edition, by LeMone, Burke, and Bauldoff.

PULMONARY EDEMA

Overview

- Pulmonary edema is an abnormal accumulation of fluid in the interstitial tissue and alveoli of the lung.

- Both cardiac and noncardiac disorders can cause pulmonary edema.

- Pulmonary edema is a medical emergency; its onset may be acute or gradual, progressing to severe respiratory distress. Immediate treatment is necessary.

- In *cardiogenic pulmonary edema,* severely impaired left ventricular function causes a sharp rise in pulmonary hydrostatic pressures; fluid leaking from pulmonary capillaries congests interstitial tissues, decreasing lung compliance and interfering with gas exchange. Eventually fluid enters the alveoli, along with red blood cells and protein molecules, severely disrupting ventilation and gas exchange.

- *Noncardiogenic pulmonary edema* occurs in response to acute lung injury and a systemic inflammatory response that damages the alveolar-capillary membrane; this allows plasma and blood cells to escape into the interstitial space and the alveoli where the fluid dilutes and inactivates surfactant; lung compliance is reduced and gas exchange is impaired.

Causes

Cardiac

- Acute myocardial infarction

- Acute heart failure
- Valvular disease

Noncardiac

- Acute respiratory distress syndrome
- Trauma, sepsis
- Drug overdose
- Neurologic damage or disorders

Manifestations

- Dyspnea, shortness of breath, and labored respirations
- Orthopnea
- Cyanosis
- Cool, clammy, diaphoretic skin
- Cough productive of pink, frothy sputum
- Crackles throughout lung fields
- Restlessness, anxiety; possible confusion or lethargy

Diagnostic Tests

- Arterial blood gases show a low PaO_2; the $PaCO_2$ may be low due to tachypnea. With increasing severity, the $PaCO_2$ rises and respiratory acidosis develops.
- Oxygen saturation shows hypoxemia.
- Chest x-ray shows pulmonary vascular congestion and alveolar edema.
- Hemodynamic monitoring shows elevated pulmonary artery wedge pressure, and possibly a low cardiac output.

Interdisciplinary Management

- Immediate treatment focuses on restoring effective gas exchange.
- Morphine is given intravenously to relieve anxiety, improve breathing, and reduce venous return. Potent loop diuretics are administered intravenously to promote rapid diuresis. Vasodilators are given to reduce afterload, and dopamine or dobutamine is administered to improve the myocardial contractility and cardiac output.

- Oxygen is administered using a positive pressure system (continuous positive airway pressure or mechanical ventilation) to increase alveolar pressures and gas exchange while decreasing fluid diffusion into the alveoli.

Selected Nursing Diagnoses with Interventions

Impaired Gas Exchange

- Ensure airway patency.
- Assess the effectiveness of respiratory efforts and airway clearance.
- Assess respiratory status frequently, including rate, effort, use of accessory muscles, sputum characteristics, lung sounds, and skin color.
- Place in high Fowler's position with the legs dangling.
- Administer oxygen as ordered by mask, continuous positive airway pressure mask, or ventilator.
- Encourage to cough up secretions; provide nasotracheal suctioning if necessary.
- Keep emergency equipment readily available in case of respiratory arrest. Be prepared to assist with intubation and initiation of mechanical ventilation.

Decreased Cardiac Output

- Monitor vital signs, hemodynamic status, and rhythm continuously.
- Assess heart sounds for possible S_3, S_4, or murmurs.
- Initiate an intravenous line for medication administration. Administer prescribed medications as ordered.
- Insert an indwelling catheter; record output hourly.
- Keep accurate intake and output records. Restrict fluids as ordered.

Fear

- Provide emotional support for the patient and family members.
- Explain all procedures and the reasons to the patient and family members. Keep information brief and to the point. Use short sentences and a reassuring tone.

- Maintain close contact with the patient and family, providing reassurance that recovery from acute pulmonary edema is often as dramatic as its onset.
- Answer questions, and provide accurate information in a caring manner.

Community-Based Care

- During the acute period, teaching is limited to immediate care. Keep information brief and to the point. Use short sentences and a reassuring tone to decrease anxiety.
- After resolution of the acute episode, teach about the underlying cause and prevention of future episodes of pulmonary edema, as well as medications, dosage, effects, and side effects.
- Provide information about coronary heart disease and heart failure as indicated.
- Discuss lifestyle alterations, such as changes in diet and physical activity, as indicated.
- Refer for home care and/or assistance with activities of daily living and prescribed medical regimen as appropriate.
- Refer to a dietitian for teaching about a low-sodium diet if indicated.
- Provide contact information for the American Heart Association for educational materials and support groups in the community.

For more information on pulmonary edema, see Chapters 31 and 37 in *Medical-Surgical Nursing,* Fifth Edition, by LeMone, Burke, and Bauldoff.

PULMONARY EMBOLISM

Overview

- Pulmonary embolism is obstruction of blood flow in the pulmonary vascular system by an embolus.
- Pulmonary embolism usually is due to a thrombus (blood clot); tumors, fat, amniotic fluid, and debris also may become emboli.
- Pulmonary embolus affects both perfusion and ventilation:
  1. Neurohumoral reflexes cause vasoconstriction and increased pulmonary artery pressures.

2. Bronchoconstriction occurs in the affected area of lung.

3. Dead space (areas that are ventilated but not perfused) increases.

4. Alveolar surfactant decreases, increasing the risk for atelectasis.

- Pulmonary embolism causes an estimated 60,000 deaths annually, and is the third leading cause of death in hospitalized patients.

Causes

- Deep venous thrombosis due to the following:
  1. Leg trauma
  2. Surgery
  3. Immobility
  4. Clotting disorders
  5. Pregnancy
  6. Oral contraceptives, especially in smokers
- Fat embolism due to fracture of large bones
- Amniotic fluid embolism
- Air embolism (scuba diving accidents)
- Foreign matter: contaminated intravenous solutions; injection drug abuse

Manifestations

- Small emboli may be asymptomatic.
- Abrupt onset of dyspnea and pleuritic chest pain.
- Anxiety, sense of impending doom.
- Cough, hemoptysis.
- Diaphoresis, cyanosis.
- Tachycardia, tachypnea.
- Crackles on auscultation.
- S_3, S_4.
- Low-grade fever.

- Fat emboli: dyspnea, tachypnea, tachycardia, confusion, delirium, and decreased level of consciousness; petechiae on chest and arms.

Diagnostic Tests

- Plasma D-dimer levels are highly specific to a thrombus, and are elevated.
- Perfusion and ventilation lung scans identify areas of the lungs that are ventilated but not perfused.
- Pulmonary angiography can detect very small emboli that may not be apparent on other studies.
- Chest x-ray often shows pulmonary infiltration and possible pleural effusion.
- Arterial blood gases usually show hypoxemia, and often respiratory alkalosis due to tachypnea and hyperventilation.
- Exhaled carbon dioxide is decreased when pulmonary perfusion is impaired.
- Coagulation studies are ordered to monitor the response to therapy.

Interdisciplinary Management

- Anticoagulant therapy is used to prevent and to treat pulmonary embolism.
- Thrombolytic therapy may be used to treat massive pulmonary embolus and hypotension.
- When pulmonary emboli are recurrent, surgical placement of a filter in the inferior vena cava may be performed.

Selected Nursing Diagnoses with Interventions

Impaired Gas Exchange

- Frequently assess respiratory status, including depth, rate, effort, and lung sounds.
- Assess level of consciousness, mental status, and skin color.
- Place in Fowler's or high Fowler's position, with the lower extremities dependent.

- Start oxygen per nasal cannula or mask as prescribed.
- Monitor oxygen saturation and arterial blood gas results, and report abnormal findings as indicated. Maintain arterial line, if in place.
- Administer vasopressors and other medications as prescribed.
- Maintain bed rest.

Decreased Cardiac Output

- Assess and record vital signs frequently as indicated.
- Auscultate heart sounds every 2 to 4 hours, and report any abnormalities.
- Monitor and record intake and output hourly.
- Assess skin color and temperature.
- Place on a cardiac monitor.
- Carefully monitor the response to prescribed vasopressors.
- Monitor pulmonary artery and wedge pressures, neck vein distention, and peripheral edema. Report findings as indicated.
- Maintain intravenous and arterial access sites as well as central lines.
- Provide frequent skin care.
- Instruct to report any chest pain or other symptoms.

Anxiety

- Assess level of anxiety.
- Provide reassurance and emotional support, listening to the patient's fears. Do not negate the fear of dying, but reassure that treatment is generally effective to restore respiratory function.
- Remain with the patient as much as possible.
- Explain procedures and treatments, using short, simple sentences.
- Reduce environmental stimuli, and use a calm, reassuring manner.
- Allow calm, supportive family members to remain with the patient as much as possible.
- Administer morphine sulfate as ordered to reduce pain and anxiety.

Community-Based Care

- Teach about the disease process, prevention, and treatment, including the importance of early ambulation and regular exercise such as walking.

- Teach about prescribed medications and monitoring for desired and adverse effects.

- Instruct patients taking anticoagulants to use a soft toothbrush, and monitor stool, urine, and sputum for blood. Advise to avoid taking aspirin without checking with the physician, and to wear a MedicAlert tag. Provide information on obtaining one.

- Discuss symptoms of recurrent pulmonary embolus, such as chest pain, shortness of breath, and possibly bloody sputum.

- Stress the need to avoid smoking; provide a referral to a smoking cessation program as appropriate.

- Consider referral for psychologic counseling to help cope with a near-death experience.

For more information on pulmonary embolism, see Chapter 37 in *Medical-Surgical Nursing,* Fifth Edition, by LeMone, Burke, and Bauldoff.

PYELONEPHRITIS

Acute

Chronic

Overview

- Pyelonephritis is inflammation of the renal pelvis and functional kidney tissue.

- *Acute pyelonephritis* is a bacterial infection of the kidney pelvis, calyces, and medulla, with white blood cell infiltration and inflammation. The kidney becomes grossly edematous and localized abscesses may develop.

- *Chronic pyelonephritis*, a common cause of chronic renal failure, involves chronic inflammation and scarring of the tubules and interstitial tissues of the kidney.

Causes

Acute

* Bacterial infection, usually ascending from lower urinary tract infection (UTI)
* Organisms: *Escherichia coli* (85%), *Proteus, Pseudomonas, Staphylococcus saprophyticus* or *aureus, Streptococcus faecalis*
* Risk factors for UTI: catheterization or instrumentation of the urinary tract; urinary stasis; vesicoureteral reflux

Chronic

* Recurrent or untreated acute pyelonephritis
* Renal damage due to hypertension or vascular conditions, severe vesicoureteral reflux, urinary tract obstruction
* Nonbacterial infections
* Inflammatory processes (metabolic, chemical, or immunologic)

Manifestations

Acute

* Manifestations of UTI: dysuria; frequency; urgency; nocturia; hematuria; pyuria
* Chills and fever
* Flank pain; costovertebral angle tenderness
* Anorexia, possible nausea
* Malaise

Chronic

* Manifestations of UTI
* Hypertension
* Manifestations of renal insufficiency or failure (*see* Renal Failure, Chronic)

Diagnostic Tests

* Urinalysis shows a bacteria count > 100,000 (10^5)/mL in acute infection.

- Urine culture and sensitivity identify the infecting organism and the most effective antibiotic.

- White blood cell count with differential may reveal leukocytosis and increased numbers of neutrophils.

- Intravenous pyelography evaluates for structural or functional abnormalities, such as vesicoureteral reflux, of the kidneys, ureters, and bladder. Cystoscopy may be done to detect underlying disorders contributing to pyelonephritis.

Interdisciplinary Management

- Acute pyelonephritis is treated with antibiotic therapy for 3 to 10 days to eradicate the infecting organism. Intravenous antibiotics may be used to treat severe illness or sepsis.

- Surgery is indicated to repair structural defects that may cause obstruction; nephrectomy may be done if the infection becomes intractable.

Selected Nursing Diagnoses with Interventions

Acute Pain

- Assess pain, including timing, quality, intensity, location, duration, and aggravating and alleviating factors.

- Provide nonpharmacologic relief measures such as warm sitz baths, warm packs or heating pads, and balanced rest and activity. Systemic analgesics, urinary analgesics, or antispasmodics may be administered as prescribed.

- Increase fluid intake unless contraindicated by therapeutic regimen.

Impaired Urinary Elimination

- Monitor urinary output and color, clarity, and character of urine, including odor.

- Provide for easy access to a bedpan, urinal, commode, or bathroom.

- Instruct to avoid caffeinated drinks and alcohol.

Community-Based Care

- Teach about the disorder, its causes, treatments, and prevention.

- Review medications and stress the importance of completing all prescribed antibiotics, even if symptoms rapidly resolve.

- Assist the patient to develop a plan for taking medications, such as taking them with meals (unless contraindicated) or setting out all doses for the day in the morning.

- If surgery was performed, provide postoperative teaching, including the importance of avoiding heavy lifting and manual labor for the prescribed time.

- Teach manifestations of recurrence and stress the importance of reporting these immediately to the healthcare provider.

- Schedule a follow-up appointment with the physician as prescribed, and stress the importance of follow-up care for any signs of recurrence.

- Information is available from the National Kidney Foundation and the American Urological Association.

For more information on pyelonephritis, see Chapter 27 in *Medical-Surgical Nursing,* Fifth Edition, by LeMone, Burke, and Bauldoff.

P

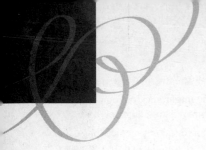

Raynaud's Disease or Phenomenon

Overview

- Raynaud's phenomenon is characterized by episodes of intense vasospasm in the small arteries and arterioles of the fingers and toes.

- Attacks are initiated by exposure to cold or stress. As the disease progresses, all digits may be affected.

- In the early, ischemic, stage, vessel spasm causes pallor of affected digits and makes them cold to the touch; as oxygen is extracted from venous blood, cyanosis develops.

- The hyperemic phase follows, as the spasm resolves, and arterioles fully dilate (reactive hyperemia), increasing perfusion so that the digits turn bright red (rubor) and feel warm.

- Raynaud's *disease* has no identifiable cause, and primarily affects young women between the ages of 20 and 40. Raynaud's *phenomenon* occurs secondarily to another disease or condition.

Causes

- Raynaud's disease may have a genetic component.

- Raynaud's phenomenon is associated with the following:

  - Collagen vascular diseases: scleroderma, rheumatoid arthritis, systemic lupus erythematosus

  - Known causes of vasospasm: atherosclerosis, thromboangitis obliterans

  - Long-term exposure to cold or machinery (such as a jackhammer)

Manifestations

Ischemic Phase

- Blanching (pallor) of fingers, possibly toes.
- Cyanosis follows blanching.

- Affected digits are cold to touch.
- Numbness, tingling, decreased sensation.

Hyperemic Phase
- Rubor
- Aching pain

Long-Term Changes
- Thickening of fingertips, brittle nails
- Ulceration and gangrene (rare)

Diagnostic Tests
- The diagnosis is usually based on history and physical examination.

Interdisciplinary Management
- Conservative treatment includes keeping the hands warm by wearing gloves when outside in cold weather and when handling cold items, stress reduction, exercise, smoking cessation, and maintaining a low-fat diet and healthy body weight.
- Vasodilators may provide symptomatic relief. A calcium channel blocker, alpha-adrenergic blocker, or transdermal nitroglycerine may be prescribed.

Selected Nursing Diagnoses with Interventions

Ineffective Tissue Perfusion: Peripheral
- Note manifestations of an episode, including color changes and swelling, and subjective reports of numbness, coldness, tingling, and pain.
- Assist to identify precipitating events and develop strategies for preventing or minimizing future occurrences.

Community-Based Care
- Review the nature of the disorder, prescribed interventions, and strategies for preventing further attacks. Include the following instructions:
    1. Dress warmly, keeping the trunk and hands warm.
    2. Avoid unnecessary exposure to cold.
    3. Stop smoking or do not start.

- Refer to smoking cessation, weight reduction, and stress management programs as appropriate.

For more information on Raynaud's disease or phenomenon, see Chapter 32 in *Medical-Surgical Nursing,* Fifth Edition, by LeMone, Burke, and Bauldoff.

RENAL CALCULI (NEPHROLITHIASIS, KIDNEY STONES)

Overview

- Nephrolithiasis is formation of stones (calculi) in the kidney.
- Renal calculi are the most common cause of upper urinary tract obstruction.
- Males are affected more often than females by a 4:1 ratio.
- Stones generally form as masses of crystals around an organic matrix or nucleus. Adequate fluid intake prevents stone growth.
- Most kidney stones are calcium stones, uric acid stones may be associated with gout, and struvite stones are associated with recurrent urinary tract infection.
- The stone can grow to fill the renal pelvis (*staghorn stones*), or may migrate into the ureter, causing pain and obstructed urine flow.

Causes

- Most are idiopathic.
- Risk factors include the following:
  - Prior personal or family history of calculi (genetic predisposition)
  - Dehydration
  - Immobility
  - Excess dietary intake of calcium, oxalate, or proteins
  - Gout, hyperparathyroidism, and urinary stasis or repeated infections

Manifestations

- May be asymptomatic when in the renal pelvis

- Dull, aching flank pain with partial obstruction of urine flow
- *Renal colic:* acute, severe flank pain on the affected side caused by acute ureteral obstruction and spasm
  1. Pain radiates to the suprapubic region, groin, and external genitals.
  2. Possible nausea; vomiting; pallor; and cool, clammy skin.
- Manifestations of urinary tract infection: chills and fever, frequency, urgency, and dysuria
- Gross or microscopic hematuria

Diagnostic Tests

- Urinalysis may show hematuria, white blood cells, and crystal fragments. Urine pH helps identify the type of stone.
- Chemical analysis of stones passed in the urine determines the type of stone. Any visible stones and sediment are sent for analysis.
- Diagnostic testing for levels of urine calcium, uric acid, serum calcium, and phosphorus as well as oxalate levels can identify the factors leading to lithiasis.
- Kidney ureter bladder x-ray and computed tomography scan can identify calculi in the kidneys, ureters, and bladder.
- Renal ultrasonography detects stones and evaluates the kidneys for hydronephrosis.
- Intravenous pyelogram may be done if less invasive tests fail to clearly demonstrate urinary calculi.

Interdisciplinary Management

R

- A narcotic analgesic, such as intravenous morphine, and indomethacin, a nonsteroidal anti-inflammatory drug, are given to relieve pain and reduce ureteral spasm in renal colic. A thiazide diuretic is frequently prescribed for calcium calculi. Potassium citrate may be ordered to prevent stones that form in acidic urine.
- Increased fluid intake is vital. For calcium stones, a diet low in calcium-rich foods and high in foods that acidify the urine is recommended. Organ meats, sardines, and other high-purine foods are eliminated to reduce the risk of uric acid stones. Foods that alkalinize urine are recommended for uric acid and cystine stones.

- Extracorporeal shock-wave lithotripsy or percutaneous ultrasonic lithotripsy may be required to destroy and remove the stone.

Selected Nursing Diagnoses with Interventions

Acute Pain

- Assess the intensity, quality, location, timing, aggravating and relieving factors, and associated symptoms with all complaints of pain.
- Administer analgesia as prescribed.
- Encourage a generous fluid intake and ambulation in the patient with ureteral colic.
- Use nonpharmacologic measures such as positioning, moist heat, relaxation techniques, guided imagery, and diversion as adjunctive therapy for pain relief.

Impaired Urinary Elimination

- Measure urinary output (hourly if catheterized). Document hematuria, dysuria, frequency, urgency, and pyuria. Strain all urine for stones, saving any recovered stones for laboratory analysis.
- If surgery or lithotripsy has been performed, monitor urinary output, catheters, incision, and wound drainage as indicated.
- Maintain patency and integrity of all catheters. Secure catheters well, label as indicated, and use sterile technique for irrigations or other procedures.

Community-Based Care

- Teach about all diagnostic and therapeutic procedures.
- Teach the patient to collect and strain all urine, saving any stones; to report stone passage to the physician and bring the stone in for analysis; and to observe the amount and character of urine, reporting any changes.
- Instruct to increase fluid intake to 2,500 to 3,500 mL per day, follow recommended dietary guidelines, remain physically active to prevent urinary stasis and bone resorption, and take medications as prescribed.
- Teach the patient and significant others how to change dressings and manage drainage systems as indicated. Instruct to contact the physician if manifestations of infection or obstructed urine output develop.

- Tell the patient to report recurrent stone symptoms to the physician immediately, and to return to the physician periodically for continued monitoring.

For more information on renal calculi (nephrolithiasis, kidney stones), see Chapter 27 in *Medical-Surgical Nursing,* Fifth Edition, by LeMone, Burke, and Bauldoff.

RENAL FAILURE

Acute

Chronic

Overview

- Renal failure is a condition in which the kidneys are unable to remove accumulated metabolites from the blood, leading to altered fluid, electrolyte, and acid–base balance.

- Renal failure may be primary or secondary to systemic disease or urologic defects. It may be either acute or chronic.

- *Acute renal failure* (ARF) has an abrupt onset and, with prompt intervention, is often reversible.

- *Chronic kidney disease* is a progressive disorder of declining kidney function. In end-stage renal failure, the kidneys are unable to meet the excretory needs of the body.

- Renal failure is characterized by *azotemia,* increased levels of nitrogenous wastes in the blood.

Acute Renal Failure

- ARF is a rapid decline in renal function with azotemia and fluid and electrolyte imbalances. Its course follows three phases: initiation, maintenance, and recovery.

  1. The initiation phase begins with the initiating event and ends when tubular injury occurs; it lasts hours to days.

  2. The maintenance phase is characterized by a significant fall in glomerular filtration rate (GFR) and tubular necrosis. The kidney cannot efficiently eliminate metabolic wastes, water, electrolytes, and acids from the body during this phase, leading to azotemia, fluid retention, electrolyte imbalances, and metabolic acidosis.

3. The recovery phase is characterized by tubule cell repair and regeneration and gradual return of the GFR to normal or pre-ARF levels. Diuresis may occur, and retained salt, water, and solutes are excreted.

Chronic Kidney Disease

- In chronic kidney disease, entire nephron units are lost and renal mass decreases, with progressive deterioration of glomerular filtration, tubular secretion, and reabsorption. The course of chronic kidney disease occurs over months to years.

  1. In the stage of *decreased renal reserve,* unaffected nephrons compensate for the lost nephrons, and the GFR is about 50% of normal.

  2. In the stage of *renal insufficiency,* the GFR is 20% to 50% of normal, and azotemia develops.

  3. *Renal failure* is characterized by a GFR of less than 20% of normal. The serum creatinine and blood urea nitrogen (BUN) levels rise sharply, and oliguria and uremia develop.

  4. In *end-stage renal disease,* the GFR is less than 5% of normal, and renal replacement therapy is necessary to sustain life.

Causes

Acute Renal Failure

- Risk factors:

  1. Major trauma or surgery, infection, hemorrhage, severe heart failure, severe liver disease, lower urinary tract obstruction, and antigen-antibody reaction

  2. Nephrotoxic drugs and radiologic contrast media

- Most common causes: ischemia and nephrotoxins

- Classification of causes:

  1. *Prerenal:* impaired renal blood flow and perfusion (e.g., hemorrhage, shock, heart failure)

  2. *Intrarenal:* acute damage to the renal parenchyma and nephrons (e.g., acute tubular necrosis, acute glomerulonephritis, malignant hypertension, rhabdomyolysis)

  3. *Postrenal:* obstruction of urine outflow (e.g., benign prostatic hypertrophy, renal or urinary tract calculi, tumors)

Chronic Kidney Disease

- Can develop from any of the causes given, if left untreated or controlled
- Leading causes: hypertension and diabetes mellitus
- Other causes: chronic glomerulonephritis, genetic kidney disorders (e.g., polycystic kidney), and other chronic kidney diseases (e.g., lupus nephritis)

Manifestations

Acute Renal Failure

- Azotemia: rising serum creatinine and BUN levels
- Oliguria, fixed specific gravity
- Edema
- Hypertension
- Anorexia, nausea, vomiting
- Decreased or absent bowel sounds
- Hyperkalemia: Muscle weakness, electrocardiogram changes
- Hyperphosphatemia, hypocalcemia
- Metabolic acidosis, Kussmaul's respirations
- Anemia
- Confusion, disorientation, agitation or lethargy
- Hyperreflexia
- Scizures, coma

Chronic Kidney Disease

- Renal insufficiency: polyuria, nocturia; proteinuria, hematuria; fixed specific gravity
- End-stage renal disease: manifestations of uremia
- Early: nausea, apathy, weakness, and fatigue
- Later: frequent vomiting, increasing weakness, lethargy, and confusion
- Fluid and electrolyte imbalances
  1. Salt and water retention with edema

2. Hyperkalemia: muscle weakness, paresthesias, and electrocardiogram changes (delayed P-R interval, widened QRS, peaked T wave)

3. Hyperphosphatemia, hypocalcemia, hypermagnesemia

4. Metabolic acidosis: Kussmaul's respirations, malaise, weakness, headache, nausea, vomiting, abdominal pain

- Cardiovascular

  1. Hypertension

  2. Manifestations of coronary heart disease, cerebrovascular disease, peripheral vascular disease

  3. Heart failure, pulmonary edema

  4. Pericarditis, pericardial friction rub; possible cardiac tamponade (muffled heart sounds, paradoxical pulse)

- Hematologic

  1. Anemia: fatigue, weakness, depression, impaired cognition

  2. Impaired platelet function, increased bleeding risk

- Immune system: increased infection risk

- Gastrointestinal

  1. Anorexia, nausea, vomiting

  2. Hiccups

  3. Peptic ulcer disease

  4. Uremic fetor: urinelike breath odor, metallic taste in the mouth

- Neurologic

  1. Changes in mentation, difficulty concentrating

  2. Fatigue, insomnia

  3. Psychotic symptoms, seizures, coma

  4. Peripheral neuropathy: crawling or creeping sensations, prickling, itching of lower legs; frequent leg movement

  5. Muscle weakness, decreased deep tendon reflexes, gait disturbances

- Musculoskeletal: osteodystrophy: bone tenderness, pain, muscle weakness

- Endocrine and metabolic

  1. Significantly elevated serum creatinine and BUN

2. Increased uric acid levels, possible gout

3. Glucose intolerance

4. High serum triglyceride levels, low high-density lipoproteins levels

5. Female: menstrual irregularity, difficulty carrying pregnancy to term

6. Male: impotence and infertility

- Dermatologic

    1. Pallor, yellowish skin tone

    2. Dry skin, poor turgor

    3. Bruising, excoriations

    4. Itching, pruritus

    5. Uremic frost, crystallized deposits of urea on the skin

Diagnostic Tests

- Urinalysis often shows a fixed specific gravity of 1.010, proteinuria, presence of red blood cells and/or white blood cells, renal epithelial cells, and cell casts.

- Serum creatinine and BUN are elevated; creatinine clearance shows a low GFR.

- Serum electrolytes may show hyperkalemia, hyponatremia, and other imbalances.

- Arterial blood gases show a metabolic acidosis.

- Complete blood count shows low red blood cells, hemoglobin, and hematocrit.

- Renal ultrasonography can identify obstructive causes of renal failure, and differentiate between acute and chronic renal failure.

- Intravenous pyelography or other x-ray studies may be used to evaluate kidney structure and function.

- Renal biopsy is done to differentiate between acute and chronic kidney disease.

Interdisciplinary Management

Acute Renal Failure

- Intravenous fluids and blood volume expanders are given to restore renal perfusion.

- All drugs that are nephrotoxic or that may interfere with renal perfusion are avoided.
- Medications: Low doses of dopamine to increase renal blood flow; loop or osmotic diuretics to reestablish urine output and manage salt and water retention; angiotensin-converting enzyme inhibitors or other antihypertensive medications to control hypertension; antacids, histamine H_2 blockers, or proton-pump inhibitors to prevent gastrointestinal bleeding.
- Hyperkalemia may be treated with intravenous calcium chloride, bicarbonate, regular insulin with glucose to move potassium into the cells, or a potassium-binding exchange resin. Aluminum hydroxide may be cautiously used to control hyperphosphatemia.
- Once renal perfusion is restored, fluid intake is usually restricted. Fluid balance is evaluated by accurate weight measurements and serum sodium levels.
- Dietary proteins are limited and should be of high biologic value; carbohydrates are increased to maintain calorie intake. Parenteral nutrition may be instituted.
- Dialysis or continuous renal replacement therapy may be required.

Chronic Kidney Disease

- Drugs eliminated by the kidney are avoided; drug dosages are adjusted to prevent toxicity. Medications: loop diuretics to reduce fluid volume and edema; antihypertensive drugs to manage hypertension; drugs to manage electrolyte imbalances and acidosis; folic acid and iron supplements to combat anemia; multiple vitamin supplement.
- Proteins are restricted and carbohydrates are increased to maintain energy requirements. Water and sodium intake are regulated. Potassium and phosphorus intake also may be restricted.
- Renal replacement therapies are considered. Dialysis options include hemodialysis or peritoneal dialysis. If the decision for transplant is made early, dialysis can potentially be avoided. Factors such as age, concurrent health problems, donor availability, and personal preference influence the choice of treatment.

Selected Nursing Diagnoses with Interventions

Excess Fluid Volume

- Maintain hourly intake and output records for the patient in ARF.

464

- Weigh daily or more frequently, as ordered. Use standard technique (same scale, clothing, or coverings) to ensure accuracy.

- Assess vital signs at least every 4 hours. Frequently assess breath and heart sounds, neck veins for distention, and back and extremities for edema. Report abnormal findings.

- If not contraindicated, place in semi-Fowler's position.

- Report abnormal serum electrolyte values and manifestations of electrolyte imbalance.

- Restrict fluids as ordered. Provide frequent mouth care and encourage using hard candies to decrease thirst. If ice chips are allowed, include the water content (approximately one-half of the total volume) as intake.

- Administer medications with meals.

- Turn frequently and provide good skin care.

Impaired Renal Perfusion

- Monitor intake and output.

- Monitor BUN, serum creatinine, pH, electrolytes, and complete blood count.

- Monitor carefully for desired and adverse effects of *all* medications.

- Administer antihypertensive medications as ordered.

Imbalanced Nutrition: Less than Body Requirements

- Monitor food and nutrient intake as well as episodes of vomiting.

- Administer antiemetic agents 30 to 60 minutes before eating.

- Assist with mouth care prior to meals and at bedtime.

- Serve small meals and provide between-meal snacks.

- Arrange for a dietary consultation. Provide preferred foods as allowed, and involve the patient in menu planning. Encourage family members to bring food as allowed.

- Monitor nutritional status by tracking weight, laboratory values such as serum albumin and BUN, and anthropometric measurements.

- Administer parenteral nutrition as prescribed. Routinely monitor blood glucose levels.

R

Risk for Infection

- Use standard precautions and good hand hygiene technique at all times.
- Use strict aseptic technique when managing ports, catheters, and incisions.
- Monitor temperature and vital signs at least every 4 hours.
- Monitor white blood cell count and differential.
- Culture urine, peritoneal dialysis fluid, and other drainage as indicated.
- Monitor clarity of peritoneal dialysate return.
- Provide good respiratory hygiene including position changes, coughing, and deep breathing.
- Restrict visits from obviously ill people. Teach the patient and family about the risk for infection and measures to reduce the spread of infection.

Disturbed Body Image

- Involve the patient in care, including meal planning; dialysis; and catheter, port, or incision care to the extent possible.
- Encourage expression of feelings and concerns, accepting perceptions and feelings without criticism.
- Include the patient in decision making and encourage self-care.
- Help the patient develop and achieve realistic goals.
- Provide positive reinforcement and feedback.
- Facilitate contact with a support group or other community members affected by renal failure.
- Refer for mental health counseling as indicated or desired.

Community-Based Care

- Teach about the disease, diagnostic tests, dietary and fluid restrictions, medications, and treatment options, including renal replacement therapies.
- Teach how to monitor weight and blood pressure, and the manifestations of complications to be reported to the physician.
- Instruct to avoid nephrotoxic drugs.

- Teach shunt or fistula care for the patient on hemodialysis. Teach peritoneal catheter care and peritoneal dialysis procedures as indicated. Include a significant other in all teaching.

- When a renal transplantation has been done, instruct about medications, adverse effects and their management, infection prevention, and the manifestations of organ rejection.

- Refer for home care services as indicated (nursing, home maintenance, etc.).

- If home hemodialysis is the treatment of choice, refer the selected dialysis assistant for training.

- Local chapters of the National Kidney Foundation and the American Association of Kidney Patients on Hemodialysis and Transplantation may be able to provide information and support for patients.

For more information about renal failure, see Chapter 26 in *Medical-Surgical Nursing,* Fifth Edition, by LeMone, Burke, and Bauldoff.

RESPIRATORY FAILURE

Overview

- Respiratory failure is a state in which the lungs are unable to oxygenate the blood and remove carbon dioxide adequately to meet the body's needs, even at rest.

- It may be identified by an arterial oxygen level (PO_2) of less than 50 to 60 mmHg and an arterial carbon dioxide level (PCO_2) of greater than 50 mmHg, or, in patients with chronic lung disease, by an acute drop in PO_2 and a significant rise in PCO_2.

- Respiratory failure can result from inadequate alveolar ventilation (hypoventilation), impaired gas exchange, or a significant ventilation-perfusion mismatch.

- Respiratory failure may be characterized by primary hypoxemia or a combination of hypoxemia and hypercapnia.

  1. *Hypoxemic* respiratory failure is a failure of oxygenation. The PO_2 is significantly reduced and the PCO_2 is at or below normal. Metabolic acidosis results from tissue hypoxia.

  2. *Hypercapnic* respiratory failure results from hypoventilation. The PCO_2 rises rapidly and respiratory acidosis develops. The PO_2 drops more slowly.

- The prognosis depends on the underlying disease process; it is less favorable when respiratory failure results from underlying lung disease.

Causes

- Chronic obstructive pulmonary disease (COPD)
- Severe asthma
- Cystic fibrosis
- Infectious lung diseases such as pneumonia
- Chest trauma: pneumothorax, pulmonary contusion
- Inhalation trauma
- Neuromuscular disorders: multiple sclerosis, amyotrophic lateral sclerosis, spinal cord injury
- Heart failure, acute pulmonary edema
- Acute respiratory distress syndrome

Manifestations

- Manifestations of the underlying disease process

Hypoxemia

- Dyspnea, tachypnea
- Restlessness, anxiety, impaired judgment, motor impairment
- Tachycardia, dysrhythmias
- Cyanosis

Hypercapnea

- Dyspnea
- Headache
- Flushed skin
- Conjunctival vasodilation, papilledema
- Muscle twitching, decreased level of consciousness
- Slowed, shallow respirations, respiratory arrest

Diagnostic Tests

- Exhaled carbon dioxide is elevated in hypoventilation and decreased when lung perfusion is impaired.

- Arterial blood gases (ABGs) show metabolic or respiratory acidosis, low PO_2, and normal (hypoxemic failure) or high (hypercapnic failure) PCO_2.

Interdisciplinary Management

- Medications may include bronchodilators to reverse airway spasm and constriction, and antibiotics to treat infection.
- Oxygen therapy is vital to reverse hypoxemia, but must be used with caution in patients with long-standing hypercapnia.
- Intubation and mechanical ventilation may be required to treat acute respiratory failure.

Selected Nursing Diagnoses with Interventions

Impaired Spontaneous Ventilation

- Assess and document respiratory rate, vital signs, and oxygen saturation every 15 to 30 minutes.
- Promptly report worsening ABG values, oxygen saturation levels, or signs of respiratory distress, including tachypnea, tachycardia, nasal flaring, use of accessory muscles, intercostal retractions, cyanosis, increasing restlessness, anxiety, or decreased level of consciousness.
- Administer oxygen as ordered, monitoring response. Observe closely for respiratory depression, especially in the patient with COPD.
- Place in Fowler's or high Fowler's position.
- Minimize activities and energy expenditures by assisting with activities of daily living, spacing procedures and activities, and allowing uninterrupted rest periods.
- Avoid sedatives and respiratory depressant drugs unless mechanically ventilated.
- Prepare for endotracheal intubation and mechanical ventilation.
- Explain the procedure and its purpose; reassure the patient and family that this is a temporary measure to reduce the work of breathing. Advise that talking is not possible while intubated, and establish a means of communication.

Ineffective Airway Clearance

- Frequently assess respiratory rate, chest movement, lung sounds, oxygen saturation, exhaled carbon dioxide, and ABGs.

- Suction as needed to maintain a patent airway. Indicators for suctioning include crackles and rhonchi on auscultation, frequent coughing or setting off the high-pressure alarm, and increasing restlessness or anxiety.
- Obtain sputum for culture if it appears purulent or is odorous.
- Perform percussion, vibration, and postural drainage as ordered.
- Firmly secure endotracheal or tracheostomy tube.
- Assess fluid balance and maintain adequate hydration.

Risk for Injury

- Assess frequently, including color, vital signs, capillary refill, and peripheral pulses; level of consciousness; condition of mucosa of mouth and nose; bowel sounds; urine output.
- Weigh daily.
- Check stool for occult blood.
- Evaluate endotracheal tube cuff pressure by measurement (should be 20 to 25 mmHg or less) or by auscultating for a hissing sound at the end of inspiration.
- Do not bypass or turn off any ventilator alarms.
- Report condition changes such as increasing air leak around the cuff and decreased breath sounds or chest movement.
- Turn and reposition frequently.
- Keep skin and linens clean, dry, and wrinkle-free. Protect pressure areas with padding, egg-crate, or heal and elbow protectors.
- Perform passive range-of-motion exercises every 4 to 8 hours.
- Keep side rails up and use soft restraints as needed.
- Administer histamine H_2 blockers and sucralfate as ordered.

Anxiety

- Remain with the patient as much as possible.
- Explain all monitors, procedures, unusual sounds, and machinery.
- Provide a simple means of communication, such as a slate or picture board. If neuromuscular blockade is used, use methods such as looking to the right for "yes" and left for "no." Reassure that endotracheal tube removal restores the ability to speak.
- Encourage frequent family visits and family participation in care.
- Provide distraction with radio or television if allowed.

- Provide sedation and antianxiety medications as needed, especially when neuromuscular blockade is used.

Community-Based Care

- Teach about the disease process. Explain all procedures, monitors, tubes, machines, and alarms.

- Teach alternative communication strategies. Explain to significant others that the patient, although not able to speak, is able to hear and understand. Emphasize the importance of talking to the patient, not above or about the patient. Explain that mechanical ventilation is a temporary measure.

- Discuss measures to prevent future episodes of respiratory failure. Teach effective coughing, and pulmonary hygiene measures such as percussion, and postural drainage.

- Patients with end-stage COPD and recurrent respiratory failure may choose terminal weaning. Discuss the terminal weaning process with the patient and significant others, and explain that support services, such as clergy and psychotherapists, are available to the patient and loved ones.

- Refer to a smoking cessation program as appropriate.

- Encourage the patient to obtain influenza and pneumococcal vaccinations.

- Provide referrals for long-term care, home health nursing, or home respiratory care services as needed.

For more information on respiratory failure, see Chapter 37 in *Medical-Surgical Nursing,* Fifth Edition, by LeMone, Burke, and Bauldoff.

R

RHEUMATOID ARTHRITIS

Overview

- Rheumatoid arthritis (RA) is a chronic, progressive, systemic inflammatory disease.

- RA has a wide variety of manifestations, and usually involves inflammatory synovitis, often in the small joints of the wrists, hands, and feet.

- In RA, T lymphocytes or T cells infiltrate and proliferate in the synovial membrane, initiating an immune response. Cytokines released in response promote inflammation and stimulate macrophage activity. B cells produce autoantibodies known as rheumatoid factors, a hallmark of the disease. The result of this immune process is the release of lysosomal enzymes that destroy joint tissue.

- Inflammation causes hyperemia and pannus formation, which erodes articular cartilage, followed by scarring, fibrosis, and bony ankylosis of the affected joint.

- RA can affect people at any age but is usually diagnosed between 30 and 50 years of age. Women are affected three times more often than men.

- The course is highly variable; in most patients the disease progresses at a moderate rate.

Causes

- Unknown, but probably autoimmune
- Possible contributing factors: genetic, environmental, hormonal, and reproductive factors; infectious agents, such as bacteria, mycoplasmas, and viruses (especially Epstein-Barr virus); heavy smoking

Manifestations

Early

- Fever, malaise
- Anorexia, weakness
- Joint swelling and pain: usually digital joints of hands and feet, wrists, and ankles, but varies; symmetric pattern; worse in morning
- Decreased range of motion
- May be accompanied by lymphadenopathy or splenomegaly
- Possible systemic manifestations: rheumatoid nodules, skeletal muscle atrophy, rheumatoid vasculitis (can lead to mono/polyneuritis), pleural fibrosis, constrictive pericarditis, scleritis, osteoporosis, Felty's syndrome (splenomegaly, neutropenia, anemia, thrombocytopenia)

Late

- Joint deformity
- Ulnar drift of fingers
- Contractures

Diagnostic Tests

- Rheumatoid factor is found in 50% of people with RA. Anti-CCP (antibodies to cyclic citrullinated peptide) blood test provides a more specific marker for RA.

- C-reactive protein levels and erythrocyte sedimentation rate (ESR) are typically elevated.

- Complete blood count often shows anemia.

- X-ray of affected joints as the disease progresses may show osteoporosis around the joint, joint space narrowing, and erosions.

- Synovial fluid examination demonstrates increased turbidity (cloudiness), decreased viscosity, increased protein levels, and 3000 to 50,000 white blood cells, indicative of inflammation.

Interdisciplinary Management

- Aspirin, other nonsteroidal anti-inflammatory drugs, and analgesics reduce inflammation and manage signs and symptoms.

- Low-dose oral corticosteroids may be used to reduce pain and inflammation, and possibly to slow the development and progression of bone erosions. Intraarticular corticosteroids may be used for temporary relief of symptoms.

- Disease-modifying anti-rheumatic drugs (DMARDs) such as gold salts, antimalarial agents, sulfasalazine, D-penicillamine, and infliximab (Remicade) may alter the course of the disease, reducing joint destruction. Immunosuppressive and cytotoxic drugs are included in this category.

- Surgeries such as synovectomy, arthrodesis, or arthroplasty may be performed for severe cases.

- Heat and cold to relieve pain.

- Physical therapy to teach and monitor exercises.

- Assistive devices, such as a cane, walker, or raised toilet seat, are helpful for patients with significant hip or knee arthritis. Splints provide joint rest and prevent contractures.

Selected Nursing Diagnoses with Interventions

Chronic Pain

- Assess the level of pain and duration of morning stiffness.

R

- Encourage the patient to relate pain to activity level and adjust activities accordingly. Teach the importance of joint and whole-body rest.

- Teach the use of heat and cold applications to provide pain relief (e.g., taking a warm shower to reduce morning pain and stiffness).

- Teach about the use of prescribed anti-inflammatory medications and the relationship of pain and inflammation.

- Encourage using other nonpharmacologic pain relief measures such as visualization, distraction, and meditation.

Fatigue

- Encourage a balance of rest and activity.

- Stress the importance of planned rest periods during the day.

- Help the patient prioritize activities, performing the most important ones early in the day.

- Encourage regular physical activity in addition to prescribed range-of-motion exercises.

- Refer to counseling or support groups.

Ineffective Role Performance

- Discuss the effects of the disease on the patient's career and other life roles. Encourage the patient to identify changes brought on by the disease.

- Encourage the patient and family to discuss feelings about role changes and grieve lost roles or abilities.

- Listen actively to concerns expressed; acknowledge the validity of concerns about the disease, prescribed treatment, and prognosis.

- Help identify strengths that can be used to cope with role changes.

- Encourage the patient to make decisions and assume personal responsibility for disease management.

- Encourage the patient to maintain life roles as far as the disease allows.

Community-Based Care

In addition to the previous instructions do the following:

- Explain the disease process, including systemic effects such as stiffness, fatigue, anorexia, and weight loss.

- Stress the importance of taking medications as prescribed, and not on an as-needed basis. Encourage the patient to take aspirin or other nonsteroidal anti-inflammatory drugs with food or milk to minimize gastric distress and to report gastrointestinal symptoms or black stools to the physician promptly.

- Discuss the use of assistive devices and provide information on where to obtain them.

- Teach the importance of keeping all follow-up appointments with the physician.

- Refer to a dietitian, physical therapist, or occupational therapist as necessary.

- The patient may require a referral to social services or a home health nurse.

For more information on rheumatoid arthritis, see Chapter 40 in *Medical-Surgical Nursing,* Fifth Edition, by LeMone, Burke, and Bauldoff.

R

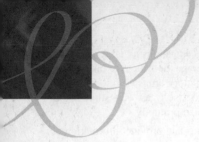

Scoliosis

Overview

- Scoliosis is a lateral deviation of the thoracic, lumbar, or thoracolumbar spine. The vertebral bodies in these regions can be rotated as well as curved to one side or the other.

- Scoliosis is classified as *postural* when the small curve corrects with bending, and *structural* when the curve does not correct with bending. Structural scoliosis, a curve caused by a fixed deformity, is more likely to require treatment.

- As scoliosis emerges, the muscles and ligaments shorten on the concave side of the curvature. Over time, progressive deformities of the vertebral column and ribs develop, causing one-sided compression of the vertebral bodies.

- A lateral curvature of less than 40 degrees at maturity carries a low risk of progression during adulthood. A lateral curvature greater than 50 degrees causes instability of the spine, with probable progression throughout the patient's lifetime.

Causes

- Structural: usually idiopathic; may have genetic link

- Secondary scoliosis: congenital and neuromuscular disorders (e.g., cerebral palsy, poliomyelitis, and muscular dystrophy)

- Functional: poor posture; inequality in limb lengths

Manifestations

- Visible curvature of spine (usually identified during pre- or early adolescence)

- Unequal hip, shoulder, elbow heights

- Asymmetric back muscles

- Backache, fatigue

- Possible dyspnea if chest volume is decreased

Diagnostic Tests

- Upright anterior-posterior and lateral x-rays of the spine will show deformity. The degree of curvature is measured by determining the amount of lateral deviation to the left or right.

Interdisciplinary Management

- Conservative treatment for adults with scoliosis may include weight reduction, active and passive exercises, and braces for support.

- Surgery for severe scoliosis involves attaching metal reinforcing rods to the vertebrae.

Selected Nursing Diagnoses with Interventions

Risk for Injury

- Assess the environment for safety hazards.

- Teach ways to reduce irritation of skin surfaces beneath the brace and to loosen the brace during meals and for the first 30 minutes after each meal.

- Emphasize the importance of maintaining body alignment.

- Following surgery:
  - Turn by using the log-rolling technique; use a fracture bedpan.
  - Teach how to apply the brace and explain ambulatory restrictions.
  - Teach to change slowly from a reclining position to sitting position and to sit on the edge of the bed for a few minutes before ambulating.

Risk for Peripheral Neurovascular Dysfunction

- Following spinal surgery, assess the movement and sensation of lower extremities every 2 hours for the first 8 hours, then every shift and as needed.

Community-Based Care

In addition to the preceding instructions, do the following:

- Explain the disease process, contributing factors, treatment, and prognosis.

- Following spinal surgery, teach activity restrictions as prescribed.

- Following surgery, the patient may require social services or a home health nurse.

For more information on scoliosis, see Chapter 40 in *Medical-Surgical Nursing,* Fifth Edition, by LeMone, Burke, and Bauldoff.

SEVERE ACUTE RESPIRATORY SYNDROME (SARS)

Overview

- **Severe acute respiratory syndrome (SARS)** is an atypical pneumonia marked by high fever, respiratory symptoms, and known exposure to the disease.

- SARS typically affects previously healthy adults aged 25 to 70 years.

- SARS appears to be spread by close person-to-person contact; potential sources of infection are direct contact with an infected person or contaminated object, and exposure of the eyes or mucous membranes to respiratory secretions.

- The incubation period for SARS is 2 to 7 days (up to 10 days in some people).

- Up to 20% of affected patients require intubation and mechanical ventilation; the fatality rate is about 11%.

Cause

- SARS is caused by a newly identified coronavirus.

Manifestations

- Fever higher than 100.4°F (38°C).
- Possible chills, headache, malaise, and muscle aches.
- After 3 to 7 days, respiratory manifestations develop, including nonproductive cough, shortness of breath, dyspnea, and possible hypoxia.

Diagnostic Tests

- Serology tests (ELISA or immunofluorescence) show the presence of antibodies to the identified coronavirus.

- Reverse-transcriptase PCR (RT-PCR) testing of respiratory and blood samples provides a rapid mechanism for identifying the virus

- Chest x-rays show focal or patchy interstitial infiltrates; consolidation may be evident.

- Pulse oximetry shows hypoxia in the respiratory phase of the illness.

- Complete blood count often identifies leukopenia and thrombocytopenia.

- CPK, ALT, and AST levels may be markedly elevated.

Interdisciplinary Management

- Healthcare providers and public health personnel should report cases of SARS to state and local health departments.

- Antibiotic and/or antiviral therapy targeted at community-acquired forms of pneumonia may be given.

- Oxygen may be administered to treat hypoxemia; intubation and mechanical ventilation may be required.

Selected Nursing Diagnoses with Interventions

Impaired Gas Exchange

- Monitor vital signs, color, oxygen saturation, and arterial blood gases. Assess for manifestations such as anxiety or apprehension, restlessness, confusion or lethargy, or complaints of headache.

- Promptly report signs of respiratory distress, including tachypnea, tachycardia, nasal flaring, use of accessory muscles, intercostal retractions, cyanosis, increasing restlessness, anxiety, or decreased level of consciousness.

- Promptly report worsening arterial blood gases and oxygen saturation levels.

- Maintain oxygen therapy and mechanical ventilation as ordered. Hyperoxygenate before suctioning.

- Place in Fowler's or high Fowler's position.

- Minimize activities and energy expenditures by assisting with activities of daily living, spacing procedures and activities, and allowing uninterrupted rest periods.

- Avoid sedatives and respiratory depressant drugs unless mechanically ventilated.

- If intubation and mechanical ventilation is necessary, explain the procedure and its purpose to the patient and family, providing reassurance that this is a temporary measure to improve oxygenation and reduce the work of breathing. Alert that talking is not possible while the endotracheal tube is in place, and establish a means of communication.

Risk for Infection

- Place the patient in a private room with air flow control that prevents air within the room from circulating into the hallway or other rooms. A negative air flow room in which air is diluted by at least six fresh-air exchanges per hour is recommended.

- Use standard precautions and respiratory and contact isolation techniques as recommended by the Centers for Disease Control and Prevention, including wearing an N95 respirator, gowns, and eye protection when caring for patients with SARS.

- Discuss the reasons for and importance of respiratory and contact isolation procedures during treatment.

- Place a mask on the patient when transporting to other parts of the facility for diagnostic or treatment procedures.

- Assist visitors to mask before entering the room.

Community-Based Care

- The disease, its origin, and how it is spread
- Manifestations of impaired respiratory status to report to the physician
- Preventing spread of the disease to others:
  1. Cover mouth and nose with tissues when coughing or sneezing. Personally dispose of tissues in a paper bag or the garbage.
  2. Wear a surgical mask during close contact with other members of the household.
  3. Limit interactions outside the home; do not go to work, school, or other public areas until free of fever for 10 days and your respiratory symptoms are resolving.
  4. Remind all members of the household to wash hands (or use an alcohol-based hand sanitizer) frequently, particularly after direct contact with body fluids.

S

5. Do not share eating utensils, towels, or bedding with others. These items can be cleaned with soap and hot water between uses. Clean contaminated surfaces with a household disinfectant.

- Instruct uninfected members of the household to report fever or respiratory symptoms to the physician.

- Refer for home health care to monitor disease status and other members of the household.

- A referral for home oxygen delivery may be appropriate.

For more information about severe acute respiratory syndrome, see Chapter 36 in *Medical-Surgical Nursing,* Fifth Edition, by LeMone, Burke, and Bauldoff.

SHOCK (HYPOVOLEMIC, CARDIOGENIC, DISTRIBUTIVE, SEPTIC)

Overview

- Shock is characterized by a systemic imbalance between oxygen supply and demand. This imbalance causes inadequate blood flow to body organs and tissues, resulting in life-threatening cellular dysfunction.

- Shock is triggered by a drop in mean arterial pressure (MAP).

- Unless effectively treated, shock progresses through predictable stages:

  1. During the early, compensatory stage, the fall in MAP triggers compensatory mechanisms to maintain cardiac output and tissue perfusion.

  2. In the progressive stage, compensatory mechanisms cannot maintain cardiac output and tissue perfusion. Cells become hypoxic and switch to anaerobic metabolism, producing a state of lactic acidosis.

  3. If shock progresses to the final refractory or irreversible stage, tissue damage is irreversible and death will ensue.

- Hypovolemic shock is caused by a 15% or more decrease in intravascular volume. Venous return is inadequate for cardiac filling, resulting in decreased stroke volume, cardiac output, and blood pressure.

- Cardiogenic shock occurs when the heart's pumping ability is compromised to the point that it cannot maintain cardiac output and adequate tissue perfusion.
- Distributive shock results from widespread vasodilatation and decreased peripheral resistance, leading to a relative hypovolemia.
- Septic shock is part of a progressive syndrome called systemic inflammatory response syndrome. It is most often the result of gram-negative bacterial infections.

Causes

Hypovolemic

- Hemorrhage
- Severe dehydration
- Third spacing or other fluid shifts

Cardiogenic

- Myocardial infarction
- Cardiac dysrhythmia/arrest
- Structural or inflammatory cardiac disorders
- Complication of cardiac surgery

Distributive

- Anaphylaxis: histamine, leukotrienes, kinins, prostaglandins
- Neurogenic: central vasomotor center malfunction

Septic

- Most often gram-negative bacteria

Manifestations

All Types

- Hypotension: MAP < 60 mmHg (nonhypertensive adult)
- Tachycardia, with weak, thready pulse
- Cool, clammy, mottled skin
- Oliguria
- Clouded sensorium

Hypovolemic

- Accompanying or previous vomiting, diarrhea, diaphoresis
- Poor skin turgor

Cardiogenic

- Dysrhythmias
- Elevated filling pressures
- Gallop rhythm
- Murmurs
- Pericardial effusion: pulsus paradoxus; muffled heart sounds

Distributive

- Anaphylactic: may have accompanying bronchoconstriction with wheezing and dyspnea
- Neurogenic: dry, warm skin; bradycardia

Septic

- Accompanying fever, chills, malaise; flushed, warm skin

Diagnostic Tests

All Types

- Early arterial blood gases reveal respiratory alkalosis; later, they will show metabolic acidosis.
- Pulmonary wedge pressure via Swan-Ganz catheter will be reduced.

Hypovolemic

- Serum electrolytes, blood urea nitrogen, hemoglobin, and hematocrit are elevated.
- Urine is concentrated with an increased specific gravity.

Septic

- Blood cultures are done to rule out or identify bacteria in blood.
- White blood cell count may be elevated early but reduced if overwhelming infection is present.
- Coagulation studies may show abnormal bleeding times.

Interdisciplinary Management

- Emergency care focuses on maintaining a level of tissue perfusion adequate to sustain life. Administration of intravenous fluids and blood is the most effective treatment for hypovolemic shock. In addition, establishing and maintaining a patent airway and ensuring adequate oxygenation are critical interventions.

- Vasoactive and inotropic drugs may also be used to treat shock. Other pharmacologic agents may be used specific to the type of shock; for example, antibiotics may be given to suppress organisms responsible for septic shock.

Selected Nursing Diagnoses with Interventions

Decreased Cardiac Output

- Assess and monitor cardiovascular status, including blood pressure, heart rate and rhythm, capillary refill, peripheral pulses, and hemodynamic monitoring.

- Maintain bed rest, and provide to the extent possible a calm, quiet environment.

- Position supine with the legs elevated to about 20 degrees, trunk flat, and head and shoulders elevated higher than the chest.

Altered Tissue Perfusion

- Monitor skin color, temperature, turgor, and moisture.

- Monitor cardiopulmonary status, including rate and depth of respirations, lung sounds, jugular vein distention, and central venous pressure measurements.

- Monitor body temperature.

- Monitor urinary output hourly, reporting output < 30mL/h.

- Monitor bowel sounds, abdominal distention, and abdominal pain.

- Assess mental status and level of consciousness.

Community-Based Care

- Provide information about the current setting.

- Provide information about resources that are available: pastoral services, social services, temporary housing, meals, and so on.

- Provide anticipatory guidance to prepare for recovery or death and to support realistic hope.

- Depending on the cause of the episode, the patient may require referrals for home health care, social services, financial assistance, rehabilitation services, a long-term care facility, or psychologic counseling.

For more information on shock, see Chapter 11 in *Medical-Surgical Nursing,* Fifth Edition, by LeMone, Burke, and Bauldoff.

SICKLE CELL ANEMIA

Overview

- Sickle cell anemia is a hereditary, chronic hemolytic anemia characterized by an abnormal form of hemoglobin (HbS) and episodes of sickling, during which red blood cells (RBCs) become abnormally crescent shaped.
- It is transmitted as an autosomal recessive genetic defect.
- People who carry one HbS gene have *sickle cell trait;* about 40% of their hemoglobin is HbS. They are asymptomatic unless stressed by severe hypoxia.
- Less than 1% of Blacks have inherited the HbS gene from both parents and have *sickle cell disease;* nearly all their hemoglobin is HbS.
- In hypoxemia, deoxygenated HbS crystallizes into rodlike structures that deform the erythrocyte into a crescent or sickle shape. Sickled cells clump together to obstruct capillary blood flow, causing ischemia and possible infarction of surrounding tissue.
- In sickle cell crisis, sickled cells and vasospasm obstruct blood flow, resulting in tissue ischemia and infarction. Vasoocclusive crises last an average of 4 to 6 days.
- *Sequestration crises,* which may affect children, are marked by pooling of large amounts of blood in the liver and spleen.
- Repeated episodes of sickling weaken RBC cell membranes, leading to hemolysis and a reduced RBC life span.

Causes

- Usually affects people of African descent; 7% to 13% of Blacks in the United States carry the defective gene.
- Conditions likely to trigger sickling include hypoxia, low environmental or body temperature, excessive exercise, anesthesia, dehydration, infections, or acidosis.

Manifestations

- Hemolytic anemia: pallor, fatigue, jaundice, irritability
- Sickle cell crisis:
  1. Painful swelling of hands, feet, large joints
  2. Priapism (persistent, painful erection of the penis)
  3. Abdominal pain
  4. Manifestations of stroke

Diagnostic Tests

- Complete blood count shows decreased RBC count with increased numbers of reticulocytes, decreased hemoglobin and hematocrit, and an elevated white blood cell count.
- Serum ferritin levels may be low as iron reserves are depleted by increased need to replace RBCs.
- Sickle cell test is positive for hemolytic anemia and HbS.
- Hemoglobin electrophoresis separates normal hemoglobin from abnormal forms. It is used to differentiate sickle cell trait from sickle cell disease.

Interdisciplinary Management

- Folic acid is given to meet the increased demands of the bone marrow.
- Hydroxyurea promotes fetal hemoglobin production and may be prescribed for those with frequent crises or severe sickle cell disease.
- Intravenous fluids are administered to patients in sickle cell crisis to improve blood flow, reduce pain, and prevent renal damage. Analgesics are given for pain.
- Blood transfusions may be necessary in severe cases and for pregnant women.
- Genetic counseling is important for patients and significant others at risk for sickle cell anemia.

Selected Nursing Diagnoses with Interventions

Acute Pain

- Assess subjective complaints of pain using a standard pain scale. Also assess objective manifestations of pain.

- Administer analgesics as ordered, assessing their effectiveness.
- Teach alternative, nonpharmacologic measures to reduce pain, such as meditation, guided imagery, and distraction.

Ineffective Tissue Perfusion

- Administer oxygen as indicated for the patient in sickle cell crisis.
- Ensure adequate hydration by offering noncaffeinated beverages and administering intravenous normal saline as prescribed.
- Encourage wearing loose, nonconstrictive clothing.
- Instruct to avoid excessive flexion of the knees and hips to promote venous return.
- Maintain a room temperature of at least 72°F.
- Maintain peripheral blood flow by avoiding external blood pressure cuffs and prolonged placement of a tourniquet for vascular access.
- Perform neurovascular checks of extremities every hour, including pulse oximetry of fingers and toes.

Community-Based Care

- Teach about the disease process, its transmission, treatment options, and measures to prevent crises.
- Discuss manifestations that signal the need for prompt medical treatment.
- Refer for genetic counseling and prenatal testing as appropriate.
- Stress the need for continuing medical management of the disease and its manifestations.
- A referral to a support group or other information resource may be helpful in increasing the patient's coping skills.

For more information on sickle cell anemia, see Chapter 33 in *Medical-Surgical Nursing,* Fifth Edition, by LeMone, Burke, and Bauldoff.

SKIN CANCER, NONMELANOMA (BASAL CELL, SQUAMOUS CELL)

Overview

- Nonmelanoma skin cancer may be classified as either basal cell or squamous cell carcinoma.

- These are the most frequently occurring cancers in the United States, with over 1 million new cases diagnosed each year; basal cell carcinoma accounts for about 80%, and squamous cell carcinoma for 20%.

- Basal cell carcinoma arises from epidermal basal cells and is locally invasive but usually does not metastasize.

- Squamous cell carcinoma arises from keratinizing epidermal cells; it invades the dermis, can grow rapidly, and can metastasize via local lymphatics.

Causes

- *Basal cell carcinoma:* Risk factors include age, fair complexion, sun (UV) exposure, immunosuppression, xeroderma pigmentosa (defective DNA repair).

- *Squamous cell carcinoma:* Risk factors include age; sun (UV) exposure; xeroderma pigmentosa (defective DNA repair); or history of ionizing radiation exposure, burns (scars), industrial carcinogen exposure, arsenic exposure, or draining lesions (fistulas, osteomyelitis).

Manifestations

Basal Cell Carcinoma

- Early: dome-shaped papule or nodule; pearly white, pink with telangiectasis on surface or plaques (may be pigmented)

- Late: painless, central ulceration with raised, rolled borders (rodent ulcer)

- Typically located on sun-exposed areas of face, chest, arms

Squamous Cell Carcinoma

- *In situ*: keratotic, scaly, red plaques

- Invasive: red, raised, ulcerative nodules with central necrosis and edematous border

- Typically located on sun-exposed areas of face, scalp, ears, lips, hands; burn scar areas; draining lesion areas

Diagnostic Test

- Skin biopsy establishes the diagnosis of either type of cancer.

Interdisciplinary Management

- Removal through surgical excision or through Mohs' micrographic surgery.
- Cryosurgery is a noninvasive technique that may be used to freeze and destroy the tumor tissue.
- Radiation for inoperable lesions because of their location or size.
- Other therapies include curettage and electrodessication, radiation, topical chemotherapy, or laser surgery.

Selected Nursing Diagnoses with Interventions (Postoperative)

Risk for Infection

- Monitor for manifestations of infection: fever, tachycardia, malaise, and incisional erythema, swelling, pain, or drainage that increases or becomes purulent.
- Keep the incision line clean and dry by changing dressings as necessary.
- Follow principles of medical and surgical asepsis when caring for the incision. Teach the importance of careful hand hygiene. Maintain standard precautions if drainage is present.
- Encourage and maintain adequate kilocalorie and protein intake in the diet.

Anxiety

- Provide accurate information about the illness, treatment, and expected length of recovery.
- Encourage discussion of expected physical changes and ways to minimize disfigurement through cosmetics and clothing.
- Provide reassurance and comfort.
- Provide interventions that decrease anxiety levels and increase coping.

Community-Based Care

- Encourage primary prevention behaviors recommended by the American Cancer Society and the Skin Cancer Foundation:
  - Minimize exposure to the sun between the hours of 10 AM and 3 PM.

- Cover up with a wide-brimmed hat, sunglasses, long-sleeved shirt, and long pants when in the sun.
- Use a waterproof sunscreen with an SPF of 15 or more.
- Avoid tanning booths.

- Explain how to conduct a monthly skin self-examination.
- Provide the patient with a brochure describing types of skin cancers and prevention behaviors, and showing photographs of lesions.
- Refer to the American Cancer Society for further information.

For more information on skin cancer, nonmelanoma, see Chapter 16 in *Medical-Surgical Nursing,* Fifth Edition, by LeMone, Burke, and Bauldoff.

SMALLPOX

Overview

- Smallpox is an infectious disease caused by the *variola* virus. It is usually spread by infected saliva droplets. Contaminated clothing or bed linen can also spread the disease.
- Routine smallpox vaccinations are no longer recommended, but the illness has been identified as a possible bioterrorism measure.
- The incubation period is 7 to 17 days following exposure.
- Most people recover, but death does occur in about 30% of cases.

Manifestations

- Initial manifestations are high fever, fatigue, headache, and backache.
- A rash that is more prominent on the face, arms, and legs follows in 2 to 3 days. The rash starts as flat red lesions, then becomes pustular and crusts form. Scabs develop and fall off after 3 to 4 weeks.

Community-Based Care

- Vaccination is not recommended, and the vaccine is not generally available to healthcare providers or the public.
- In the event of an outbreak, the Centers for Disease Control and Prevention has established guidelines to provide vaccine to exposed persons. If the vaccine is given within 4 days after

exposure, the disease is less serious or does not occur. The vaccine does have some associated risks.

For more information about smallpox see Chapter 12 in *Medical-Surgical Nursing,* Fifth Edition, by LeMone, Burke, and Bauldoff.

Sodium Imbalance

Hyponatremia

Hypernatremia

Overview

- Sodium is the most plentiful electrolyte in extracellular fluid (ECF).
- Normal serum sodium levels are 135 to 145 mEq/L.
- Sodium is the primary regulator of ECF volume, osmolality, and distribution, and is important for neuromuscular activity.
- Sodium imbalances affect the osmolality of ECF and water distribution between the fluid compartments.
    1. In hyponatremia, water is drawn into the cells of the body, causing them to swell.
    2. In hypernatremia, water is drawn out of body cells, causing them to shrink.
- Most sodium in the body comes from dietary intake. It is primarily excreted by the kidneys, which regulate sodium balance by excreting or conserving sodium in response to changes in vascular volume.
    1. The renin-angiotensin-aldosterone system regulates sodium reabsorption in the renal tubules and cortical collecting tubules of the kidney.
    2. Antidiuretic hormone from the posterior pituitary regulates sodium and water reabsorption in the distal tubules of the kidney.
    3. The glomerular filtration rate affects the rate at which water and sodium is filtered and excreted.
    4. Atrial natriuretic peptide, a hormone produced by cells in the atria of the heart, increases sodium excretion by the kidneys.

Causes

Hyponatremia (Serum Sodium < 135 mEq/L)

Loss of Sodium and Water

- Renal losses: diuretic use, kidney diseases, or adrenal insufficiency
- Gastrointestinal losses: vomiting, diarrhea, gastrointestinal suction, repeated tap water enemas
- Skin losses: excessive sweating, extensive burns

Loss of Sodium with Normal or Excess Water

- Systemic diseases: heart failure, renal failure, cirrhosis
- Syndrome of inappropriate secretion of antidiuretic hormone
- Excessive water through oral intake or hypotonic intravenous (IV) fluids

Hypernatremia (Serum Sodium > 145 mEq/L)

- Water deprivation, inability to respond to thirst
- Excess water loss: diarrhea, fever, hyperventilation, excessive perspiration, or massive burns, diabetes insipidus
- Excess sodium intake: ingestion of excess salt, hypertonic IV solutions
- Near-drowning in seawater, heatstroke

Manifestations

Hyponatremia

- Early: muscle cramps, weakness, and fatigue; anorexia, nausea, vomiting, abdominal cramping, and diarrhea
- Later: headache, depression, dulled sensorium, personality changes, irritability, lethargy, hyperreflexia, muscle twitching, and tremors
- Severe: convulsions and coma
- Manifestations of fluid volume deficit or fluid volume excess

Hypernatremia

- Thirst
- Lethargy, weakness, and irritability
- Seizures, coma

Diagnostic Tests

- Serum sodium levels will be abnormal.
- Serum osmolality will be either increased or decreased.
- Urine sodium levels may be abnormal.
- Urine specific gravity may be high or lower than normal.

Interdisciplinary Management

- Treatment for sodium imbalances focuses on restoring normal fluid and sodium balance.
- Sodium-containing fluids are administered for hyponatremia. If the disorder is associated with fluid volume excess, diuretics may be ordered.
- Diuretics may be used to promote sodium excretion in hypernatremia. Water is replaced using IV infusions of dextrose in water.

Selected Nursing Diagnoses with Interventions

Hyponatremia
Risk for Imbalanced Fluid Volume

- Monitor intake and output, weigh daily, and calculate 24-hour fluid balance.
- Carefully monitor patients receiving sodium-containing IV solutions for signs of hypervolemia (increased blood pressure and central venous pressure, tachypnea, tachycardia, gallop rhythm, shortness of breath, crackles).
- Use an IV flow-control device to administer hypertonic saline (3% and 5% NaCl) solutions; carefully monitor flow rate and response.
- If fluids are restricted, explain the reason for the restriction, the amount of fluid allowed, and how to calculate fluid intake.

Risk for Ineffective Cerebral Tissue Perfusion

- Monitor serum electrolytes and serum osmolality. Report abnormal results to the care provider.
- Assess for neurologic changes, such as lethargy, altered level of consciousness, confusion, and convulsions. Monitor mental status and orientation. Compare baseline data with continuing assessments.

- Assess muscle strength and tone, and deep tendon reflexes.
- Maintain a quiet environment, and institute seizure precautions in patients with severe hyponatremia.

Hypernatremia
Risk for Injury

- Monitor and maintain fluid replacement to within the prescribed limits. Monitor serum sodium levels and osmolality; report rapid changes to the care provider.
- Monitor neurologic function, including mental status, level of consciousness, and other manifestations such as headache, nausea, vomiting, elevated blood pressure, and decreased pulse rate.
- Institute safety precautions as necessary: Keep the bed in its lowest position, side rails up and padded, and an airway at the bedside.
- Keep clocks, calendars, and familiar objects at the bedside. Orient to time, place, and circumstances as needed. Allow significant others to remain with the patient as much as possible.

Community-Based Care

- Discuss the need for dietary restrictions or increases of sodium and how to incorporate them.
- Teach about the cause of the sodium imbalance and strategies to prevent recurrences.
- Stress the importance of drinking liquids containing sodium and other electrolytes at frequent intervals when perspiring heavily or when experiencing diarrhea.
- If the patient is taking a potent diuretic or other medication affecting sodium and water balance, stress the importance of regular laboratory testing for electrolyte levels.
- Provide a referral to a dietitian for further teaching as appropriate.
- Home nursing services may be appropriate for the patient unable to respond to the thirst mechanism.

For more information about sodium imbalances, see Chapter 10 in *Medical-Surgical Nursing,* Fifth Edition, by LeMone, Burke, and Bauldoff.

Stroke (Cerebrovascular Accident, Brain Attack)

Overview

- A stroke is a sudden reduction in cerebral perfusion secondary to a thrombus, embolus, or hemorrhage.

- Reduced blood flow reduces available oxygen and can result in cerebral ischemia with temporary deficits (a transient ischemic attack) or cerebral infarction with permanent brain damage.

- Stroke is a leading cause of disability and death in the United States.

Causes

- *Thrombosis* is the most common cause in middle-aged and older persons; it results from occlusion of a cerebral vessel with atheromatous plaques. This type of stroke often is preceded by transient ischemic attacks. Risk factors include smoking, sedentary lifestyle, and atherosclerosis.

- *Embolus* is the second most common cause. Embolic stroke can occur at any age, and is associated with disorders predisposing to clot formation, for example, atherosclerosis, endocarditis, valve disease, cardiac dysrhythmias, or heart surgery. Risk factors include smoking, oral contraceptive use, and a sedentary lifestyle.

- *Hemorrhage* is the least common cause. Hemorrhagic stroke can occur at any age, caused by vessel rupture secondary to aneurysm, hypertension, or trauma. Clotting disorders also are a risk factor.

Manifestations

- Vary with location and extent of each type of lesion.

- General manifestations include weakness; dizziness; contralateral hemiparesis or hemiplegia; changes in cognition or level of consciousness; seizures; communication difficulties (agnosia, aphasia, apraxia); coma.

- Onset and prognosis vary according to type:
  - Thrombotic—gradual development, onset over minutes, hours, days; prognosis good
  - Embolic—sudden onset, not related to activity; usually immediate maximum deficits; prognosis fair to good

- Hemorrhagic—sudden onset, often associated with activity, continued symptom progression; headache and nuchal rigidity (stiff neck due to meningeal irritation of blood); may rapidly progress with deepening coma; poor prognosis

Diagnostic Tests

- Lumbar puncture may be bloody, if hemorrhagic type.
- Computed tomography scan shows edema, lesions, structural details with high accuracy.
- Positron emission tomography scan gives blood flow and metabolic activity data; especially useful for thrombotic or embolic cerebrovascular accident (CVA).
- Magnetic resonance imaging delineates size and location of lesion only.
- Angiography shows arterial vessel shadow and can identify narrowing, blockage, or rupture.
- Electroencephalogram can assess localized damage.

Interdisciplinary Management

- Antiplatelet agents and antithrombotic drugs are often used as a preventive measure for patients at risk for embolic and thrombotic CVA.
- Fibrinolytic and anticoagulant drug therapy is often prescribed for thrombotic CVA during the stroke-in-evolution phase, but is contraindicated in complete stroke because it may increase the risk of cerebral hemorrhage.
- Calcium channel blockers may be used to reduce cerebral vasospasm.
- Surgery (e.g., atherectomy or thrombectomy) may be performed to prevent CVA or to restore blood flow when a CVA has already occurred.
- Various types of interdisciplinary therapy are necessary for post-stroke rehabilitation.

Selected Nursing Diagnoses with Interventions

Ineffective Tissue Perfusion: Cerebral

- Monitor respiratory status and airway patency. Suction as necessary, place in side-lying position, and administer oxygen as prescribed.

- Monitor neurologic status.
- Continuously monitor cardiac status, observing for dysrhythmias.
- Monitor body temperature.
- Maintain accurate intake and output records.
- Monitor for seizures. Pad the side rails, and administer prescribed anticonvulsants.

Impaired Physical Mobility

- Encourage active range-of-motion (ROM) exercises for unaffected extremities and perform passive ROM exercises for affected extremities every 4 hours during the day and evening shifts and once during the night shift. Support the joint during passive ROM exercises.
- Turn at least every 2 hours around the clock. Maintain body alignment, and support extremities in proper position with pillows.
- Monitor for manifestations of venous thrombosis. Assess for increased warmth and redness in calves. Measure the circumference of the calves and thighs.
- Do not use a footboard. Use hand splints only as prescribed to prevent flexion contractures of the fingers and wrists.
- Collaborate with the physical therapist as the patient gains mobility, using consistent techniques to move the patient from the bed to the wheelchair or to help the patient ambulate.

Self-Care Deficit

- Encourage use of the unaffected arm to bathe, brush teeth, comb hair, dress, and eat.
- Teach the patient and significant others to put on clothing by first dressing the affected extremities and then dressing the unaffected extremities.
- Collaborate with the occupational therapist in scheduling times for training for upper-extremity functioning necessary for activities of daily living. Encourage the use of assistive devices if required for eating, physical hygiene, and dressing.

Impaired Verbal Communication

- Approach and treat the patient as an adult. Do not assume that the patient who does not respond verbally cannot hear. Allow adequate time for the patient to respond. Face the patient and speak slowly. When you do not understand what the patient has said, be honest and say so. Use short, simple statements and questions.

- Accept frustration and anger as a normal reaction to the loss of function.

- Try alternate methods of communication, including writing tablets, flash cards, and computerized talking boards.

Community-Based Care

- Explain the illness, its causes, treatment, and prevention.

- Discuss strategies for self-care, mobility, and coping skills. Provide teaching as appropriate.

- Teach about medications, including dosage, effects, and side effects.

- Review home and equipment modifications and advise, as appropriate, use of a wheelchair, walker, bath chair, vise lid opener, and long-handled shoe horn, and/or installation of raised toilet seat and grab bars in the bathroom.

- Referral to a home health nurse and physical and occupational therapy may be appropriate.

- Initiate communications with a long-term care facility about the established plan of care if the patient is going to such a setting for rehabilitation or care.

- Refer the patient to Meals on Wheels, eldercare groups, social services, the National Stroke Association, stroke clubs, support groups, and respite care, as appropriate.

For more information on stroke, see Chapter 42 in *Medical-Surgical Nursing,* Fifth Edition, by LeMone, Burke, and Bauldoff.

S

SUBSTANCE ABUSE

Overview

- Substance abuse is the use of any chemical in a manner inconsistent with medical or culturally defined social norms despite physical, psychological, or social adverse effects.

- Substance abuse affects over 9% of Americans aged 12 and older.

- More than 90% of people who commit suicide have a depressive or substance abuse disorder.

- The reinforcing properties of drugs can create a pleasurable experience and reduce the intensity of unpleasant experiences.

- Substance dependence or addiction is the uncontrolled use of a chemical substance for at least 3 months, persisting despite adverse physical, psychologic, and interpersonal effects.

- Tolerance is a progressive decrease in the response to a drug.

- Withdrawal occurs when a person physically addicted to a drug stops taking it; it is an uncomfortable state lasting several days, manifested by tremors, diaphoresis, anxiety, high blood pressure, tachycardia, and possibly convulsions.

- Detoxification is the process of removing the physiologic effects of a drug from an addicted person. Repeated detoxifications cause long-term changes in brain neurotransmission, increase neuron sensitivity, and may intensify obsessive thoughts or cravings for a substance.

Causes

- Unknown; may involve the endogenous opioid system.

- Adolescent males with the D2 dopamine receptor gene (DRD2 A1 allele) have increased risk for alcohol abuse.

- Risk factors: genetic (heredity), biologic (particularly the neurotransmitters dopamine, serotonin, endorphin, enkephalin, dynorphin, and norepinephrine), psychologic, and sociocultural (ethnicity, religion, culture).

Manifestations

- Compulsive preoccupation with obtaining the substance, loss of control over consumption, and development of tolerance and dependence

- Impaired social and occupational functioning

- Impulsive, risk-taking behaviors

- Low tolerance for frustration and pain

Withdrawal:

- Caffeine (stimulant): headaches and irritability.

- Nicotine (stimulant in low doses): craving, nervousness, restlessness, irritability, impatience, increased hostility, insomnia, impaired concentration, increased appetite, and weight gain.

- Cannabis (marijuana, also known as grass, weed, pot, dope, joint, and reefer; and hashish): unknown.

- Alcohol and other central nervous system depressants: Early signs of withdrawal appear within a few hours, peak in 24 to 48 hours, and then rapidly disappear. Delirium tremens or severe withdrawal is a medical emergency; it usually occurs 2 to 5 days following alcohol withdrawal and persists 2 to 3 days. Delirium tremens manifestations include disorientation, paranoid delusions, visual hallucinations, and marked withdrawal symptoms. Seizures also may occur.

- Psychostimulants (cocaine and amphetamines): dysphoria and craving with fatigue, prolonged sleep, excessive eating, and depression; suicide a risk during cocaine withdrawal.

- Opiates (narcotic analgesics, including morphine, meperidine, codeine, hydrocodone, and oxycodone): Initial—drug craving, lacrimation, rhinorrhea, yawning, and diaphoresis for up to 10 days; second phase—(months) insomnia, irritability, fatigue, and potential gastrointestinal hyperactivity and premature ejaculation.

- Hallucinogens (psychedelics; includes PCP, MDMA or Ecstasy, LSD, mescaline, DMT, and psilocin): No apparent physical dependence or withdrawal symptoms. However, may induce continuing psychosis or "flashbacks."

- Inhalants: withdrawal symptoms unknown; brain damage or sudden death ("sudden sniffing death") can occur during use.

Diagnostic Tests

- A urine drug screen is the preferred method for detecting substances in the body. Saliva, perspiration, and hair also can be tested.

- A Breathalyzer is the simplest method of detecting blood alcohol content.

- Serum drug levels are useful in the emergency department and other hospital settings to treat drug overdoses or complications. The length of time that drugs can be found in blood and urine varies according to dosage and metabolic properties of the drug.

Interdisciplinary Management

- Effective treatment requires an interdisciplinary team specializing in the treatment of psychiatric and substance abuse disorders.

- Therapies may include detoxification, aversion therapy to maintain abstinence, group and/or individual psychotherapy, psychotropic medications, cognitive-behavioral strategies, family counseling, and self-help groups.

- An overdose is a life-threatening emergency requiring stabilization of the patient before treatment of the abuse. Respiratory depression may require mechanical ventilation. A seizure is a serious complication requiring emergency treatment.

- Medications such as benzodiazepines are used to minimize discomfort during alcohol withdrawal and to prevent serious adverse effects, in particular seizures. Other drugs used in treating withdrawal include vitamins, antidepressants and mood stabilizers, anticonvulsants, and drugs to promote abstinence, such as disulfiram (Antabuse) and naltrexone (ReVia, Depade).

Selected Nursing Diagnoses with Interventions

Risk for Injury

- Place in a quiet, private room to decrease excessive stimuli, but do not leave patient alone if excessive hyperactivity or suicidal ideation is present.

- Frequently orient to reality and the environment, ensuring that potentially harmful objects are stored outside the patient's access.

- Monitor vital signs every 15 minutes until stable and assess for signs of intoxication or withdrawal.

Ineffective Coping

- Establish trusting relationship.

- Set limits on manipulative behavior and maintain consistency in responses.

- Encourage to verbalize feelings, fears, or anxieties. Use attentive listening and validate feelings with observations or statements that acknowledge feelings.

- Explore methods of dealing with stressful situations other than resorting to substance use. Provide encouragement for changing to a healthier lifestyle. Teach healthy coping mechanisms (e.g., physical exercise, progressive muscle relaxation, deep breathing exercises, meditation, and imagery).

Imbalanced Nutrition: Less than Body Requirements

- Administer vitamins and dietary supplements as ordered by the physician.

- Monitor lab work (e.g., total albumin, complete blood count, urinalysis, electrolytes, and liver enzymes) and report significant changes to physician.

- Collaborate with dietitian to determine number of calories needed to provide adequate nutrition and realistic weight gain. Document intake, output, and calorie count. Weigh daily if condition warrants.

- Teach the importance of adequate nutrition by explaining the food guide pyramid and relating the physical effects of malnutrition on body systems.

Chronic or Situational Low Self-Esteem

- Spend time with patient and convey an attitude of acceptance. Encourage to accept responsibility for own behaviors and feelings.

- Encourage to focus on strengths and accomplishments rather than weaknesses and failures.

- Encourage participation in therapeutic group activities. Offer recognition and positive feedback for actual achievements.

- Teach assertiveness techniques and effective communication techniques such as the use of "I feel" rather than "You make me feel" statements.

Disturbed Sensory Perceptions

- Observe for withdrawal symptoms. Monitor vital signs. Provide adequate nutrition and hydration. Place on seizure precautions.

- Assess level of orientation frequently. Orient and reassure patient of safety in presence of hallucinations, delusions, or illusions.

- Explain all interventions before approaching patient. Avoid loud noises and talk softly to patient. Decrease external stimuli by dimming lights.

- Administer medications according to detoxification schedule.

Disturbed Thought Processes

- Give positive reinforcement when thinking and behavior are appropriate or when patient recognizes that delusions are not based in reality.

- Use simple, step-by-step instructions and face-to-face interaction when communicating.

- Express reasonable doubt if patient relays suspicious or paranoid beliefs. Reinforce accurate perception of people or situations.

- Do not argue with delusions or hallucinations. Convey acceptance that the patient believes a situation to be true, but that the nurse does not see or hear what is not there.

- Talk to patient about real events and real people. Respond to feelings and reassure patient that he or she is safe from harm.

Community-Based Care

Following withdrawal, teaching for the patient and family includes the following:

- The negative effects of substance abuse including physical and psychological complications of substance abuse.

- The signs of relapse and the importance of after-care programs and self-help groups to prevent relapse.

- Information about specific medications, including the potential side effects, possible drug interactions, and any special precautions to be taken.

- Ways to manage stress including techniques such as progressive muscle relaxation, abdominal breathing techniques, imagery, meditation, and effective coping skills.

In addition, suggest the following resources:

- Alcoholics Anonymous, Narcotics Anonymous, and other self-help groups

- Employee assistance programs

- Individual, group, and/or family counseling

- Community rehabilitation programs

- National Alliance for the Mentally Ill

For more information about substance abuse, see Chapter 6 in *Medical Surgical Nursing*, Fifth Edition, by LeMone, Burke, and Bauldoff.

Syndrome of Inappropriate Antidiuretic Hormone Secretion

Overview

- Syndrome of inappropriate antidiuretic hormone secretion (SIADH) is characterized by excess antidiuretic hormone (ADH) (vasopressin) secretion despite low plasma osmolality.

- Excess ADH causes water to be retained. Blood volume expands, but the plasma is diluted. Aldosterone is suppressed, resulting in increased renal sodium excretion. Water moves from the hypotonic plasma and the interstitial spaces into the cells.

Causes

- The usual cause of SIADH is ectopic production of ADH by malignant tumors, including oat cell carcinoma of the lung, pancreatic carcinoma, leukemia, and malignant lymphoma.

- Transient SIADH may follow a head injury, lung disorders, pituitary surgery, or medications such as barbiturates, anesthetics, or diuretics.

Manifestations

- Anorexia, nausea, vomiting
- Increased body weight
- Tachycardia
- Hypothermia
- Cerebral edema: headache, changes in mental status or personality, lethargy, and irritability
- Decreased deep tendon reflexes

Diagnostic Tests

- Serum sodium will be less than 135 mEq/L and falling.
- Serum osmolality will be < 275 mOsm/L.
- Plasma or urine arginine vasopressin levels will be elevated.

Interdisciplinary Management

- Medical care is aimed at treating the underlying causes, treating the hyponatremia with intravenous hypertonic saline, and restricting oral fluid intake to less than 800 mL per day.

- Diuretics may be prescribed for manifestations of heart failure from fluid overload.

Selected Nursing Diagnoses with Interventions

Excess Fluid Volume

- Restrict fluid intake as instructed, typically to less than 800 mL per day. Provide ice chips (if allowed, as part of the fluid allowance), hard candy, and/or lemon-glycerin swabs to relieve mouth dryness. Provide frequent mouth care.

- Carefully monitor intake and output and report any abnormalities.

- Weigh daily at the same time of day and in the same clothes; report any weight gain.

- Administer diuretics and other medications as prescribed.

Risk for Injury

- Monitor neurological status, including level of consciousness, and motor and sensory functions. Institute seizure precautions, providing interventions for patient safety (such as padding bed rails, keeping bed in low position). In the event of a seizure, provide interventions to maintain a patent airway.

Community-Based Care

- Explain the disease process, treatment, medication regimen, and prognosis.

- Show how to recognize signs of recurrence and how to cope with seizure activity. Stress the importance of maintaining a safe home environment.

- Explain how to maintain prescribed fluid restrictions, and explain the rationale to increase compliance.

- Emphasize the importance of weighing the patient daily at the same time of day and in the same clothing, and of reporting any weight gain to the physician.

- Tell the patient to avoid nonsteroidal anti-inflammatory drugs and aspirin, which may contribute to hyponatremia.

For more information on syndrome of inappropriate antidiuretic hormone secretion, see Chapter 19 in *Medical-Surgical Nursing, Fifth Edition,* by LeMone, Burke, and Bauldoff.

S

SYPHILIS

Overview

- Syphilis is a sexually transmitted infection caused by the spirochete *Treponema pallidum,* which begins locally and causes a systemic infection.

- The incubation period averages about 3 weeks.

- Untreated syphilis develops in three stages:

  1. Primary lesion (chancre) occurs on genitalia.

  2. Secondary lesions form on skin and mucous membranes.

  3. Tertiary lesions form in the central nervous system; granulomatous lesions (gummas) form in blood vessels (especially the thoracic aorta), visceral organs, and skin.

- If not treated, syphilis can lead to blindness, paralysis, mental illness, cardiovascular damage, and death.

- Congenital syphilis is passed transplacentally to the embryo or fetus.

Cause

- Sexually or congenitally transmitted spirochete, *T. pallidum*

Manifestations

- Primary: chancre, a painless, raised, indurated papule with an ulcerated center on external genitalia, within the rectum, or on the cervix; spontaneously resolves; latency period follows

- Secondary syphilis:

  - Generalized skin rash: nonitchy; symmetric; macular/papular, possibly pustular; on face, scalp, trunk, palms, soles

  - Condyloma lata: broad, moist, white/gray lesions, surrounded by redness; found on mucous membranes or wet skin areas

  - Alopecia: scalp, eyebrows, beard

  - Lymphadenopathy

  - Headache, fever, malaise; sore throat, weight loss

- Tertiary syphilis:

  - Neurosyphilis: paresis, ataxia, meningeal syphilis, cranial neuropathies, incontinence, impotence, optic atrophy with blindness

S

- Cardiovascular syphilis: aortic vasculitis with medial necrosis; aneurysm formation, aortic regurgitation
- Gumma formation: multiple, diffuse or solitary inflammatory, granulomatous lesions of skin, skeletal system; mucosa of respiratory, gastrointestinal tracts or any visceral organ; locally destructive

Diagnostic Tests

- Venereal disease research laboratory serology test will be positive (false positives are possible).
- Rapid plasma reagin serology test will be positive.
- Fluorescent treponemal antibody-absorbed serum test will be positive.

Interdisciplinary Management

- The treatment of choice for syphilis is benzathine penicillin G, given intramuscularly. It is very effective in the early stages, less so in later stages.
- Tetracycline or doxycycline is used in penicillin-sensitive patients.

Selected Nursing Diagnoses with Interventions

Readiness for Enhanced Self-Health Management

- Encourage referral of all partners for evaluation and treatment.
- Instruct to abstain from sexual contact until patient and partner(s) are cured and to use condoms to prevent future infections.
- Emphasize the importance of returning for follow-up testing at 3- and 6-month intervals for early syphilis, and 6- and 12-month intervals for late latent syphilis.
- Provide information about the manifestations of reinfection.

Noncompliance

- Stress the importance of taking all prescribed medication.
- Emphasize that syphilis can be effectively treated, thus preventing the serious complications of late-stage disease.
- Teach the pregnant patient that taking medications as directed and returning each month for follow-up testing will help ensure the well-being of her baby.

Community-Based Care

- Discuss untreated syphilis as a chronic disease that can be spread to others even when no symptoms are present.
- Stress the importance of the following:
  - Referring sexual partners for evaluation and treatment
  - Abstaining from all sexual contact for a minimum of 1 month after treatment
  - Using a condom to avoid transmitting or contracting infections in the future
  - Returning for follow-up testing at 3- and 6-month intervals for early syphilis, and 6- and 12-month intervals for late latent syphilis
- Provide a referral to social services, a psychologic counselor, or a couples counselor as appropriate.

For more information on syphilis, see Chapter 50 in *Medical-Surgical Nursing,* Fifth Edition, by LeMone, Burke, and Bauldoff.

SYSTEMIC LUPUS ERYTHEMATOSUS

Overview

- Systemic lupus erythematosus (SLE) is a chronic inflammatory connective-tissue disease that affects multiple body systems.
- In SLE, a large variety of autoantibodies are produced against normal body components such as nucleic acids, erythrocytes, coagulation proteins, lymphocytes, and platelets.
- SLE autoantibodies react with their corresponding antigen to form immune complexes, which are then deposited in the connective tissue of blood vessels, lymphatic vessels, joints, kidneys, and other tissues. The deposits trigger an inflammatory response that damages local tissue.
- The manifestations of SLE vary considerably. In some patients, only one or two systems are affected, while in others, many systems are affected.
- The disease course is highly variable, ranging from mild and intermittent to rapidly fulminating; most patients have multiple exacerbations and remissions, spread over years.

Causes

- Etiology unknown; genetic, environmental, and hormonal factors play a role.
- Risk factors:
  - Female gender: 90% of cases, usually those in the reproductive years.
  - Race: more common in Blacks, Hispanics, and Asians than in Whites.
  - Family history of other connective tissue disorders.
  - Environmental factors: viruses, bacterial antigens, chemicals, drugs, or ultraviolet light may play a role in activating pathologic mechanisms of the disease.

Manifestations

- General: fever, malaise, fatigue, anorexia, weight loss
- Dermatologic: "butterfly" rash, a fixed, red, macular or papular rash over malar surface is classic; may be generalized, or may also occur in areas of sun exposure (photosensitive), usually seen during an exacerbation; alopecia accompanies
- Musculoskeletal: arthralgia, symmetric joint swelling, synovitis, myalgia
- Hematologic: anemia (pallor, fatigue, shortness of breath, tachycardia), thrombocytopenia (abnormal bleeding, ecchymosis, petechiae)
- Neurologic: headache, changes in cognition and/or mood, personality changes, cranial neuropathy, retinal vasculitis, blindness, ataxia, seizures, stroke
- Endocrinologic: Syndrome of inappropriate antidiuretic hormone secretion
- Vascular: vasculitis, thrombosis
- Cardiac: pericarditis with effusion or tamponade, dysrhythmias; myocardial infarction, sudden cardiac arrest, heart failure
- Pulmonary: pneumonitis; pleuritis with effusion; pulmonary hypertension; acute respiratory distress syndrome
- Renal: glomerulonephritis, with manifestations of renal insufficiency/failure such as proteinuria, polyuria, nocturia, hypertension, azotemia, oliguria

- Gastrointestinal: nausea, vomiting, diarrhea, cramping, obstruction, perforation

Diagnostic Tests

- ANA testing is positive in more than 95% of patients with SLE.
- Anti-DNA antibody testing reveals these antibodies, rarely found in other disorders, in SLE.
- Eosinophil sedimentation rate is typically elevated.
- Serum complement levels are usually decreased.
- Complete blood count abnormalities include moderate to severe anemia, leukopenia and lymphocytopenia, and possible thrombocytopenia.
- Urinalysis shows mild proteinuria, hematuria, and blood cell casts when the kidneys are involved.
- Serum creatinine, eGFR, and BUN may be done to evaluate for renal disease.
- Kidney biopsy assesses the severity of renal lesions.

Interdisciplinary Management

- Aspirin and other nonsteroidal anti-inflammatory drugs can manage mild arthralgia, fatigue, fever, and arthritis. Skin and arthritis manifestations may be treated with antimalarial drugs. Severe SLE requires corticosteroid therapy. Immunosuppressive agents also may be employed.
- Patients with SLE who progress to end-stage renal disease are treated with dialysis and kidney transplantation.

Selected Nursing Diagnoses with Interventions

Impaired Skin Integrity

- Assess knowledge of the disease and its possible effects.
- Discuss the relationship between sun exposure and disease activity, both dermatologic and systemic. Help identify strategies to limit sun exposure.
- Keep the skin clean and dry. Apply therapeutic creams or ointments to lesions as prescribed.

Ineffective Protection (for the hospitalized patient)

- Wash hands on entering the room and before providing care.

- Use strict aseptic technique in caring for intravenous lines and indwelling catheters or performing any wound care.

- Assess for manifestations of infection. Monitor vital signs every 4 hours. Assess for signs of cellulitis, including tenderness, redness, swelling, and warmth. Report signs of infection to physician promptly.

- Monitor laboratory values, including complete blood count and tests of organ function.

- Initiate protective isolation procedures as indicated by the immune status.

- Instruct visitors to avoid contact with the patient when they are ill.

- Help ensure an adequate nutrient intake, offering supplementary feedings as indicated or maintaining parenteral nutrition if necessary.

- Teach the importance of good hand hygiene after using the bathroom and before eating.

- Provide good mouth care.

- Monitor for potential adverse effects of medications.

Community-Based Care

- Explain the disease and its potential effects. Promote an optimistic outlook, stressing that the majority of patients do not require long-term corticosteroid therapy and that the disease may improve over time.

- Teach the importance of skin care, including avoiding harsh chemicals and sun exposure.

- Review the importance of avoiding exposure to infection, and getting adequate rest and nutrition.

- Stress the importance of following the prescribed treatment plan, including medication regimen and follow-up appointments. Instruct to report the following to the physician: fever, chills, rash, increased fatigue and malaise, arthralgias, arthritis, urinary manifestations, chest pain, cough, or neurologic symptoms.

S

- Encourage to wear a MedicAlert tag and provide information on how to obtain one.

- Discuss family planning with the patient and spouse as appropriate. Oral contraceptive use may be contraindicated. The pregnant patient requires close monitoring for acute episodes.

- A referral to national and community agencies for support and education is important.

For more information on systemic lupus erythematosus, see Chapter 40 in *Medical-Surgical Nursing,* Fifth Edition, by LeMone, Burke, and Bauldoff.

S

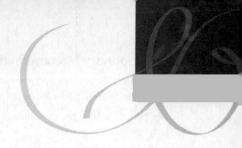

TESTICULAR CANCER

Overview

- Testicular cancer is a primary malignant tumor of the testis, usually of germ cells (sperm cell precursors).

- Local spread to the epididymis or spermatic cord is inhibited by the outer covering of the testicles; distant disease (spread by lymphatic and vascular channels) often is present before large masses develop in the scrotum.

- Testicular cancer usually affects only one testicle.

- Testicular cancer is the most common cancer in men between the ages of 15 and 40; the cure rate is nearly 100% for men with early-stage disease.

Causes

- Risk factors: cryptorchidism, age 15 to 40, European ancestry, family history, cancer of the other testicle

Manifestations

- Palpable mass in testis
- Swollen testis
- Pain and/or pulling sensation, may be sporadic

Diagnostic Tests

- Biopsy will identify and classify malignancy.
- Serum levels of human chorionic gonadotropin and alpha-fetoprotein typically are elevated.

Interdisciplinary Management

- Radical orchiectomy is the definitive treatment used in all forms and stages of testicular cancer.

- The patient with advanced disease may receive platinum-based combination chemotherapy.

- Radiation therapy may be used to treat metastasis in retroperitoneal lymph nodes.

Selected Nursing Diagnoses with Interventions

Deficient Knowledge: Postoperative Care

- Provide both verbal and written instructions for pain control, wound care, and signs of complications, as most patients are discharged within 24 hours of the procedure.

- Prepare the patient for an extensive surgical procedure when retroperitoneal lymph node dissection is to be performed.

- Assess frequently for complications of surgery, including vital signs and wound care.

Ineffective Sexuality Patterns

- Assess the patient's prediagnosis sexual functioning.

- Clarify possible effects of treatment on sexual functioning.

- Discuss the possibility of preserving sperm in a sperm bank. If the patient has chemotherapy and retroperitoneal surgery, the chance of preserving reproductive function is remote.

- Help the patient to cope with feelings about possible changes in sexual function. Use active listening skills and recommend male support groups and couples counseling.

Community-Based Care

- Explain the disease process, treatment options, and prognosis.

- Explain methods to control pain. In addition to analgesics, ice bags may be applied to the scrotum. A scrotal support provides relief, especially when the patient ambulates.

- Teach the signs of complications. If the incision gapes open, or if there is bleeding beyond slight oozing after 24 hours, the patient should call the physician. Scrotal edema, which may be caused by bleeding from the stump of the spermatic cord, also requires prompt intervention.

- Review the effects of treatment on sexuality. A radical orchiectomy alone should have no lasting effects on sexual or reproductive function. Chemotherapy and retroperitoneal surgery significantly reduce the chance of preserving reproductive function. Include the patient's sexual partner as appropriate in discussions of sexual and reproductive function.

- Explain the importance of surveillance with periodic physical examinations, chest x-rays, tumor marker tests, and computed tomography scans. Stress the importance of monthly testicular self-examination on remaining testis.

- Provide the names and addresses of local cancer support groups. Refer the patient to the American Cancer Society for information and support services.

- A referral for psychologic or sexual therapy may be important.

For more information on testicular cancer, see Chapter 48 in *Medical-Surgical Nursing,* Fifth Edition, by LeMone, Burke, and Bauldoff.

TETANUS

Overview

- Tetanus (commonly called *lockjaw*) is a disorder caused by a toxin secreted from the anaerobic bacteria, *Clostridium tetani,* which lives in soil. Spores enter the body through open wounds contaminated with dirt, street dust, or feces.

- Following an incubation period of 5 days to 15 weeks (average 8 to 12 days), tetanospasmin toxin ascends nerves leading to the spinal cord and blocks neurons that inhibit muscle contraction. As a result, even minor stimuli cause uncontrolled muscle spasms.

- Tetanus has a high mortality rate, with death occurring more commonly in older adults.

Causes

- Infection with the anaerobic bacteria, *Clostridium tetani.*

- Risk factors:
  - Contaminated wounds (particularly of the head and face) such as scratches or abrasions, bee stings; abortions, surgery, trauma, burns; or intravenous drug use.
  - Incidence is highest among people who have never been immunized, older adults whose immunity has been lost, and women.

Manifestations

- Pain at the site of the infection
- Stiffness of the jaw and neck and dysphagia
- Profuse perspiration and drooling from increased salivation
- Hyperreflexia, painful spasms of the jaw muscles (*trismus*) or facial muscles, and rigidity and painful spasms of the abdominal, neck, and back muscles
- Generalized tonic seizures (caused by even minor stimuli); opisthotonic position with the head retracted, back arched, and feet extended, during the seizures
- Possible respiratory arrest from spasms of the glottis and respiratory muscles

Diagnostic Tests

- There are no specific diagnostic tests for tetanus; diagnosis is based on manifestations.

Interdisciplinary Management

- Tetanus is completely preventable by active immunization with diphtheria-pertussis-tetanus series in children and tetanus toxoid series in adults; booster every 10 years or at the time of a major injury if the last booster dose was given more than 5 years previously.
- Passive immunization with tetanus immune globulin for major or contaminated wounds or uncertain immunization status.
- Medications for patients with tetanus include antibiotics to destroy the organism and chlorpromazine or diazepam to control muscle spasms and seizures. Anticoagulants may be given to

T

prevent venous thrombosis. Neuromuscular blocking agents may be used to treat severe spasms and seizures.

- Intensive care in an environment with minimal stimulation is required. Intubation and mechanical ventilation may be necessary to support respirations.

Selected Nursing Diagnoses with Interventions

Risk for Injury

- Place in a quiet, darkened room to decrease stimuli that cause muscle spasms and seizures.
- Provide only necessary physical care, and do so during periods of maximal sedation to decrease tactile stimulation that causes muscle spasms.

Ineffective Breathing Pattern

- Monitor respiratory and cardiovascular status and provide immediate interventions for respiratory or cardiovascular failure.
- Maintain oxygenation through mechanical ventilation and frequent suctioning of secretions.
- Maintain intravenous access for the administration of fluids and medications.
- Administer prescribed antibiotics, anticonvulsants, and sedatives.

Imbalanced Nutrition: Less than Body Requirements

- Provide adequate nutrition through prescribed nutritional support. Monitor fluid and electrolyte status. Ensure adequate fluid intake to maintain hydration and urinary output.
- Monitor urinary output, which should be maintained at 1.5 to 2 L per day.
- Monitor for the hazards of immobility, including constipation, pneumonia, deep venous thrombosis, and pressure ulcers.

Community-Based Care

- Review the disease process, treatments (including medication regimen), and prognosis.

- Promote immunizations for children and adults; emphasize the need for booster doses.

- Teach proper wound care: Thoroughly wash all wounds, no matter how small, with soap and water; flush out or remove all foreign material from the wound; keep wound clean while healing. Promptly seek medical care for large or contaminated wounds.

- Teach the patient with tetanus and significant others about safety measures, seizure precautions, and symptoms that require further medical attention.

- Explain how to take the prescribed antibiotic (e.g., either with food or on an empty stomach, the dosage and timing, and potential side effects).

- Monitor the wound site for signs and symptoms of infection.

- Review seizure precautions with the patient and significant others before discharge.

For more information on tetanus, see Chapter 43 in *Medical-Surgical Nursing,* Fifth Edition, by LeMone, Burke, and Bauldoff.

THROMBOANGIITIS OBLITERANS (BUERGER'S DISEASE)

Overview

- Thromboangiitis obliterans is an inflammatory, occlusive vascular disease that affects small and midsize peripheral arteries.

- Inflammation is accompanied by thrombus formation and vasospasms of arterial segments that impair blood flow.

- Affected vessels eventually become scarred and fibrotic.

- It may affect the upper or lower extremities, but often affects a leg or foot.

- Prolonged periods of tissue hypoxia increase the risk for tissue ulceration and gangrene.

Causes

The exact etiology is unknown. Risk factors are as follows:

- Male gender

- Cigarette smoking
- Asian or eastern European descent
- Presence of HLA-B5 and 2A9 antigens

Manifestations

- Intermittent claudication, cramping pain in calves and feet or the forearms and hands.
- Rest pain in the fingers and toes.
- Diminished sensation.
- Thin, shiny skin; thickened, malformed nails.
- Involved extremities are pale, cyanotic, or ruddy; cool or cold to touch.
- Diminished or absent peripheral pulses.
- Painful ulcers, gangrene.

Diagnostic Tests

- Doppler ultrasonography may show diminished peripheral perfusion.
- Arteriography or magnetic resonance imaging may be done to determine the extent of the disease.

Interdisciplinary Management

- Smoking cessation is the single most important treatment for thromboangiitis obliterans.
- Measures to prevent vasoconstriction (warmth, stress management, dependent positioning of affected extremities) and injury are recommended.
- Walking for 20 or more minutes several times a day is recommended.
- A calcium channel blocker or pentoxifylline (Trental) may be prescribed for symptom relief.
- Surgical approaches may include sympathectomy or arterial bypass graft. Amputation of an affected digit or extremity may be necessary if gangrene develops.

Selected Nursing Diagnoses with Interventions

Ineffective Tissue Perfusion: Peripheral

- Assess peripheral pulses, capillary refill, temperature, and color of extremities every shift or home or office visit; more often if changes occur.
- Emphasize the importance of smoking cessation.
- Assist to develop a plan for regular physical exercise.

Acute/Chronic Pain

- Assess pain every shift or home or office visit.
- Position with affected extremities dependent; frequently change positions. Encourage activity to tolerance.
- Provide time for the patient to discuss issues related to pain.

Impaired Physical Mobility

- Explain the physiologic basis for balanced rest and exercise.
- During acute exacerbations of the disease, provide diversional activities to combat boredom associated with bed rest.

Risk for Injury

- Inspect extremities every shift, office, or home visit. Note and report changes in color, sensitivity, or skin continuity as appropriate.
- Teach the importance of meticulous foot care.

Community-Based Care

Include the following topics in patient and family teaching:

- The absolute necessity of smoking cessation.
- Foot care and protecting affected extremities from injury.
- The purpose, dose, desired and adverse effects, interactions, and any precautions associated with prescribed medications.
- Signs and symptoms to report to the physician.

- Discuss the importance of regular exercise as prescribed and complying with long-term medical follow-up care.

- Referral to home health services may be appropriate.

For more information on thromboangiitis obliterans, see Chapter 32 in *Medical-Surgical Nursing,* Fifth Edition, by LeMone, Burke, and Bauldoff.

THROMBOCYTOPENIA

Overview

- Thrombocytopenia is a platelet count of less than 100,000/µI.

- A platelet count of < 20,000/µL can lead to spontaneous bleeding and hemorrhage; potentially fatal bleeding occurs with a platelet count of < 10,000/µL.

- Bleeding usually occurs in small vessels; mucous membranes of the nose, mouth, gastrointestinal tract, and vagina often bleed.

- There are two types of primary thrombocytopenia: immune thrombocytopenic purpura (ITP) and thrombotic thrombocytopenic purpura (TTP).

- ITP is an autoimmune disorder in which antibodies to the platelet membrane are produced, leading to accelerated platelet destruction. The chronic form typically affects young adults; acute ITP is more common in children.

- TTP is a rare disorder of platelet aggregation and thrombosis in the microcirculation.

- Secondary thrombocytopenia develops due to either decreased platelet production or increased platelet destruction.

- Heparin-induced thrombocytopenia (HIT) occurs when (1) heparin reacts directly with platelets, causing them to agglutinate (clump) and be removed from circulation by phagocytosis; or (2) heparin forms an immune complex with a platelet protein, stimulating antibody production with subsequent platelet aggregation and thrombocytopenia.

T

Causes

- ITP: autoimmune; may follow acute viral illness

- Secondary thrombocytopenia: aplastic anemia, bone marrow malignancy, infection, radiation therapy, or drug therapy. Heparin therapy is the most common drug-induced thrombocytopenia.

Manifestations

- Petechiae and purpura (purple bruising) on anterior chest, arms, neck, and oral mucous membranes

- Epistaxis (nosebleed), bleeding gums

- Hematuria

- Excess menstrual bleeding

- Weight loss, fever, and headache

- Possible altered level of consciousness

Diagnostic Tests

- Complete blood count with platelet count reveals a decreased platelet count and possible hemolytic anemia.

- Antinuclear antibodies are used to assess for autoantibodies and identify possible contributing disorders such as systemic lupus erythematosus.

- Serologic studies to identify possible viral infection and when HIT is suspected.

- Bone marrow examination evaluates for aplastic anemia and megakaryocyte production.

Interdisciplinary Management

- Oral glucocorticoids or immunosuppressive drugs are prescribed to suppress the autoimmune response. Prompt withdrawal of heparin therapy reverses HIT.

- Platelet transfusions may be required to treat acute bleeding. Plasma exchange therapy may be done to remove autoantibodies, immune complexes, and toxins, and is the treatment of choice for TTP.

- Splenectomy is the treatment of choice for ITP if glucocorticoids are ineffective to maintain remission.

Selected Nursing Diagnoses with Interventions

Ineffective Protection

- Monitor vital signs, heart, and breath sounds every 4 hours.
- Frequently assess for bleeding: petechiae, ecchymoses, and hematomas; obvious or occult blood in emesis, urine, or stool; epistaxis, bleeding gums, or vaginal bleeding; prolonged bleeding from puncture sites; neurologic changes; evidence of intra-abdominal bleeding.
- Avoid rectal temperatures, urinary catheterization, and parenteral injections.
- Apply pressure to puncture sites for 3 to 5 minutes; apply pressure to arterial blood gas sites for 15 to 20 minutes.
- Instruct to avoid forcefully blowing or picking the nose, straining during defecation, and forceful coughing or sneezing.

Impaired Oral Mucous Membranes

- Frequently assess the mouth for bleeding, oral pain, or tenderness.
- Encourage use of soft-bristle toothbrush or sponge to clean teeth and gums.
- Instruct to rinse the mouth with saline every 2 to 4 hours. Apply petroleum jelly to lips as needed.
- Instruct to avoid alcohol-based mouthwashes, very hot foods, alcohol, and crusty foods. Teach to drink cool liquids at least every 2 hours.

Community-Based Care

Include the following topics in patient and family teaching:

- The nature of the disorder, its usual course, and the treatment plan.
- Use, desired effects, and potential adverse effects of prescribed medications.

- Risks and benefits of surgery or treatments such as plasma replacement therapy.
- The importance of follow-up tests and visits for care.
- Measures to reduce the risk of bleeding: safety measures such as a soft-bristle toothbrush, electric razor, avoidance of contact sports and hazardous activities, and avoiding medications that further interfere with platelet function.
- Emphasize the need for long-term follow-up care with the hematologist for continued management.
- Refer for home health or other community services as indicated.

For more information on thrombocytopenia, see Chapter 33 in *Medical-Surgical Nursing,* Fifth Edition, by LeMone, Burke, and Bauldoff.

TONSILLITIS

Overview

- Tonsillitis is acute inflammation of the palatine tonsils.
- It usually is due to streptococcal infection, but may be viral.
- Both bacterial and viral tonsillitis are communicable by droplet nuclei. Symptoms usually resolve within 3 to 10 days after onset.
- Peritonsillar abscess (quinsy) is a potential complication of tonsillitis.

Causes

- *Streptococcus* bacteria, often beta-hemolytic
- Other bacterial or viral infections

Manifestations

- Sore throat, difficulty swallowing
- General malaise
- Fever

- Otalgia (pain referred to the ear)
- Tonsils bright red and edematous, with white exudate
- Uvula may be reddened and swollen
- Tender cervical lymphadenopathy

Diagnostic Tests

- Throat swab may demonstrate streptococcus antigen or presence of the infecting bacteria on culture.
- The white blood cell count is usually normal or low in viral infections and elevated in bacterial infections.

Interdisciplinary Management

- Antipyretics and mild analgesics such as aspirin or acetaminophen provide symptomatic relief. Penicillin is the drug of choice for group A streptococci. Erythromycin, amoxicillin, or cefuroxime may be used.
- Peritonsillar abscess is drained by needle aspiration or by incision and drainage.
- Tonsillectomy is indicated for recurrent or chronic infections, hypertrophy of the tonsils with risk of airway obstruction, peritonsillar abscess, repeated attacks of purulent otitis media, and tonsil malignancy. Bleeding is the most significant postoperative complication of tonsillectomy.

Selected Nursing Diagnoses with Interventions

Health-Seeking Behaviors

- Encourage all patients with persistent sore throat, fever, lymphadenopathy, and myalgias to seek evaluation and treatment.
- Home care is appropriate for acute uncomplicated tonsillitis.

Acute Pain

- Encourage rest and mild analgesics for symptom relief.
- Instruct to consume a liquid or soft diet with increased fluid intake.

- Advise that warm saline gargles, moist inhalations, and application of an ice collar may help relieve throat pain.

Risk for Ineffective Airway Clearance

- Following tonsillectomy, place in semi-Fowler's position with the head turned to the side.

- Keep oral or nasopharyngeal airway in place until the gag and swallowing reflexes have returned.

- Apply an ice collar to reduce swelling and pain.

- Observe for spontaneous swallowing as a possible indication of bleeding; assess the oropharynx for the presence of blood if noted.

- Notify the surgeon immediately if excessive bleeding or hemorrhage occurs.

- Assist with warm saline mouthwashes to remove thick oral secretions following tonsillectomy.

Community-Based Care

Discuss the following topics when preparing the patient for home care:

- The importance of completing the full 10 days of antibiotic therapy if prescribed

- Using warm saline gargles or throat lozenges for symptomatic relief

- Manifestations of possible complications of streptococcal infection such as glomerulonephritis or rheumatic fever

- Monitoring temperature in the morning and evening until well to ensure that the infection has not spread to deeper tissues

- Proper use and disposal of tissues and frequent hand hygiene to prevent spreading the infection to others

Following peritonsillar abscess drainage or tonsillectomy, provide the following instructions:

- Postoperative mouth and throat care

- No aspirin for 2 weeks to reduce the risk of postoperative bleeding

- Manifestations of bleeding to report to the physician (delayed hemorrhage may occur for up to 1 week postsurgery)

For more information on tonsillitis, see Chapter 35 in *Medical-Surgical Nursing,* Fifth Edition, by LeMone, Burke, and Bauldoff.

TRIGEMINAL NEURALGIA

Overview

- Trigeminal neuralgia (also called tic douloureux) is a mononeuropathy of one or more of the three branches of the trigeminal nerve. It causes severe facial pain.

- Trigeminal neuralgia occurs in attacks of excruciating pain, usually following the maxillary and mandibular branches of the nerve; sometimes the ophthalmic branch is affected.

- Attacks are generally of short duration (a few seconds to a few minutes) but are extremely intense, producing a facial tic.

- Attacks occur sporadically, and may be initiated when "trigger zones" on the face, such as lips, cheeks, chin, or tongue, are stimulated, as by washing the face or brushing the teeth.

Causes

- The actual cause of trigeminal neuralgia is unknown, but generally follows vascular compression and demyelination of the trigeminal nerve.

- Contributing factors: trauma, dental or jaw infections, flulike illnesses, aneurysm, tumor, and multiple sclerosis.

Manifestations

- Brief, repetitive episodes of excruciating pain along the route of the nerve; appears in paroxysmal attacks; triggered by facial stimulation.

- Pain usually unilateral; often begins near one side of the mouth and rises toward the ear, eye, or nostril on the same side.

- Pain episodes may recur for several weeks or months, followed by spontaneous remission.

- Shorter periods of remission with aging; may have a dull ache between episodes of acute pain.

Diagnostic Tests

- There are no specific diagnostic tests; x-rays and computed tomography scan may be done to rule out other causes.

Interdisciplinary Management

- Medications used to control the pain include the anticonvulsants carbamazepine (Tegretol), phenytoin (Dilantin), or gabapentin (Neurontin). Baclofen, a skeletal muscle relaxant, also may be used.

- Surgery may be performed when drug therapy is ineffective. Percutaneous rhizotomy destroys part of the trigeminal nerve. When a blood vessel compresses the nerve, decompression and separation of a blood vessel from the nerve root produces lasting relief of the pain.

Selected Nursing Diagnoses with Interventions

Acute Pain

- Identify factors that trigger an attack and discuss strategies to avoid precipitating factors.

- Determine usual response to pain.

- Assess factors that affect the patient's ability to tolerate pain, including knowledge of the cause of the pain and pain management options, cultural factors, and support system.

- Monitor the effects of the medication prescribed for the neuralgia.

Risk for Imbalanced Nutrition: Less than Body Requirements

- Monitor dietary intake and weight loss at each visit, and ask the patient to keep a record of weekly weight.

- Discuss the effect of food temperature and consistency on pain.

- Suggest chewing on the unaffected side of the mouth.

- If the patient is unable to tolerate oral food, enteral feedings may be necessary.

Community-Based Care

- Explain the disease process, medications, and methods of reducing the incidence of attacks.

- Teach proper eye, face, and mouth care for patients treated with surgery:

  - Do not rub eyes. Use artificial tears if the eyes are dry or irritated.

  - Wear an eyepatch at night, and sunglasses or goggles when outside or working in areas where dust or other eye irritants may be present.

  - Remember to blink frequently.

  - Check the eyes for redness or swelling each day.

  - Schedule regular eye examinations.

  - Chew on unaffected side of mouth.

  - Avoid eating hot foods or drinking hot liquids.

  - Brush the teeth and inspect the mouth for food that may collect between the gums and cheek after each meal.

  - Have regular dental examinations.

  - Use an electric razor to shave.

  - Protect the face from cold and wind.

- Following surgery, referral to a physical therapist may be appropriate.

For more information on trigeminal neuralgia, see Chapter 44 in *Medical-Surgical Nursing,* Fifth Edition, by LeMone, Burke, and Bauldoff.

TUBERCULOSIS

Overview

- Tuberculosis (TB) is a chronic, infectious disease caused by *Mycobacterium tuberculosis.*

- *M. tuberculosis* is an aerobic, acid-fast bacillus that spreads through inhalation of droplet nuclei, implanting in an upper lobe.

- A local inflammatory response isolates the bacilli, preventing their spread. *M. tuberculosis* multiplies slowly; bacilli entering the lymphatic system stimulate cellular immune responses. A tubercle forms, encasing the bacilli. If the immune response is effective, the disease does not develop.

- In *primary tuberculosis,* granulomatous tissue erodes a bronchus or blood vessel, allowing the disease to spread throughout the lung or other organs.

- *Reactivation tuberculosis* occurs when the immune system is suppressed and tubercles rupture, spreading bacilli into the airways to form satellite lesions and produce TB pneumonia.

- When primary disease or reactivation allows live bacilli to enter the bronchi, the disease may spread through the blood and lymph system to other organs. Types of extrapulmonary TB are as follows:

  1. Miliary TB results from hematogenous spread of the bacilli throughout the body.

  2. Genitourinary TB can destroy portions of the kidney and cause scarring and strictures of the ureters and bladder. The prostate, seminal vesicles, epididymis, fallopian tubes, and ovaries also may be involved.

  3. TB meningitis, with potentially permanent neurologic effects, results from infection of the subarachnoid space.

  4. Skeletal TB, affecting the vertebrae, ends of long bones, and joints, usually affects children. The hips and knees are most often affected by tuberculous arthritis.

- In the United States, Asians and Pacific Islanders have the highest rates of TB; Blacks, Hispanics, and Native Americans are affected more frequently than Whites. People with altered immune function (older adults, homeless people, and people with human immunodeficiency virus) are at particular risk for TB.

- Some strains of *M. tuberculosis* have become resistant to drugs used to treat the disease.

Cause

- Infection with *M. tuberculosis*

Manifestations

Primary Infection

- Usually asymptomatic; subsides spontaneously
- Positive response to injection of purified protein derivative (PPD)

Primary Progressive Tuberculosis or Reactivation Tuberculosis

- Weight loss, anorexia
- Fatigue
- Low-grade afternoon fever, night sweats
- Cough that is dry initially and later becomes productive of purulent and/or blood-tinged sputum
- Fever, night sweats

Diagnostic Tests

- Positive tuberculin test (PPD); the induration surrounding the injection site determines infection. A positive response indicates infection and a cellular (T-cell) response; it does not necessarily indicate active disease or infectiousness.
- Sputum smear is positive for acid-fast bacilli.
- Sputum culture is positive for *M. tuberculosis*.
- Polymerase chain reaction detects DNA from *M. tuberculosis*.
- Chest x-ray shows dense lesions in the apical and posterior segments of the upper lobe and possible cavity formation in pulmonary TB.

Interdisciplinary Management

- Combination chemotherapy with two, three, or four antituberculosis drugs is used to prevent and treat TB.

Selected Nursing Diagnoses with Interventions

Risk for Infection

- Place in a private room with negative airflow that prevents room air from circulating into the hallway or other rooms. Multiple fresh-air exchanges dilute the concentration of droplet nuclei within the room.

- Use standard precautions and TB isolation techniques as recommended by the Centers for Disease Control and Prevention.

- Use personal protective devices to reduce the risk of transmission during care. Occupational Safety and Health Administration requires use of a HEPA-filtered respirator.

- Inform the patient of the reasons for and importance of respiratory isolation procedures during hospitalization. For patients treated in the community, teach to avoid crowds and close physical contact, and maintain good ventilation in living facilities, particularly during the first 3 weeks of treatment.

- Place a mask on the patient when transporting to other parts of the facility.

- Inform all personnel having contact with the patient of the diagnosis.

- Assist visitors to mask before entering the room.

Ineffective Therapeutic Regimen Management

- Assess self-care abilities and support systems.

- Assess level of knowledge and understanding of the disease, its complications, its treatment, and risks to others. Provide additional teaching and reinforcement as indicated.

- Assist the patient to identify barriers or obstacles to managing the prescribed treatment.

- Help develop a plan for managing the prescribed regimen.

- Provide verbal and written instructions that are at the patient's level of knowledge, literacy, and understanding.

Community-Based Care

- Teach about the disease process, treatment, respiratory isolation and its purpose, and the medication regimen.

- Emphasize the importance of eating a nutritious diet, balancing exercise with rest, and avoiding crowds and people with respiratory infections.

- Stress the importance of avoiding alcohol and other substances that damage the liver while taking antituberculosis drugs.

- Encourage fluid intake of 2.5 to 3 quarts of fluid per day.

- Teach measures to limit the transmission of TB:

  1. Always cough and expectorate into tissues.

  2. Dispose of tissues personally in a closed bag.

  3. If unable to control respiratory secretions, as when sneezing, wear a mask.

- Teach how to collect sputum specimens.

- Stress the importance of complying with prescribed treatment for the entire course of the regimen.

- Instruct to report to the physician chest pain, hemoptysis, or dyspnea; anorexia, nausea, or vomiting; yellow tint to skin or sclera; sudden weight gain, swollen feet, ankles, legs, or hands; hearing loss, tinnitus, or vertigo; and change in vision or difficulty discriminating colors.

- Refer as appropriate to smoking cessation programs, alcohol and drug treatment groups or facilities, and hospice or residential care facilities.

- Provide active intervention for homeless people, including shelter placement or other housing, and ongoing follow-up by easily accessed healthcare providers.

- Refer patients who are unlikely to comply with the treatment regimen to the public health department for supervised medication administration and follow-up care.

For more information on tuberculosis, see Chapter 36 in *Medical-Surgical Nursing,* Fifth Edition, by LeMone, Burke, and Bauldoff.

T

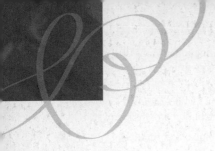

ULCERATIVE COLITIS

Overview

- Ulcerative colitis is a chronic inflammatory bowel disease that affects the mucosa and submucosa of the colon and rectum.

- Chronic intermittent colitis is the most common form; it has an insidious onset with recurrent attacks that last 1 to 3 months occurring at intervals of months to years.

- The inflammatory process begins in the anal canal and progresses proximally. It usually is confined to the rectum and sigmoid colon but may involve the entire colon.

- The inflammatory process affects the mucosa and submucosa of the bowel in a continuous pattern, leading to necrosis and sloughing of bowel mucosa.

- Chronic inflammation causes atrophy, narrowing, and shortening of the colon, with loss of its normal haustra.

- The peak incidence of inflammatory bowel disease is in young adults between the ages of 15 and 35 years. A second peak occurs between the ages of 60 and 80.

- Ulcerative colitis significantly increases the risk for colorectal cancer.

- Acute complications of ulcerative colitis include hemorrhage, toxic megacolon (acute motor paralysis and dilation of the colon), and perforation.

U

Causes

- The etiology of ulcerative colitis is unknown.

- Heredity, infectious agents, autoimmunity, environment, and lifestyle factors such as smoking contribute to its development.

Manifestations

Mild Disease

- Diarrhea: fewer than four stools per day
- Abdominal pain, cramping, and urgency
- Intermittent rectal bleeding and mucus

Severe Disease

- GI: diarrhea—more than 6 to 10 bloody stools per day; fecal urgency, tenesmus, anemia, malnutrition, lower left quadrant cramping relieved by defecation, hypovolemia
- Skeletal/muscular: possible arthritis of one or more joints, skin and mucous membrane lesions, uveitis
- General: fatigue, anorexia, weakness, increased risk for gallstones, cirrhosis, kidney stones, and ureteral obstruction

Diagnostic Tests

- Sigmoidoscopy or colonoscopy shows edema, inflammation, mucus and pus, mucosal ulcers or abscesses, and a continuous pattern of involvement.
- Barium enema demonstrates ulcerations, shortening and loss of colon haustra, and possible complications such as toxic megacolon.
- Stool examination shows blood and mucus.
- Serum albumin may be decreased due to protein loss and chronic inflammation.

Interdisciplinary Management

- Locally acting and systemic anti-inflammatory drugs are the primary medications used to manage ulcerative colitis. Balsalazide and olsalazine are especially useful to treat ulcerative colitis. Mesalamine (Canasa, Rowasa) is orally or rectally administered drug that provides topical anti-inflammatory action in the colon of patients with ulcerative colitis.
- Corticosteroids may be administered rectally or intravenously to treat acute exacerbations; oral preparations are used for less severe manifestations and long-term therapy.
- Immunosuppressive agents such as mercaptopurine azathioprine, methotrexate, and cyclosporine can be used to treat patients who have not responded to other treatments.

- Antidiarrheal agents may be given with caution during chronic manifestations to slow gastrointestinal motility and reduce diarrhea, but not during an acute attack.

- Dietary management may restrict milk products, caffeine, and raw fruits and vegetables. Bulk-forming agents may be prescribed.

- Surgical removal of the colon cures the disease, and may be recommended when the disease resists more conservative treatment or when the risk for colon cancer is significant.

Selected Nursing Diagnoses with Interventions

Diarrhea

- Monitor the character and frequency of bowel movements using a stool chart.

- Observe and test stools for the presence of obvious or occult blood.

- Maintain accurate fluid intake and output records; weigh daily.

- Assess and document vital signs every 4 hours.

- Assess for orthostatic hypotension to identify possible fluid volume deficit.

- Assess for manifestations of fluid deficit: warm, dry skin; poor skin turgor; dry, shiny mucous membranes; weakness, lethargy; complaints of thirst.

- Administer anti-inflammatory and antidiarrheal medications as prescribed.

- Maintain fluid intake by mouth or parenterally as indicated.

- Assess the perianal area for irritation or denuded skin from the diarrhea. Protect perianal skin, using gentle cleansing and a zinc oxide-based cream.

Disturbed Body Image

U

- Accept the patient's feelings and perception of self.

- Encourage discussion of physical changes and their consequences on the patient's self-concept and close personal relationships.

- Encourage the patient to make choices and decisions regarding care.

- Discuss possible effects of treatment options openly and honestly.

- Involve the patient in care, providing teaching and instruction as needed.

- Arrange for interaction with other patients or groups of persons with ulcerative colitis or ostomies.

- Teach coping strategies (odor control, dietary modifications, and so on), and support their use.

Community-Based Care

Teach the patient and family about the following topics:

- The nature of the disease, its short- and long-term effects, the relationship of stress to disease exacerbations, and manifestations of complications.

- Prescribed medications, including drug names, desired effects, schedules for tapering the doses if ordered, and possible adverse reactions and their management.

- The recommended diet and the rationale for any specific restrictions.

- Use of nutritional supplements such as Ensure to maintain weight and nutritional status.

- The importance of maintaining a fluid intake of at least 2 to 3 quarts per day, increasing fluid intake during warm weather, exercise or strenuous work, and when fever is present.

- The increased risk for colorectal cancer and importance of regular bowel exams.

- Risks and benefits of various treatment options.

If surgery is planned or has been done, include the following topics:

- Ostomy care as indicated.

- Where to obtain ostomy supplies.

- Use of nonprescription drugs, such as enteric-coated and timed-release capsules that may not be adequately absorbed before elimination through the ileostomy.

- Community and national ostomy support groups.

- Provide referrals to a dietary consultant or nutritionist, a community healthcare agency, home care services, and home intravenous care services as indicated.

For more information on ulcerative colitis, see Chapter 24 in *Medical-Surgical Nursing,* Fifth Edition, by LeMone, Burke, and Bauldoff.

URINARY TRACT INFECTION

Overview

- Urinary tract infection (UTI) may affect either the lower or upper urinary tract. The infection may involve superficial tissues (e.g., bladder mucosa) or may invade other tissues such as prostate or renal tissues.

- UTIs also are classified as community-acquired or nosocomial, associated with catheterization.

- Pathogens usually ascend into the urinary tract from the mucous membranes of the perineal area.

- Cystitis, inflammation of the urinary bladder, is the most common UTI. The infection tends to remain superficial, involving the bladder mucosa.

- Catheter-associated UTI is common, affecting 10% to 15% of hospitalized patients with indwelling urinary catheters.

- Acute pyelonephritis is a bacterial infection of the kidney. It usually results from an ascending infection from the lower urinary tract.

Causes

- Bacteria that have colonized the urethra, vagina, or perineal tissues, including *E. coli, Proteus, Pseudomonas, Klebsiella,* and others

- Risk factors: female gender; aging; sexual intercourse; use of a diaphragm for birth control; pregnancy; prostatic hypertrophy; obstruction or structural abnormalities; chronic diseases such as diabetes mellitus; instrumentation

Manifestations

- UTI may be asymptomatic.

Cystitis

- Dysuria, urgency

- Frequency, nocturia

- Hematuria, pyuria (cloudy, foul-smelling urine)

- Suprapubic discomfort

Pyelonephritis

- Manifestations of cystitis

- Acute: rapid onset with chills, fever, malaise, vomiting, flank pain/costovertebral angle tenderness
- Chronic: can be asymptomatic or similar to mild manifestations of cystitis; hypertension may result

General Manifestations
- Fever, chills
- Malaise, anorexia
- Possible nausea, vomiting

Diagnostic Tests
- Urinalysis reveals the presence of bacteria, white blood cells, pus, and cell casts.
- Culture and sensitivity establishes the causative organism and effective antibiotic for treatment.
- White blood cell count may be elevated.
- Intravenous pyelogram to evaluate for structural or functional abnormalities.
- Cystoscopy to diagnose prostatic hypertrophy, urethral strictures, bladder calculi, tumors, polyps or diverticula, and congenital abnormalities.

Interdisciplinary Management
- Uncomplicated cystitis usually is treated with a short, 3-day course of antibiotic therapy with follow-up cultures to verify cure.
- A 10- to 14-day course of antibiotics is prescribed for pyelonephritis or recurrent UTI.
- Surgery may be indicated for the presence of calculi, structural anomalies, or strictures that contribute to the risk of infection.

Selected Nursing Diagnoses with Interventions

Acute Pain
- Assess pain: timing, quality, intensity, location, duration, and aggravating and alleviating factors.
- Be alert for manifestations of UTI such as incontinence or cloudy or malodorous urine in the older adult.
- Teach or provide comfort measures, such as warm sitz baths, warm packs or heating pads, and balanced rest and activity.

U

Systemic analgesics, urinary analgesics, or antispasmodic medication may be used as ordered.

- Increase fluid intake unless contraindicated.

Impaired Urinary Elimination

- Monitor (or instruct the patient to monitor) color, clarity, and odor of urine.

- Provide for easy access to a bedpan, urinal, commode, or bathroom. Make sure that lighting is adequate and that pathways are free of obstacles.

- Instruct to avoid caffeinated drinks, including coffee, tea, and cola; citrus juices; drinks containing artificial sweeteners; and alcoholic beverages.

- Use strict aseptic technique and a closed urinary drainage system when inserting a straight or indwelling urinary catheter.

- When possible, use intermittent straight catheterization to relieve urinary retention. Remove indwelling urinary catheters as soon as possible.

- Maintain the closed urinary drainage system, and use aseptic technique when emptying catheter drainage bag. Maintain gravity flow, preventing reflux of urine into the bladder from the drainage system.

- Provide perineal care on a regular basis and following defecation. Use antiseptic preparations only as ordered.

Readiness for Enhanced Self Health Maintenance

- Teach how to obtain a midstream clean-catch urine specimen.

- Assess knowledge about the disease process, risk factors, and preventive measures.

- Discuss the prescribed treatment plan and the importance of taking all prescribed antibiotics.

- Help develop a plan for taking medications, such as taking them with meals (unless contraindicated) or setting out all doses for the day in the morning.

- Instruct to keep appointments for follow-up and urine culture.

- Teach measures to prevent future UTI.

   1. Empty the bladder at least every 2 to 4 hours while awake. Avoid voluntary urinary retention.

2. Maintain intake of 2 to 2.5 quarts, or 8 to 10 glasses, of fluid per day.

3. For women: cleanse perineal area front to back after voiding and defecating; void before and after sexual intercourse; avoid bubble baths, feminine hygiene sprays, and douches; wear cotton (not nylon) undergarments.

4. Unless contraindicated, teach measures to maintain acidic urine; for example, drink two glasses of cranberry juice per day; take ascorbic acid (vitamin C); avoid excess intake of milk and milk products, other fruit juices, and sodium bicarbonate (baking soda).

Community-Based Care

- Teach about the disease process, causes, treatment, and prevention strategies. Patients should be able to identify the early manifestations of UTI and state the importance of seeking medical intervention promptly.

- Discuss the role of good general health and stress management in preventing infection.

- Stress the importance of completing all of the prescribed antibiotic regimen.

- Advise to refrain from sexual intercourse until infection and inflammation have cleared.

- Instruct to return for follow-up as recommended, usually 10 to 14 days after initial treatment, and to seek medical care for any signs of recurrence.

- Refer to a urologist or urology clinic for recurrent UTI.

For more information on urinary tract infection, see Chapter 27 in *Medical-Surgical Nursing,* Fifth Edition, by LeMone, Burke, and Bauldoff.

UTERINE LEIOMYOMAS (FIBROIDS)

Overview

- Leiomyomas (fibroids) are benign tumors of the uterine smooth muscle (myometrium).

- Fibroid tumors are the most common of all female genital tract tumors (20%–25% of women over 35), are usually multiple, and can vary in size from tiny to very large.

- Most form in the body of the uterus; the tumors may be intramural, subserous, or submucous.

- The incidence of fibroids in Black women is three times higher than in White women.

- Fibroids are estrogen-dependent, increasing in size during pregnancy and regressing after menopause.

Cause

- Unknown but there is a strong association with estrogen stimulation.

Manifestations

- Menorrhagia, dysmenorrhea
- Pelvic pain
- Uterine enlargement on examination
- Urinary bladder compression: frequency, urgency, nocturia
- Bowel compression: constipation, obstruction
- Anemia: pallor, fatigue

Diagnostic Tests

- Complete blood count may show decreased hemoglobin, hematocrit.
- Pelvic ultrasound helps differentiate leiomyoma from endometriosis.
- Laparoscopy may be done to identify subserosal tumors.

Interdisciplinary Management

- Leuprolide acetate (Lupron) or fluocinolone (Synaral) may be used to decrease tumor size if surgery is not an option. Long term use of these medications is limited because of their side effects (hot flashes, vaginal dryness, and headaches) and significant risk of bone loss if treatment continues 6 months or more.

- Myomectomy, removal of the tumor only, is the surgical procedure of choice for young women who wish to retain reproductive capability. A hysterectomy may be done if tumors are large, and if bleeding or other problems continue in perimenopausal women.

- Uterine fibroid embolization may be done to cut off the fibroid's blood supply.

Selected Nursing Diagnoses with Interventions

Chronic Pain

- Provide information about pain management, including use of nonnarcotic analgesics, a heating pad, acupuncture, meditation, or other stress reduction techniques.

Fatigue

- Encourage iron-rich foods in the diet, such as lean meats; dark, leafy green vegetables; eggs; whole grain and enriched breads and cereals; dried fruits; legumes; shellfish; and molasses.
- Suggest extra periods of rest and relaxation to relieve the fatigue, particularly when symptoms are most acute.

Community-Based Care

- Review the disease process, treatment options, and prognosis.
- Suggest use of protective pads to absorb urine leakage, and reduction of caffeine intake to decrease urinary urgency and frequency.
- Explain the need for regular follow-up assessments to monitor tumor growth.
- Emphasize that fibroids are benign and that there often are alternatives to hysterectomy.
- If surgery is chosen, teaching emphasizes pain control techniques and appropriate preoperative and postoperative instruction.
- Recommend increased intake of fresh fruits and vegetables and other high-fiber foods.

For more information on uterine leiomyoma (fibroids), see Chapter 49 in *Medical-Surgical Nursing,* Fifth Edition, by LeMone, Burke, and Bauldoff.

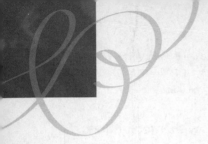

VAGINITIS

Overview

- Vaginitis is an inflammation of the vaginal mucosa.

- In younger patients, vaginitis is usually a sexually transmitted infection. The most common are bacterial vaginosis, candidiasis, and trichomonas.

- The low pH of vaginal secretions, normal vaginal flora, and estrogen provide protection against vaginal infections. Alterations in these factors are conducive to the development of vaginal infection.

- In older women, atrophic vaginitis results from estrogen withdrawal at menopause.

- Less commonly, vaginitis may be due to parasites (pediculosis pubis) or to a hypersensitivity to feminine hygiene products.

Causes

- Bacteria: *Escherichia coli, Staphylococcus, Streptococcus*
- Protozoa: *Trichomonas vaginalis*
- Fungi: *Candida albicans*
- Parasites: pediculus pubis
- Atrophic: lack of estrogen
- Hypersensitivity
- Risk factors: use of oral contraceptives or broad-spectrum antibiotics, obesity, diabetes, pregnancy, unprotected sexual intercourse, multiple sexual partners, and poor personal hygiene

Manifestations

- Burning, itching

V

- Edema
- Discharge (color and odor often specific to causative organism)

Diagnostic Tests
- Vaginal smear with microscopy can identify trichomoniasis and candidiasis.
- Culture and sensitivity can identify specific bacterial species.

Interdisciplinary Management
- Medical intervention is aimed at identifying the causative organism and prescribing a regimen of the appropriate antibiotic or antifungal agent.

Selected Nursing Diagnoses with Interventions

Acute Pain
- Suggest the use of cool compresses and sitz baths to alleviate discomfort and cleanse the perineal area.
- Recommend cotton underwear to reduce irritation and absorb secretions.

Disturbed Body Image
- Discuss sexual concerns openly and honestly.
- Assess for high-risk behaviors.

Community-Based Care (Include Partner as Appropriate)
- Explain how the infection is transmitted. Most vaginal infections are transmitted during sexual contact; the male partner often is asymptomatic.
- Emphasize the need for both to complete the full course of treatment and to abstain from sexual intercourse until treatment is completed. Incomplete treatment allows for recurrence of infection and reinfection of the partner.
- Discuss safer sex practices and improved genital hygiene techniques to reduce the risk of recurrence. Unless contraindicated, encourage the patient with repeated mild candidiasis infections

V

to consume daily 8 oz of yogurt containing live active cultures to help restore normal vaginal flora. Encourage the patient to avoid douches, feminine hygiene sprays, and perfumed powders in the genital area. Instruct to cleanse the perineum from front to back after urine and bowel elimination and to wear cotton underwear.

- Encourage postmenopausal women with atrophic vaginitis to talk to healthcare provider about the use of topical estrogen creams or hormone replacement therapy to restore vaginal tissue. Discuss use of water-soluble lubricants for comfort during sexual intercourse.

- Encourage follow-up visits for recurrence of symptoms.

- Stress the importance of regular Pap smears.

For more information on vaginitis, see Chapter 50 in *Medical-Surgical Nursing,* Fifth Edition, by LeMone, Burke, and Bauldoff.

VALVULAR HEART DISEASE

Mitral Stenosis

Mitral Insufficiency (Regurgitation)

Mitral Valve Prolapse

Aortic Stenosis

Aortic Insufficiency (Regurgitation)

Overview

- Valvular heart disease is characterized by alterations in the structure and function of heart valves.

- Normal valves direct blood flow within the heart. The atrioventricular valves (mitral on the left and tricuspid on the right) allow blood to flow from the atria into the ventricles during diastole but prevent retrograde (backward) flow during ventricular systole. The aortic (left) and pulmonic (right) valves permit blood to flow from the ventricles into the great vessels during ventricular systole, but prevent retrograde flow back into the ventricles during diastole.

- Two major types of valve defects are seen:

   1. A *stenotic valve* has a constricted opening and restricts forward blood flow, increasing pressures behind the defective valve.

V

2. An *insufficient (regurgitative) valve* does not close completely and allows retrograde blood flow.

- Valve disorders increase the cardiac workload and may impair the cardiac output.

- Compensatory cardiac mechanisms such as dilation and hypertrophy accommodate increased workloads, but may eventually lead to heart failure.

- The valves on the left side of the heart, which are subjected to high pressures, are more often affected. Mitral valve lesions are most common; aortic, second; tricuspid, third; pulmonic lesions, rare.

- More than one valve may be affected.

- Left-sided heart failure with decreased cardiac output, pulmonary hypertension, congestion, and possible edema are common consequences of severe mitral and aortic valve disorders.

- Right-sided heart failure with decreased cardiac output and peripheral vascular congestion and edema are possible consequences of severe tricuspid and pulmonic valve disorders.

Mitral Stenosis

- Mitral stenosis impairs flow from the left atrium to the left ventricle.

- Pressures in the left atrium increase, leading to dilation and hypertrophy. Eventually, pressure increases in the pulmonary system, leading to pulmonary congestion and pulmonary hypertension.

Mitral Insufficiency (Regurgitation)

- Mitral insufficiency allows retrograde blood flow from the left ventricle into the left atrium during ventricular systole.

- Pressures in the left atrium increase, leading to dilation and hypertrophy.

- The left ventricular workload increases, causing it to dilate and hypertrophy. Left-sided heart failure may result.

Mitral Valve Prolapse

- This congenital condition is characterized by increased compliance (floppiness) of valve leaflets.

- During ventricular systole, valve leaflets bulge backward into the left atrium, slightly increasing its volume.

Aortic Stenosis
- Aortic stenosis obstructs blood flow from the left ventricle to the aorta during systole.
- Left ventricular work increases, leading to dilation and hypertrophy.
- Cardiac output falls as a result of impaired flow into the aorta.

Aortic Insufficiency (Regurgitation)
- Aortic insufficiency allows blood to flow from the left ventricle to the aorta during systole. Impaired valve closure allows retrograde flow from the aorta back to the left ventricle during diastole.
- The volume and pressures in the left ventricle increase, leading to dilation and hypertrophy. The left atrium also may dilate and hypertrophy as higher pressures in the left ventricle impair diastolic blood flow.
- Left-sided heart failure may develop.

Causes
- Rheumatic heart disease
- Congenital anomaly
- Calcification
- Endocarditis
- Papillary muscle rupture
- Connective tissue disease: Marfan's syndrome
- Hypertension
- Syphilis

V

Manifestations

Mitral Stenosis
- Exertional dyspnea, fatigue
- Cough, hemoptysis

- Frequent respiratory infections
- Paroxysmal nocturnal dyspnea, orthopnea, weakness
- Palpitations
- Manifestations of right-sided heart failure: jugular vein distention, ascites, peripheral edema
- Murmur: loud S_1, opening snap, low-pitched, rumbling, crescendo-decrescendo systolic murmur heard best in apical region; possible palpable thrill
- Manifestations of atrial fibrillation: irregular pulse rate and magnitude

Mitral Insufficiency (Regurgitation)
- Often asymptomatic
- Fatigue, weakness, exertional dyspnea, orthopnea
- Manifestations of left-sided heart failure and pulmonary congestion; possible manifestations of right heart failure
- Murmur: loud, high-pitched (cooing or musical), rumbling, holosystolic heard best at apex; may be accompanied by palpable thrill

Mitral Valve Prolapse
- Usually asymptomatic
- Midsystolic ejection click; possible high-pitched late systolic murmur
- Atypical chest pain (fatigue related)
- Tachydysrhythmias with palpitations, lightheadedness, syncope
- Anxiety

Aortic Stenosis
- Possibly asymptomatic
- Dyspnea on exertion, angina, exertional syncope
- Narrowed pulse pressure (≤ 30 mmHg)
- Harsh systolic murmur heard best at right sternal border, second intercostal space; crescendo-decrescendo; may radiate to carotid arteries; possible palpable thrill

- Displacement of cardiac impulse to the left of the midclavicular line
- Manifestations of left- and possibly right-sided heart failure
- Risk for sudden cardiac death

Aortic Insufficiency (Regurgitation)

- Often asymptomatic
- Persistent palpitations, especially at rest
- Visible arterial pulse in neck; characteristic head bob with pulse (Musset's sign)
- Dizziness, exercise intolerance, angina
- Fatigue, exertional dyspnea, orthopnea, paroxysmal nocturnal dyspnea
- Blowing, high-pitched diastolic murmur heard best at left third intercostals space; palpable thrill and ventricular heave may accompany
- Apical impulse displaced to left
- Widened pulse pressure
- Water-hammer pulse with rapid upstroke and quickly collapsing downstroke to arterial pressure waveform

Diagnostic Tests

- Chest x-ray shows cardiac hypertrophy and possible pulmonary congestion, valvular calcifications.
- Electrocardiogram shows changes of atrial and ventricular hypertrophy and possible dysrhythmias.
- Echocardiogram shows thickened valve leaflets, valve and ventricular wall function, and heart chamber size.
- Cardiac catheterization allows assessment of contractility, pressure gradients, and chamber and pulmonary pressures.

Interdisciplinary Management

- Medications such as diuretics, vasodilators, anticoagulants, and cardiac glycosides are used to manage heart failure, maintain cardiac output, and prevent clot formation. Antibiotics are used to prevent infection prior to dental work and other invasive procedures.

- Percutaneous balloon valvuloplasty may be used to dilate stenotic heart valves. Surgery to repair or replace the diseased valve is the definitive treatment.

Selected Nursing Diagnoses with Interventions

Decreased Cardiac Output

- Monitor and record vital signs and hemodynamic parameters, reporting changes from the baseline or negative trends.
- Assess for manifestations of decreased cardiac output: decreased level of consciousness; jugular venous distention; respiratory crackles and dyspnea; decreased urine output; cool, clammy, mottled skin; peripheral edema; and decreased peripheral pulses and capillary refill. Notify the physician of significant changes.
- Monitor intake and output; weigh daily, reporting any gain of 3 to 5 lb within 24 hours.
- Maintain fluid restriction as ordered.
- Elevate the head of the bed. Administer supplemental oxygen as prescribed.
- Monitor oxygen saturation continually and arterial blood gases as prescribed.
- Ensure physical, emotional, and mental rest.

Activity Intolerance

- Obtain vital signs before and during activities.
- Encourage gradual increases in activity and self-care, as tolerated. Ensure adequate rest periods, uninterrupted sleep cycles, and adequate nutrition.
- Provide assistance with activities of daily living as needed. Suggest use of a shower chair, sitting while brushing teeth, and so on.
- Consult with a physical therapist for in-bed exercises and a progressive activity plan of care.
- Discuss ways to decrease energy requirements at home with the patient and significant others.

V

Risk for Infection

- Maintain aseptic technique for all invasive procedures.

- Monitor temperature every 4 hours. Notify physician if the temperature exceeds 100.5°F (38.5°C).

- Assess wounds and catheter sites for redness, swelling, warmth, pain, or drainage.

- Administer antibiotics as prescribed. Ensure completion of the full course.

- Monitor white blood cell counts and notify the physician of counts below 5000/μL or above 10,000/μL.

Community-Based Care

- Explain the disorder and all tests and procedures, including surgery.

- Discuss symptom management, including activity restrictions, diet restrictions, and medication regimen.

- Stress the importance of notifying all healthcare providers about the valve disorder or surgery so prophylactic antibiotics can be given before any procedure that might allow bacterial invasion, including dental procedures.

- Provide referrals to community resources and the address and phone number of the American Heart Association prior to discharge.

- Alert the patient and significant others to manifestations that should be reported immediately to the physician.

For more information about these and other cardiac valve disorders, see Chapter 31 in *Medical-Surgical Nursing,* Fifth Edition, by LeMone, Burke, and Bauldoff.

VARICELLA ZOSTER VIRUS INFECTION (CHICKENPOX, HERPES ZOSTER [SHINGLES])

Overview

- Varicella zoster virus (VZV) causes two discrete clinical diseases: chickenpox and herpes zoster, also called shingles.

- Chickenpox is a primary infection with the highly contagious VZV that usually occurs during childhood, between 5 and 9 years of age.

- Primary VZV infection is acquired via the respiratory system, and produces a systemic viremia; vesicular lesions form in a disseminated pattern.

- The incubation period is 10 to 21 days; the infectious period is from 48 hours before onset of rash until all lesions are crusted over.

- The virus remains latent in the dorsal root ganglia of cranial or peripheral nerves.

- Herpes zoster is a reinfection that usually reappears after age 60, or in immunocompromised individuals; it presents as painful vesicles in a dermatomal pattern.

- A disseminated form, usually involving the lung and/or brain, can also occur in neonates or in the immunocompromised.

Cause

- Infection with the VZV, a DNA-containing herpes virus

Manifestations

Primary Infection

- Prodromal manifestations may precede rash: headache, anorexia, malaise.

- Rash: successive groups of erythematous pruritic maculopapules, evolving to vesicles and crusts over hours to days; trunk and face usually affected first, then other areas and mucous membranes of the mouth, pharynx, and vagina. Number of lesions varies from several to many, depending on age and immune status.

- Other manifestations include the following:
  - Fever 37.8°C to 39.4°C (100°F to 103°F)
  - Malaise
  - Anorexia

- Complications of primary VZV include secondary infection of lesions (usually with *Streptococcus pyogenes* or *Staphylococcus aureus*), meningitis, VZV pneumonia, ulcerative keratitis, myocarditis, nephritis, arthritis, hepatitis, and Reye's syndrome.

Herpes Zoster (Shingles)

- Pain: severe, deep; continuous; often debilitating; usually precedes rash by 48 to 72 hours
- Rash: unilateral, erythematous vesicles; dermatomal pattern; most common at T3 to L3; crust over after 10 days
- Fever
- Malaise
- Complications of herpes zoster: postherpetic neuralgia, central nervous system infection, disseminated infection

Diagnostic Tests

- Viral culture can identify the VZV.
- Immunofluorescent methods can identify varicella in skin cells.

Interdisciplinary Management

- The antiviral medication acyclovir is the drug of choice for herpes zoster infections. Although it does not cure the infection, it decreases the severity and the pain.
- Corticosteroids may be used to decrease inflammation; however, they also slow healing and suppress the immune response.
- Narcotic and nonnarcotic analgesics are prescribed for pain management.

Selected Nursing Diagnoses with Interventions

Acute Pain

- Assess and monitor the location, duration, and intensity of the pain.
- Administer prescribed medications regularly and evaluate their effectiveness.
- Use measures to relieve pruritus: Administer prescribed medications, apply calamine lotion or wet compresses as prescribed, keep the room temperature cool, and use a bed cradle to keep sheets off affected areas.
- Encourage the use of distraction and relaxation techniques.

Risk for Infection

- Monitor for signs of infection: vital signs every 4 hours; assess skin lesions for erythema, pustules, discharge; monitor white blood cell count; assess for lymph gland enlargement.

- Use interventions to decrease the itch-scratch-itch cycle, thereby decreasing the possibility of excoriation.

- Institute infection control procedures.

Community-Based Care

- Discuss the risks and benefits of varicella vaccine with patients concerned about chickenpox or herpes zoster.

- Discuss the disease process, medications, dosage, effects and side effects, and prognosis. Explain that the disease is self-limiting and typically heals completely. Second occurrences of herpes zoster are rare.

- Teach to avoid contact with children or pregnant women until crusts have formed over the blisters. The disease is contagious to those who have not had chickenpox.

- Follow the previous suggestions to help control pain and itching.

- Tell the patient to report to the physician any increase in pain, fever, chills, drainage that smells bad or has pus, or a spread in the blisters.

For more information on varicella zoster virus infection, see Chapter 16 in *Medical-Surgical Nursing,* Fifth Edition, by LeMone, Burke, and Bauldoff.

VARICOSE VEINS

Overview

- Varicose veins are weak, dilated veins that become tortuous and lead to valve incompetence and venous insufficiency, increasing the risk for venous thrombosis and chronic venous stasis ulcers.

- Varicosities may affect peripheral vessels such as the saphenous veins in the leg or mucosal tissues such as the esophagus (varices), scrotum (varicocele), or rectum (hemorrhoids).

- Varicose veins are classified as primary (with no involvement of deep veins) or secondary (caused by the obstruction of deep veins).
- They are more common in females and are associated with occupations in which long periods of standing are required.

Causes

- Inherent vein weakness (genetic predisposition)
- Obesity
- Pregnancy
- Long periods of standing
- Venous thrombosis

Manifestations

- Visible dilated, tortuous veins
- Leg heaviness, fatigue
- Manifestations of venous thrombosis: leg pain, edema; erythema and warmth
- Long term: venous stasis ulcers

Diagnostic Tests

- Doppler ultrasonography or duplex Doppler ultrasound helps to identify specific locations of incompetent valves.
- The Trendelenburg test helps differentiate between incompetent valves of deep or superficial veins.

Interdisciplinary Management

- Conservative measures include antiembolism stockings and regular, daily walking and leg elevation.
- Mild analgesics may relieve the pain associated with varicose veins.
- Compression sclerotherapy and vein stripping are surgical techniques that may alleviate the major symptoms of varicose veins; however, there is no real cure.

V

Selected Nursing Diagnoses with Interventions

Chronic Pain

- Teach and reinforce methods of pain relief that do not require analgesic drugs.
- Collaborate with the patient to establish a plan of pain control.
- Regularly evaluate the effectiveness of interventions used to minimize pain.

Ineffective Tissue Perfusion: Peripheral

- Assess peripheral pulses, capillary refill, skin temperature, and degree of edema.
- Teach how to apply properly fitted supportive or antiembolic stockings and to remove them each day for 30 to 60 minutes.
- Discuss the importance of regular exercise.
- Advise elevating legs 15 to 20 minutes several times per day and sleeping with legs elevated above the heart level.

Risk for Impaired Skin Integrity

- Assess the skin on the lower extremities for warmth, erythema, moisture, and signs of breakdown as part of an initial examination.
- Teach daily skin hygiene. Use nondrying soaps and lotions to prevent skin dryness and cracking.
- Instruct to protect the extremities from trauma that may lead to skin breakdown.
- Encourage adequate nutrition and fluid intake.

Community-Based Care

- Teach about the disease process, symptom management, pain management, and the importance of avoiding injury to the extremities.
- Instruct to report signs of neurovascular dysfunction, including numbness, coldness, pain, or tingling of an extremity.
- Stress the importance of daily walks and of elevating the legs and avoiding standing or sitting in one place for prolonged periods.

- Teach correct technique for applying antiembolism stockings.
- Stress the importance of follow-up care with the physician or surgeon as recommended.

For more information on varicose veins, see Chapter 32 in *Medical-Surgical Nursing,* Fifth Edition, by LeMone, Burke, and Bauldoff.

VENOUS INSUFFICIENCY, CHRONIC

Overview

- Chronic venous insufficiency is a disorder of inadequate venous return over a prolonged period.
- Increased pressure distends peripheral veins, separating valve leaflets and impairing their ability to close. This impairs normal unidirectional blood flow and deep vein emptying.
- Venous blood collects and stagnates in the lower leg (*venous stasis*), increasing venous pressures and impairing arterial circulation to the lower extremities. This impairs delivery of oxygen and nutrients to the cells and metabolic waste product removal.
- Cells die, leading to necrosis of subcutaneous fat and development of venous stasis ulcers. Inflammatory and immune defenses are impaired, increasing the risk for infection.

Causes

- Deep venous thrombosis
- Varicose veins, leg trauma
- May be idiopathic

Manifestations

- Lower leg edema, itching, and discomfort that increase with prolonged standing
- Cyanosis of the extremity
- Recurrent stasis ulcers, usually on the medial surface above the ankle
- Shiny, atrophic tissue surrounding the ulcer

V

- Brownish skin pigmentation
- Leg feels hard, leathery to touch

Diagnostic Tests

- There are no specific diagnostic tests for chronic venous insufficiency.

Interdisciplinary Management

- Care focuses on symptom relief, promoting adequate circulation and healing, and preventing tissue damage.
- Prolonged standing or sitting is discouraged. Graduated compression hose and frequent elevation of the legs and feet during the day is recommended. The foot of the mattress is elevated to raise the feet above the level of the heart.
- Stasis ulcers are treated with wet compresses followed by a topical corticosteroid. Bed rest is prescribed during the acute period. A semirigid boot (Unna's boot) may be applied to the foot and lower leg.

Selected Nursing Diagnoses with Interventions

Ineffective Health Maintenance

- Keep the legs and feet clean, soft, and dry.
- Avoid clothing that constricts the legs (such as knee-high hose, garters, or girdles).

Ineffective Tissue Perfusion: Peripheral

- Elevate the legs while resting and during sleep.
- Walk as much as possible, but avoid sitting or standing for long periods of time. When sitting, do not cross the legs or put pressure on the back of the knees.
- Wear elastic hose as prescribed.

Community-Based Care

- Home and community-based care is primarily educative and supportive. Include the previously discussed nursing interventions in patient teaching as appropriate.

For more information about chronic venous insufficiency, see Chapter 32 in *Medical-Surgical Nursing,* Fifth Edition, by LeMone, Burke, and Bauldoff.

VENOUS THROMBOSIS (THROMBOPHLEBITIS)

Overview

- Venous thrombosis (thrombophlebitis) is a condition of venous inflammation, thrombus formation, and obstructed venous blood flow.
- Venous thrombosis is associated with Virchow's triad: venous stasis, vessel damage, and increased blood coagulability.
- The thrombus propagates in the direction of blood flow; pieces of it may break loose to become emboli.
- Thrombi can form in either superficial or deep veins.
- Deep vein thrombosis (DVT) usually begins in the deep veins of the calf, propagating into the popliteal and femoral veins; pelvic veins also may be affected by DVT.
- DVT can lead to chronic venous insufficiency and pulmonary embolism. Pulmonary embolism occurs when emboli from the clot enter the pulmonary circulation to occlude arterial flow to a portion of the lungs.

Causes

Deep Vein Thrombosis

- Immobilization: myocardial infarction, heart failure, stroke, postoperative
- Surgery: orthopedic, thoracic, abdominal, genitourinary
- Cancer: pancreatic, lung, ovary, testes, urinary tract, breast, stomach
- Trauma: fractures of the spine, pelvis, femur, tibia; spinal cord injury
- Pregnancy and delivery

- Hormone therapy: oral contraceptives, hormone replacement therapy
- Coagulation disorders

Superficial Vein Thrombosis
- Venous catheters and infusions
- Thromboangiitis obliterans, varicose veins
- Post partum
- Abdominal or pancreatic cancer

Manifestations

Deep Vein Thrombosis
- Usually asymptomatic
- Dull, aching pain in affected extremity, especially when walking
- Possible tenderness, warmth, erythema along affected vein
- Cyanosis of affected extremity
- Edema of affected extremity

Superficial Vein Thrombosis
- Localized pain and tenderness over the affected vein
- Redness and warmth along the course of the vein
- Palpable cordlike structure along the affected vein
- Swelling and redness of surrounding tissue

Diagnostic Tests
- Duplex venous ultrasonography shows decreased velocity of blood flow.
- Plethysmography also measures changes in blood flow through the veins.
- Magnetic resonance imaging is used to diagnose thrombosis of the vena cavae or pelvic veins.
- Ascending contrast venography identifies the location and extent of venous thrombosis.

V

Interdisciplinary Management

- Prophylaxis for venous thrombosis includes low-molecular-weight heparins, oral anticoagulation, early mobilization, leg exercises, intermittent pneumatic compression devices, and elastic stockings for patients at risk.

- Anticoagulants to prevent clot propagation and reduce the risk of pulmonary embolism are the primary treatment for venous thrombosis.

- Nonsteroidal anti-inflammatory drugs may be ordered to reduce venous inflammation and relieve symptoms.

- For superficial vein thrombosis, warm, moist compresses over the affected vein and extremity rest are ordered.

- For DVT, bed rest with the legs elevated, and elastic antiembolism stockings (TEDS) or pneumatic compression devices are frequently ordered.

- Surgery may be required to remove the thrombus (venous thrombectomy), prevent its extension into deep veins, or prevent pulmonary embolism.

Selected Nursing Diagnoses with Interventions

Acute Pain

- Regularly assess location, characteristics, and level of pain. Report increasing pain or changes in its location or characteristics.

- Measure calf and thigh diameter of the affected extremity on admission and daily thereafter. Report increases promptly.

- Apply warm, moist heat to affected extremity at least four times daily, using warm, moist compresses or an aqua-K pad.

- Maintain bed rest as ordered.

Ineffective Tissue Perfusion: Peripheral

- Assess peripheral pulses, skin integrity, capillary refill times, and color of extremities at least every 8 hours. Report changes promptly.

- Assess skin of the affected lower leg and foot at least every 8 hours; more often as indicated.

- Elevate extremities at all times, keeping knees slightly flexed and legs above the level of the heart.

- Remove antiembolic stockings or pneumatic compression device for 30 to 60 minutes during daily hygiene.

- Use mild soaps, solutions, and lotions to clean the affected leg and foot daily. Pat dry after washing, and apply a non-alcohol-based lotion or moisturizing cream.

- Use egg-crate mattress or sheepskin on the bed as needed.

- Encourage frequent position changes, at least every 2 hours while awake.

Ineffective Protection

- Assess for and promptly report evidence of bleeding such as petechiae; bruising; bleeding gums; obvious or occult blood in vomitus, stool, or urine; and unexplained back or abdominal pain.

- Monitor laboratory results, including the INR (prothrombin time), aPTT, hemoglobin, and hematocrit as indicated. Report values outside the normal or desired range.

Impaired Physical Mobility

- Encourage active range-of-motion exercises at least every 8 hours; provide passive range of motion as needed.

- Encourage frequent position changes, deep breathing, and coughing.

- Encourage increased fluid and dietary fiber intake.

- Assist with and encourage ambulation as allowed.

- Encourage diversional activities such as reading, handwork or other hobbies, television or video games, and socializing.

Risk for Ineffective Tissue Perfusion: Cardiopulmonary

- Frequently assess respiratory status, including rate, depth, ease, and oxygen saturation levels.

- Immediately report complaints of chest pain and shortness of breath, anxiety, or a sense of impending doom.

- Initiate oxygen therapy, elevate the head of the bed, and reassure the patient who is experiencing manifestations of pulmonary embolism.

Community-Based Care

Include the following topics when teaching the patient and family:

- Explanation of the disease process.
- Treatment measures, including laboratory tests and their purposes, medications, and adverse effects that should be reported.
- Appropriate methods of heat application.
- Prescribed activity restrictions.
- Measures to prevent future episodes of venous thrombosis.
- The importance of follow-up visits and laboratory tests as scheduled.
- Refer for community nursing services for continued assessment and reinforcement of teaching.
- Provide referrals for assistance with activities of daily living and home maintenance services as indicated. Consider referral for physical therapy if needed.

For more information on venous thrombosis, see Chapter 32 in *Medical-Surgical Nursing,* Fifth Edition, by LeMone, Burke, and Bauldoff.

V

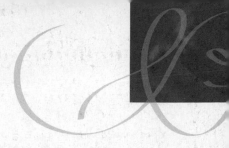

Table 1　Normal ABG Values

	Range	Average
pH	7.35–7.45	7.4
$PaCO^2$	35–45 mmHg	40 mmHg
HCO_3	22–26 mEq/L	24 mEq/L
PaO_2	80–100 mmHg	95 mmHg
SaO_2*	94%–100%	96%
O_2 Content	15–25 mL%	19 mL% (Hg = 15 g)

Percent hemoglobin saturated with O_2.

Key: ABG, arterial blood gas.

Table 2　ABG Changes in Acid–Base Disorders

	pH	$PaCO_2$	HCO_3
Respiratory acidosis			
Uncompensated	decreased	increased	normal
Compensated	normal	increased	increased
Respiratory alkalosis			
Uncompensated	increased	decreased	normal
Compensated	normal	decreased	decreased
Metabolic acidosis			
Uncompensated	decreased	normal	decreased
Compensated	normal	decreased	decreased
Metabolic alkalosis			
Uncompensated	increased	normal	increased
Compensated	normal	increased (limited)	increased

Key: ABG, arterial blood gas.

Table 3 Types of Anemia

Name	Mechanism	Laboratory Indicators	Specific S/S
Hypoproliferative			
Pernicious	↓Serum B$_{12}$	Macrocytic RBCs, (↓MCV), negative Schilling test	Dyspepsia, glossitis, stomatitis, numbness, tingling, clumsiness
Folate deficiency	↓Serum folic acid	Macrocytic RBCs, (↓MCV), ↓serum folate	Similar to pernicious anemia
Iron deficiency	↓Serum iron (Fe), chronic bleeding	↓RBCs, ↓[Hgb], ↓HCT, microcytic/hypochromic RBCs, ↓MCV, ↓MCHC, ↓serum Fe, ↑TIBC	Stomatitis, brittle hair/nails, koilonychia, pica, heart murmurs
Aplastic	Bone marrow damage • radiation • chemotherapy • infection	↓RBCs, ↓[Hgb], ↓HCT, normocytic RBCs, ↓RBCs, ↓platelets	S/S of anemia, frequent infection, bleeding disorders
Hemorrhagic			
Acute	Blood loss/short time course (i.e., minutes, hours, days)	↓RBC, ↓[Hgb], ↓HCT, normocytic/chromic RBCs, ↓reticulocytes, ↓nucleated RBCs	Hypotension, dizziness, vertigo, restlessness, thirst, rapid/thready pulse. May progress to shock, coma, and death.

Chronic	Blood loss/long course (i.e., weeks, months, years)	Similar to iron-deficiency anemia	Similar to iron-deficiency anemia
Hemolytic			
G6PD deficiency	Genetic, autosomal-recessive	↓G6PD enzyme in RBCs, ↓G6PD, ↓HCT, ↓bilirubin, positive for Heinz bodies	S/S anemia and jaundice
Sickle cell disease	Genetic, autosomal-recessive, defective Hgb molecule	Positive for sickle cells, target cells, RBC count/morphology depend on stage	Multiple organ-system ischemia, pain, and dysfunction
Transfusion reaction	Acquired, immune-mediated RBC destruction	Varying degrees of anemia, ↓bilirubin	Fever, S/S hypersensitivity, S/S shock, jaundice

Key: ↓ = decreased; G6PD = glucose-6-phosphate deficiency; RBC = red blood cell; Hgb = hemoglobin; MCV = mean corpuscular volume; [Hgb] = hemoglobin concentration; HCT = hematocrit; MCHC = mean corpuscular hemoglobin concentration; TIBC = total iron binding capacity; WBC = white blood cell.

Table 4   Expected Laboratory Values

Hematology

Red blood cells	Male: 4.6–6.2 mil/mm^3
	Female: 4.2–5.4 mil/mm^3
MCV	85–100 μm^3
MCH	27–34 pg/cell
MCHC	31–35 g/dL
Hemoglobin (Hgb)	Male: 13–18 g/dL
	Female: 12–16 g/dL
Hematocrit (Hct)	Male: 40%–52%
	Female: 37%–47%
White blood cells	5,000–10,000/mm^3
Neutrophils	60%–70%
Eosinophils	1%–3%
Basophils	0.3%–0.5%
Lymphocytes	20%–30%
Monocytes	3%–8%
Platelets	250,000–400,000/mm^3

Coagulation Studies

Prothrombin time (Protime or PT)	9.5–13 seconds
Therapeutic range (international normalized ratio or INR)	1.5–4.5
Activated partial thromboplastin time (APTT or PTT)	22.0–32.0 seconds
Therapeutic range (heparin)	2.0–2.5 × normal limit
Thrombin clotting time (TCT)	7.0–12 seconds
Bleeding time	2–9.5 minutes
Activated coagulation time (ACT)	150–180 seconds

Serum Electrolytes

Sodium (Na$^+$)	135–145 mEq/L
Potassium (K$^+$)	3.5–5.0 mEq/L
Calcium (Ca^{2+})	8.5–10 mg/dL
Magnesium (Mg^{2+})	1.6–2.6 mg/dL (1.3–2.1 mEq/L)
Chloride (Cl$^-$)	98–106 mEq/L
Bicarbonate (HCO$_3^-$)	22–26 mEq/L
Phosphate/phosphorus (PO$_4^{2-}$)	2.5–4.5 mg/dL (1.7–2.6 mEq/L)
Serum osmolality	275–295 mOsm/kg

Blood Chemistries

Blood urea nitrogen (BUN)	5–20 mg/dL

(continued)

Table 4   Expected Laboratory Values (Continued)

Creatinine	Male: 0.6–1.2 mg/dL
	Female: 0.5–1.1 mg/dL
Bilirubin (Total)	0.3–1.2 mg/dL (SI 5–21 μmol/L)
Direct bilirubin	0–0.2 mg/dL (SI < 3.4 μmol/L)
Indirect bilirubin	< 1.1 mg/dL (SI < 19 μmol/L)
Glucose	70–110 mg/dL
Protein (total)	6.0–8.0 g/dL
Albumin	3.2–5 g/dL
	Older adult: 3.2–4.8 g/dL
Cholesterol (Total) (desirable values)	140–199 mg/dL
LDL	< 100–129 mg/dL
HDL	≥ 60mg/dL
Triglycerides	< 150–199mg/dL
VLDL	25%–50% of total triglyceride level
Creatine kinase (CK or CPK)	Male: 12–80 U/L
	Female: 10–70 U/L
CK-MB	0–3% of total CK
Cardiac muscle troponins	
cT_nt	< 0.2 μg/L
cT_nI	< 3.1 μg/L
Alanine aminotransferase (ALT)	5–40 U/L
Aspartate aminotransferase (AST)	5–40 U/L
Alkaline phosphatase	30–95 U/L
Gamma-glutamine transferase (GGT)	Male: 5–85 U/L
	Female: 5–55 U/L
Lactic dehydrogenase (LDH)	120–300 U/L
Amylase	25–125 U/L
Lipase	< 200 U/L
Thyroxine (T_4)	5–12 μg/dL
Triiodothyronine (T_3)	800–200 ng/dL
TSH	0–5 μIU/mL
Uric acid	Male: 3.4–7.0 mg/dL
	Female: 2.4–6.0 mg/dL
Urinalysis	
Color	Yellow, clear
Specific gravity	1.010–1.035

(continued)

Table 4 Expected Laboratory Values (Continued)

pH	4.5–7.8
Protein	Negative
Glucose	Negative
Ketones	Negative

Key: MCH, mean corpuscular hemoglobin; MCHC, mean corpuscular hemoglobin concentration; MCV, mean corpuscular volume.

INDEX

in ulcerative colitis, 536–537
in vaginitis, 545
Body temperature imbalance:
in encephalitis, 162
in endocarditis, 165
Bone marrow aspiration, in aplastic
anemia, 29
Bone marrow studies:
in multiple myeloma, 338
in polycythemia, 431
Bone marrow suppression, 28
Bone marrow transplantation, 83, 307
Bone mineral density (BMD), in osteoporosis, 372
Bone scan:
in fracture, 194
in melanoma, 324
in multiple myeloma, 338
in osteomyelitis, 369
Bone tumor, primary:
cause, 55
CBFC, 67
diagnostic tests, 56
interdisciplinary management, 56
manifestations, 55
nursing diagnoses with interventions,
56–57
overview, 55
Boniva. *See* Ibandronate
Bordella pertussis, 407
Borrelia burgdorferi, 310
Botulism, 202
Bouchard's nodes, 364
BPH. *See* Benign prostatic hyperplasia
Bradykinesia, 387
Brain attack. *See* Stroke
Brain tumor:
causes, 58
community-based care, 61–62
diagnostic tests, 59
interdisciplinary management, 59
manifestations, 56
nursing diagnoses with interventions,
60–61
overview, 57–58
Breast cancer:
causes, 62–63
community-based care, 66
diagnostic tests, 64
interdisciplinary management, 64
manifestations, 63
nursing diagnoses with interventions,
64–66
overview, 62

Breast self-examination, in fibrocystic
breast disease, 179–180
Breathing pattern, ineffective:
in acid–base disorders, 5
in asthma, 45
in bronchiectasis, 68
in cardiomyopathy, 92
in emphysema, 157
in hypermagnesemia, 322
in influenza, 292
in intestinal obstruction, 296
in occupational lung disease, 362
in pericarditis, 399
in pneumonia, 420
in poliomyelitis, 426
in tetanus, 517
Bronchial provocation testing, in asthma, 43
Bronchiectasis:
causes, 67
community-based care, 69
diagnostic tests, 68
interdisciplinary management, 68
manifestations, 67
nursing diagnoses with interventions,
68–69
overview, 67
Bronchitis, acute:
causes, 70
community-based care, 71
diagnostic test, 70
interdisciplinary management, 70
manifestations, 70
nursing diagnoses with interventions,
70–71
overview, 69
Bronchitis, chronic:
causes, 71–72
community-based care, 73–74
diagnostic tests, 72
interdisciplinary management, 72–73
manifestations, 72
nursing diagnoses with interventions, 73
overview, 71
Bronchodilators:
in bronchiectasis, 68
in chronic bronchitis, 73
in COPD, 107
in cystic fibrosis, 132
in emphysema, 157
in Legionnaires' disease, 304
in pneumonia, 419
in respiratory failure, 469
Bronchopneumonia, 418

Bronchoscopy:
in bronchiectasis, 68
in flail chest, 183
in Legionnaires' disease, 304
in occupational lung disease, 362
in pneumonia, 419
Brudzinski sign, 161, 331
Buerger's disease. *See* Thromboangiitis obliterans
Buffers, 1
BUN. *See* Blood urea nitrogen
Bupropion, in COPD, 107
Burkitt's lymphoma, 336
Byssinosis, 362

C

CA 19–9, 381
CA-125, 378
CA-MRSA *See* Community-associated MRSA infection
Calcimimetics, in hyperparathyroidism, 265
Calcipotriene, in psoriasis, 441
Calcitonin:
in calcium balance, 75
in hyperparathyroidism, 264
in osteoporosis, 372
Calcitriol, 75
Calcitrol, 75
Calcium, 75–76. *See also* Hypercalcemia; Hypocalcemia
Calcium channel blockers:
in angina pectoris, 36
in hypertension, 275
in Raynaud's disease, 455
in stroke, 496
in thromboangiitis obliterans, 519
Calcium gluconate:
in hyperkalemia, 435
in magnesium imbalance, 322
Canasa. *See* Mesalamine
Cancer:
causes, 82
community-based care, 86
diagnostic tests, 82
grading, 82–83
interdisciplinary management, 83
manifestations, 82
nursing diagnoses with interventions, 84–85
overview, 81
staging, 83
Cancer, types:
basal cell cancer, 487–490
bladder, 52–55

bone tumors, 55–57
brain tumors, 57–62
breast, 62–66
cervical, 97–100
colorectal, 116–118
endometrial (uterine), 167–169
Kaposi's sarcoma, 300–302
leukemia, 305–310
melanoma, 323–327
multiple myeloma, 337–341
non-Hodgkin's lymphoma, 312–316
ovarian, 377–379
pancreatic, 380–382
prostate, 437–440
skin cancer, nonmelanoma, 487–490
squamous cell cancer, 487–490
testicular, 513–515
Candida albicans, 87
Candida organisms, 86, 87
Candidemia, 87
Candidiasis:
causes, 87
community-based case, 89
diagnostic tests, 88
interdisciplinary management, 88
manifestations, 87–88
nursing diagnoses with interventions, 88–89
overview, 86–87
Cannabis withdrawal, 500
Capnography, 2, 72, 107
Carbamazepine, in trigeminal neuralgia, 528
Carbimazole, in hyperthyroidism, 278
Carbonic acid, 1
Carcinoembryonic antigen, 117
Carcinoma, 81
Carcinoma *in situ*, 52
Cardiac catheterization:
in cardiomyopathy, 91
in valvular heart disease, 550
Cardiac enzymes, in pericarditis, 398
Cardiac glycosides, in valvular heart disease, 550
Cardiac ischemia. *See* Acute coronary syndrome
Cardiac output, decreased:
in acid–base disorders, 5
in acute respiratory distress syndrome, 12
in anaphylaxis, 26
in anemia, 30
in cardiomyopathy, 92
in heart failure, 224, 226
in hypermagnesemia, 322
in hypersensitivity, 270–271

587

Insulin shock, 280
Interferon:
    in melanoma, 325
    in multiple sclerosis, 343
Interleukin, in melanoma, 325
Intermittent claudication, 401
Interstitial edematous pancreatitis, 383
Intestinal obstruction:
    causes, 294
    community-based care, 296–297
    diagnostic tests, 295
    interdisciplinary management, 295
    manifestations, 294–295
    nursing diagnoses with interventions,
        295–296
    overview, 293–294
Intracranial hypertension. *See* Increased
    intracranial pressure
Intraocular pressure (IOP), 206. *See also*
    Glaucoma
Intravenous pyelography:
    in bladder cancer, 53
    in kidney stones, 457
    in pyelonephritis, 452
    in renal failure, 463
    in urinary tract infection, 539
Invasive carcinoma, 97
Iron-deficiency anemia, 29, 566
Irritable bowel syndrome (IBS):
    causes, 297
    community-based care, 298–299
    diagnostic tests, 298
    interdisciplinary management, 298
    manifestations, 297
    nursing diagnoses with interventions,
        298–299
    overview, 297
ISMO. *See* Isosorbide
Isosorbide, in cirrhosis, 113
ITP. *See* Immune thrombocytopenic purpura

J

Jacksonian march, 173

K

Kaposi's sarcoma (KS):
    causes, 300
    community-based care, 302
    diagnostic tests, 301
    interdisciplinary management, 301
    manifestations, 300–301
    nursing diagnoses with interventions,
        301–302
    overview, 300

Kayexalate. *See* Sodium polystyrene
    sulfonate
Kernig's sign, 161, 331
Ketoacidosis. *See* Diabetic ketoacidosis
Ketoconazole:
    in candidiasis, 88
    in Cushing's syndrome, 129
Kidney stones. *See* Renal calculi
KS. *See* Kaposi's sarcoma
Kussmaul's respiration, 146
Kussmaul's sign, 398

L

Lactic dehydrogenase, normal values, 569
Lactulose, in cirrhosis, 113
Laënnec's cirrhosis, 111
Lansoprazole, in gastritis, 199
Laparoscopy:
    in fibroids, 542
    in pelvic inflammatory disease, 391
Large bowel obstruction, 294–295
Late onset Alzheimer's disease, 16
Latex allergy, 267, 268, 269
LDL, normal values, 569
Left-sided heart failure, 223, 547, 548
Legionella pneumophila, 303
Legionnaires' disease:
    causes, 303
    community-based care, 305
    diagnostic tests, 303–304
    interdisciplinary management, 304
    manifestations, 303
    nursing diagnoses with interventions, 304
    overview, 303
Leiomyomas, uterine. *See*
        Uterine leiomyomas
Lentigo maligna, 324. *See also* Melanoma
Leukemia, 81
    causes, 306–307
    community-based care, 309–310
    diagnostic tests, 307
    interdisciplinary management, 307
    manifestations, 307
    nursing diagnoses with interventions,
        308–309
    overview, 305–306
Leuprolide acetate:
    in fibroids, 542
    in prostate cancer, 438
Levamisole, in colorectal cancer, 117
Ligase chain reaction tests, in chlamydial
        infection, 101
Lipase, normal values, 569
Liver failure, 112

Y

Z